W

DATE DUE

MAR 2 8 2003		
MAR 2 1 2005		
JUN 2 3 2005		
JUL 0 4 2005		
DEC 1 4 2005		
MAR 2 7 2006		
MAY 1 6 2006		
APR 2 4 2009		
DEC 1 2010		

DEMCO

643-1234

NORMAL AND ABNORMAL BEHAVIOR IN CHINESE CULTURE

CULTURE, ILLNESS, AND HEALING

Studies in Comparative Cross-Cultural Research

VOLUME 2

NORMAL AND ABNORMAL BEHAVIOR IN CHINESE CULTURE

Edited by

ARTHUR KLEINMAN

University of Washington, Seattle

and

TSUNG-YI LIN

University of British Columbia, Vancouver, Canada

D. REIDEL PUBLISHING COMPANY

DORDRECHT : HOLLAND / BOSTON : U.S.A.

LONDON : ENGLAND

Library of Congress Cataloging in Publication Data (Rev.)

Main entry under title:

Normal and abnormal behavior in Chinese culture.

(Culture, illness, and healing ; v. 2)
Includes bibliographies and index.
1.   Psychology, Pathological—China.   2.   Personality and
culture—China.   3.   National characteristics, Chinese.   I.   Kleinman,
Arthur.   II.   Lin, Tsung-yi.   III.   Series.   [DNLM: 1.   Cross-cultural
comparison.   2.   Anthropology, Cultural—China.   3.   Anthropology,
Cultural—Taiwan.   4.   Mental disorders.   5.   Socioeconomic factors.
WM31 K64n]
RC451.C6N67   616.89'07'0951   80–19489
ISBN 90–277–1104–6

Published by D. Reidel Publishing Company,
P.O. Box 17, 3300 AA Dordrecht, Holland.

Sold and distributed in the U.S.A. and Canada
by Kluwer Boston Inc.,
190 Old Derby Street, Hingham, MA 02043, U.S.A.

In all other countries, sold and distributed
by Kluwer Academic Publishers Group,
P.O. Box 322, 3300 AH Dordrecht, Holland.

D. Reidel Publishing Company is a member of the Kluwer Group.

Printed in The Netherlands

TABLE OF CONTENTS

SECTION I: HISTORICAL AND CULTURAL BACKGROUND OF BELIEFS AND NORMS GOVERNING BEHAVIOR

SECTION II: CHILD DEVELOPMENT AND CHILDHOOD PSYCHOPATHOLOGY

SECTION III: FAMILY STUDIES

To our families. And to the one-fourth of mankind who are Chinese about whose individual lives and emotional problems so much more remains to be described, compared, and understood.

PREFACE

Our purpose in assembling the papers in this collection is to introduce readers to studies of normal and abnormal behavior in Chinese culture. We want to offer *a sense of* what psychiatrists and social scientists are doing to advance our understanding of this subject, including what findings are being made, what questions researched, what conundrums worried over. Since our fund of knowledge is obviously incomplete, we want our readers to be aware of the limits to what we know and to our acquisition of new knowledge. Although the subject is too vast and uncharted to support a comprehensive synthesis, in a few areas – e.g., psychiatric epidemiology – enough is known for us to be able to present major reviews. The chapters themselves cover a variety of themes that we regard as both intrinsically interesting and deserving of more systematic evaluation. Many of the issues they address we believe to be valid concerns for comparative cross-cultural studies. No attempt is made to artificially integrate these chapters, since the editors wish to highlight their distinctive interpretive frameworks as evidence of the rich variety of approaches that scholars take to this subject.

We see this volume as a modest and self-consciously limited exploration. Here are some accounts and interpretations (but by no means all) of normal and abnormal behavior in the context of Chinese culture that we believe fashion a more discriminating understanding of at least a few important aspects of that subject. We ask our readers to join us in thinking through the tough questions they raise, such as what are the universal and what are the culture-specific dimensions of pathology and deviance among Chinese. We recognize that certain readers may discover that we have omitted contributions that they regard as essential. While others may decide that some of our choices for inclusion are idiosyncratic. But on the whole we do believe we have represented in this book examples of much of the major work that is presently being conducted. Of course, being psychiatrists we have tipped the balance in favor of studies of abnormality. But this emphasis also reflects the particular way the field has developed.

Compared with research on Western cultures and even certain non-Western ones, China studies have paid remarkably little attention to individual behavior. Kinship, community organization, large scale sociopolitical and economic change have dominated the interest of scholars. While the Chinese family has been an abiding focus of concern, only infrequently has it been studied in terms of its crucial influences on individual development and the genesis and control of deviance. Studies of Chinese cultural influences on cognition, affects, coping processes, and other psychological issues, though admittedly in an early stage, have already generated considerable data, but this information has not enjoyed a wide circulation. In fact it is the editors' experience that "China scholars"

ix

A. Kleinman and T.-Y. Lin (eds.), Normal and Abnormal Behavior in Chinese Culture, ix–xi.
Copyright © 1980 by D. Reidel Publishing Company.

often disparage psychological findings and the theories developed to explain them, making use in their stead of common sense assumptions about human nature that are naive, ethnocentric, and sometimes downright mistaken. This bias may reflect Chinese culture's own reticence about psychological and especially psychiatric matters. It also smacks of the "orientalism" manufactured by Western scholars to render Chinese and other Asian cultures simultaneously "different" and "exotic" yet "understandable" (cf. E. W. Said: Orientalism. New York: Pantheon, 1978). Such scholars have maintained *both* that there is no individuality (in the Western sense), or mentally ill persons, in Asian cultures *and* that Asian individuals and the mentally ill are exactly the same as in the West. Each position, readers of this volume will soon discover, is wrong. It is our intention, then, to correct this distortion by contributing substantially to the advancement of psychocultural analyses and comparisons in the China field.

We believe many of the chapters in this volume will be of direct interest to students of Chinese culture. But we also hope that they will be read by psychiatrists and psychologists who are more generally concerned with elaborating a comparative science of human behavior and psychopathology. For most of what we know about these subjects has come from studies of Western populations, and thereby can only be generalized at great risk. Research on Chinese and other non-Western groups is absolutely essential if psychiatry and psychology are to become universal sciences. Finally, certain of the contributions to this volume should be of practical significance to clinicians who treat Chinese patients and plan services for Chinese communities. Clinical work among Chinese has lacked just the kind of research foundation to which this book hopes to contribute.

Much of the data presented in the chapters in this collection comes from research in Chinese communities outside of China. The editors are keenly aware of this imbalance, but there was nothing that could be done to correct it since it reflects reality. Up to the present, only a very limited amount of psychiatric and behavioral science research on Chinese has been reported for the People's Republic of China. We hope that this volume will be of use to our colleagues in the People's Republic as an outline of the present status of research in this field and that some of the chapters may even be of practical help in their own research and clinical work. We also hope that it will foster further communication and possibly future collaboration. We want our colleagues in China as well as other readers to understand why we are not using the *pinyin* Romanization system for rendering Chinese terms into English. These chapters were written and collected before the widespread changeover to *pinyin* in North America occurred and the editors decided after carefully reviewing the issues to retain the Wade-Giles Romanization system in this volume.

The editors wish to acknowledge help from many sources: the Department of Psychiatry and Behavioral Sciences, University of Washington; the Department of Psychiatry, University of British Columbia; the World Federation of Mental Health; the Foundations' Fund for Research in Psychiatry; the National Institute of Mental Health; to mention just a few. Specific individuals who have contributed in one way or another to this volume are simply too numerous to list, but several deserve our special thanks. We greatly appreciate the secretarial assistance of Marge Healy and Nora Curiston; Leslie Morris's contributions to editing individual chapters and help in preparing the index; Paul Anders' work on the index; and as always the general support of our wives during the several years it has taken us to complete the book. To Arthur Evans and Blake Vance of the D. Reidel Publishing Co. we owe thanks for seeing us through a venture that came to occupy so much more time than we had originally planned that at several points it appeared as if we would never finish the job. The contributors deserve our particular praise not only for the high quality of their contributions, but also for bearing with us during a long and drawn out editorial process. Finally, we thank our Chinese patients and research subjects, who, by leading us to realize how very much we needed to learn to better understand their problems and offer them appropriate care, made it essential for us to put together this work.

THE EDITORS

ARTHUR KLEINMAN AND TSUNG-YI LIN

INTRODUCTION

We may regard Chinese culture as exerting different influences on the normal and abnormal behavior of its members. These influences can be more or less separated for analytic purposes into the following categories of cultural influences on: cognition, affect, and communication; management of interpersonal transactions; perception of and reaction to universal stressors; creation of and coping with culture-specific stressors; susceptibility, epidemiological rates, symptomatology, illness behavior, help seeking, and treatment response associated with particular psychiatric disorders; labeling of and societal reaction to social deviance; and indigenous and professional systems for treating mental illness and the psychosocial concomitants of physical illness. While other cultural influences on behavior surely can be described, we believe that the more important ones are subsumed under these categories. In this chapter we will briefly review each of these different cultural influences on the behavior of Chinese and outline their potential clinical consequences.

The crux of our argument is that psychocultural interactions relate core symbolic meanings and behavioral norms to universal psychophysiological processes in such a way as to constitute a biosocial bridge between different phenomenological levels of reality (i.e., biological, psychological, social). This meaning-centered biopsychosocial connection should become the focus of research if we are to understand the genesis of normal and abnormal behavioral patterns that possess both universal and culture-specific aspects. But in order to adequately assess this psychocultural interrelationship psychiatric and psychological studies must develop methodologies that are anthropologically oriented toward meanings and norms and anthropological research must include psychobiological measurements.

(1) CULTURAL INFLUENCES ON COGNITIVE, AFFECTIVE AND COMMUNICATIVE PROCESSES

The key influence here is the reliance on cognitive coping processes to manage dysphoric affects by articulating them in certain culturally approved idioms. By focusing on how depression, anxiety and other dysphoric affects are articulated as somatic (not psychological) distress in Chinese culture, we will be able to study a core cultural influence on cognitive, affective, communicative and behavioral processes that is of great clinical significance. It is simply beyond the scope of this chapter to examine the many other ways that Chinese culture affects each of these psychological phenomena (cf. Hsu 1971a, 1971b; Kleinman 1979: 119–178; and Chapters 1, 7, 8, and 13 in this volume). But the particular

A. Kleinman and T.-Y. Lin (eds.), Normal and Abnormal Behavior in Chinese Culture, xiii–xxiii.
Copyright © 1980 by D. Reidel Publishing Company.

psychocultural phenomenon analyzed below should indicate to readers how other Chinese psychocultural processes too can be discussed from this perspective.

In our view, affects are universal psychobiological states of response to internal and external stimuli. Culture shapes affects, and affective disorders, through the mediation of cognitive coping processes such as denial, suppression, displacement, dissociation. These coping responses most frequently are universal ones that are utilized in culturally specific patterns of hierarchical resort. Hence among traditionally-oriented Chinese it has been repeatedly found that *externalizing* coping responses are drawn on to manage dysphoric affects to a much greater extent than are *internalizing* ones, whereas among middle-class Caucasian-Americans the reverse is true. Moreover, even among externalizing coping responses, these cultures (and others) differ as to which responses are selected most frequently to manage particular affects in particular settings. Obviously, within Chinese and other cultures individuals also vary in their coping patterns (cf. Kleinman 1979: 119–178).

Our current measures of cognitive coping strategies are relatively crude. It is to be expected that in future more refined assessments of coping processes will yield more discriminating understanding of these different cultural patterns of coping response and how they shape the perception, experience and behavioral correlates of universal affective states into culturally-specific "final common pathways" (Carr 1978). It is also reasonable to expect that certain cognitive coping processes may be unique to particular cultures, even though the evidence for them is at present meager. For example, *amae*, an integration of universal affect and culture-specific coping response among Japanese, is held by Doi (1973) to create a unique, personnally and socially valued patterning of dependency. This is a question that demands much more cross-cultural psychological research before it is resolved. The moral articulation of affect along specifically Confucian lines depicted by Metzger in the next chapter could be an example of such a culturally unique coping response among Chinese and for this reason should be investigated by psychologists working in traditional Chinese settings.

Somatization among Chinese appears to be brought about through the systematic channeling of depression, anxiety and other dysphorias by externalizing cognitive coping responses into somatically experienced and expressed distress (cf. Kleinman 1979: 119–178; Tseng 1975). The very terms Chinese apply to dysphoric states *mên* (depressed, sad), *fan-tsao* (troubled, worried, anxious), *kan-huo* (irritable, angry), *shen-k'uei* (kidney weakness or deficiency), *shen-ching shuai-jo* (neurasthenia) are semantic networks that convey psychological meaning through somatic symbols (heart, liver, kidney, nerves, respectively).[1] Since affective states are psychobiological conditions in which emotion (psychological state) and autonomic nervous system response (physiological state) occur together, we can see how Chinese cultural meanings and behavioral norms create "final common pathways" of somatized behavior by blocking overt expression of the former, while simultaneously sanctioning preoccupations with the latter (cf. Chapters 13, 17, and 18 in this volume and Kleinman 1979: 119–178 for examples of this culturally constituted pattern of somatization.)

Somatized affects (e.g., headaches, backaches, weakness, impotence, etc.) are not the only externalizing channels along which dysphoric emotions travel in the process of being culturally shaped. Moral, cosmological, social and other culturally sanctioned idioms for experiencing and expressing distress are also commonly resorted to by Chinese. But we know very little about these other coping responses. Clearly there are culture-specific forms of somatization and other externalizing patterns of managing dysphoria such as *shen-k'uei* discussed in Chapter 18 and the Chinese culture-bound syndromes covered in Chapter 19 in this volume. But in addition to these extreme examples, doubtless there are more subtle distinctions between the ways Chinese and members of other cultures employ culturally constituted mechanisms for coping with difficult emotions and emotional disorders. It is not our purpose here to detail these mechanisms, but we do wish to bring this subject to the attention of readers in the hope that it will be more adequately investigated in future. However, it is important to stress the fact that these processes also structure communication, such that patients, families and practitioners speak a somatic (or moral or cosmological), but not a psychological language to name, discuss, decide on treatment choices and apply therapy to these culturally shaped problems.

The clinical significance of the cultural patterning of cognition, affects and communication is easily seen. Problems that might be labeled as depression or anxiety in contemporary Western cultures are labeled as physical, moral, or cosmological problems in traditional Chinese culture and are so treated. This creates special forms of "clinical reality" in Chinese societies that are built up from cultural definitions and expectations that are particular to these settings. This process and its consequences for the practice of medicine and psychiatry among Chinese have been described in detail elsewhere (cf. Kleinman 1979). Clearly such cultural influences may create problems for clinicians in terms of misdiagnosis of unusual presentations of common disorders, patient and practitioner conflicts over treatment styles and objectives, poor compliance, patient and family dissatisfaction with care, and culturally inappropriate treatment leading to poor therapeutic outcome. For example, Chinese patients with somatized depression will not go to psychiatrists for care since they believe *and* experience their problem as a physical one. Rather they will go to general practitioners or traditional healers where they are likely not to receive adequate treatment of a disorder now effectively treated with psychiatric interventions. If they do go to a psychiatrist for care, their somatic orientation is likely to render psychotherapy inappropriate and ineffective, unless it is conducted with particular cultural strategies (Hsu and Tseng 1972). Such patients may drop out of care before they receive an adequate therapeutic trial because of the cultural expectation that Western medicine should be effective in one or two sessions or not at all and because the ubiquitous minor side-effects of tricyclic antidepressant medication may be unacceptable to them owing to the Chinese cultural belief that when Western medicine creates side-effects they are powerful and dangerous necessitating the medicine be stopped. Of course their entire pattern of help seeking will also be affected, so that virtually every aspect of clinical care can be strongly influenced by Chinese illness beliefs and treatment norms.

(2) CULTURAL INFLUENCES ON THE MANAGEMENT OF INTERPERSONAL TRANSACTIONS

Since this topic has received extensive coverage by social scientists in the literature (cf. Hsu 1971a, 1971b; Hu 1944; Solomon 1971: 1–133; and Chapters 1, 2, 3, 4, 7, 8, 10, and 11 in this volume), we simply wish to underline its potential clinical significance. Obviously somatization and other culturally constituted idioms of distress are used not just to express troubles, but also to manipulate interpersonal relations so as to produce desired change in these social situations. That is to say, these coping responses possess social efficacy. For example, in clinical cases we have seen patients complain of pain or possession as ways of complaining about untenable social situations that could not be complained of directly in a socially sanctioned way. Such complaints also manipulate these situations to the advantage of the patient. Hence in one case, a Taiwanese patient was possessed by both a god and a ghost. The ghost angrily complained of the patient's difficult home life and accused her husband and other family members as being the source of her trouble, while the god demanded that they alter their behavior toward her and give in to particular requests she had made. In Chapters 1 and 4 below, Metzger and Seaman discuss typical literati and peasant patterns of negotiating relationships of authority in Chinese society. Other aspects of the management of interpersonal relations in Chinese culture are covered in Harrell's chapter on patterns of drinking (Chapter 3) and in the chapters on childhood socialization (Chapters 7 and 8) and family structure and relations (Chapters 10 and 11).

It has been argued by Hsu (1971b), among others, that traditionally-oriented Chinese regard interpersonal relations as more important than intrapsychic affairs, that the maintenance of harmonious relations ("psychosocial homeostasis") within the family and social network is their major psychosocial preoccupation, and that their situation-orientation and other salient psychological features are particularly suited to the management of interpersonal problems. This core cultural theme we believe cannot be overemphasized. The specific techniques Chinese employ to manage important social relations, the stresses and tensions that these relations generate, and the clinical consequences of their breakdown are important points for future studies. We do not know at present if Chinese can be shown to be more heavily invested in such relations than members of Western cultures, if this investment changes with Westernization, and if this has any significant effect on types and prevalence rates of psychopathology as well as on patterns of help seeking and the nature of therapeutic interactions. But these are the kinds of researchable questions that are raised by ethnographic description and clinical impression.

(3) CULTURAL INFLUENCES ON THE PERCEPTION OF AND REACTION TO UNIVERSAL STRESSORS

Culture can influence whether a ubiquitous environmental stimulus is perceived as stressful or not, how stressful it is ranked among other stressors, and the kinds of coping processes brought into play to deal with particular stressors. For example, both Hsu (1971b) and Kleinman (1979: 134–135) report that traditionally oriented Chinese perceive interpersonal stress as more significant than financial stress, which in turn is rated as more stressful than intrapsychic stress, whereas Caucasian-Americans appear to reverse this order of perceived significance. Not enough work has been done with common life event changes to see if significant cross-cultural differences exist in their perceived severity for Chinese compared with other groups, or if Chinese experience different rates of illness onset at the same levels of life event change. This is such an obviously important area for comparative cross-cultural research that it is surprising and disappointing how little research has been carried out to date. Research in this area to be culturally valid clearly must take into account the specific cultural significance of particular life events, and hence this is an instance of the importance of meaning-oriented studies in cultural psychiatry. Now that scales are being developed to measure the psychological impact of particular events (Horowitz et al. 1979), special care must be taken to determine what Schweder (in press), in a massive review of studies in psychological anthropology, has called the major determinants of behavior: namely, " . . . 'idiosyncratic' or 'interactive' effects, the particular 'meaning' that a particular situation has for a particular person . . ."

(4) CULTURAL INFLUENCES ON CREATION OF AND COPING WITH CULTURE-SPECIFIC STRESSORS

In Chapter 13, Lin, Kleinman and Lin note that in a cross-cultural perspective on alcoholism, Chinese culture appears to "immunize" its members against this enormous public health problem. But whereas Chinese culture may be associated with more adaptive behaviors in this and perhaps other instances, it also may predispose to other behaviors that are maladaptive. For example, the traditional mother-in-law/daughter-in-law relationship has been a special source of culturally constituted stress that has yielded high rates of psychological problems and suicide for young married women. Similarly, the fact that the eldest son and youngest daughter positions in the birth order of siblings have been associated with the highest rates of psychopathology in Chinese culture suggests that family members who occupy these birth order ranks and the social roles that go with them are subjected to culturally constituted stressors that predispose them to mental illness. It has even been suggested of Chinese culture that in channeling behavior away from alcohol abuse it merely pushes deviant careers in the direction of pathological gambling and drug abuse.

If we take the broadest possible view of culture, then any special environmental stimulus can be discussed here. For example, the ecology of particular Chinese communities may expose their members to specific pathogens that affect behavior, e.g., infections or toxic agents that produce organic psychoses. Schistosomiasis, epidemic hemorrhagic fever, toxin induced nasophoryngeal carcinomas, etc., can produce central nervous system effects in Chinese residing in particular local environments in the People's Republic where these problems are found, whereas overseas Chinese are not at risk because they are not exposed to the same causative agents.

The fact that in traditional Chinese communities dissociative states are routinely sanctioned as individual coping mechanisms for handling personal stress may predispose to the development of hysterical reactions and even reactive psychoses in these settings. Although the epidemiological data to support this suggestion are not available, it illustrates a potentially significant maladaptive effect of culturally constituted coping processes.

(5) CULTURAL INFLUENCES ON SUSCEPTIBILITY, EPIDEMIOLOGICAL RATES, SYMPTOMATOLOGY, ILLNESS BEHAVIOR, HELP SEEKING, AND TREATMENT RESPONSE ASSOCIATED WITH PARTICULAR PSYCHIATRIC DISORDERS

This long list of variables boils down to Chinese cultural influences on psychiatric disorder and its treatment. Differential susceptibility to disease may result from genetically-based racial differences. To date we have no evidence of such an effect on mental disorders among Chinese populations. Indeed, survey findings demonstrate that schizophrenia and mental retardation have roughly comparable prevalence rates in Chinese and Western societies (see Chapter 13). Putting the still controversial culture-bound psychiatric syndromes and alcoholism aside, there is no evidence that any other form of psychopathology has either an extremely low or high rate among Chinese.

The same major ecological factors that increase susceptibility to mental illness in other societies seem to exert similar influences in Chinese communities. Hence increased rates of mental disorders are associated with lower socioeconomic status, migration, and urbanization. But finer analyses are needed to determine more subtle influences such as whether marriage in Chinese society as in the West protects men from depression but is a risk factor for women or whether the absence of a confiding relationship is a major risk factor for depression for married Chinese women as it has been shown to be for married women in the West. In Chapter 13, Lin, Kleinman and Lin review the available literature on the epidemiology of mental illness among Chinese and discuss research on the influence of ecological factors (see also Lee's discussion of influence of sex role and social class on psychiatric epidemiology in Chinese settings in Chapter 14).

In the preceding section, we reviewed culturally constituted stressors that appear to heighten risk for mental disorder for Chinese, but more research is needed to firmly establish this association and it must be compared cross-culturally to determine if it is specific to Chinese culture or not. Such cross-cultural comparisons must take into account other Asian as well as Western populations before unique patterns of susceptibility among Chinese can be adequately assessed.

Cross-cultural differences in epidemiological rates of neuroses and other minor psychopathology have been repeatedly demonstrated in surveys, and this is the case for Chinese populations that have been studied as well (cf. Chapter 13), though we cannot as of yet quantitate these differences for disorders like depression, hysteria, anxiety neurosis, and personality problems. Preliminary data on family pathology is only now becoming available (see Chapter 12).

In our discussion of cultural influences on affects and affective disorders in the first section of this chapter, we described how Chinese cultural meanings and behavioral norms shape the symptomatology of depression as well as the illness behavior associated with that disorder. As we best understand what occurs, depression, a universal psychiatric *disease* with a psychobiological basis, is transformed into a type of *illness* behavior that is culturally-specific. The experience of depressive illness among most Chinese is vegetative not intrapsychic as it tends to be in the West. Moreover, the experience of somatization that is constructed among Chinese is organized around *culture-specific* symptom terms, patterns of resort to coping mechanisms, "final common" behavioral pathways, and types of help seeking. The patterns of illness behavior associated with other psychiatric disorders among Chinese are not as well understood as that associated with depression, but in our view the illness behavior associated with all diseases are culture-specific. What we now need are careful descriptions of the types of different illness behaviors in Chinese culture, comparisons of illness behaviors associated with the same diseases across different Chinese and other populations, and determination of what are universal and culture-specific features of the sick role. Obviously this approach leads to a reassessment of the culture-bound syndromes, which become only extreme examples of a common cultural transformation.

The clinical significance of the cultural patterning of illness behavior is discussed in Chapters 13, 15, 17, 18, and 20 in this volume. As we have already noted it affects patterns of help seeking, doctor-patient interactions, clinical judgment, and sometimes therapeutic response as well. For example, in the WHO International Pilot Study of Schizophrenia, outcome from schizophrenia has been found to vary inversely with social development, i.e., outcome was better for schizophrenic patients in less developed societies (Sartorius, Jablensky and Shapiro 1978). A leading explanation of this finding is that the illness behavior associated with schizophrenia varies in these settings such that, in spite of the serious nature of the disease, it (the illness behavior) is treated as limited in more traditional societies and interminable in modern Western societies. These cultural expectations, it is argued, become self-fulfilling prophecies. Hence culture may exert a major effect on outcome through its influence on illness behavior.

Lin and Lin (1978, and Chapter 20 below) have shown that Chinese ethnicity is associated with a unique help-seeking pathway to the mental health center in Vancouver that contrasts strikingly with the pathways associated with Caucasian-Canadian and other ethnic groups. This Chinese help-seeking pathway is associated with significant delay in obtaining professional services that may well exert a negative effect on therapeutic response. We have already discussed other potentially negative clinical consequences of Chinese cultural beliefs and values. An additional one that can be extremely important is differential evaluation of therapeutic outcome owing to distinctive cultural perceptions of what constitutes *efficacy*. Both the professional culture of mental health workers and Chinese popular culture set out criteria by which to assess outcome. These criteria reflect beliefs about cause, pathophysiology and appropriate treatment. Where disease is viewed in narrow biomedical terms by psychiatrists, while illness is articulated in the indigenous categories of Chinese medicine or folk religion by patients, two distinctive sets of criteria are elaborated to judge therapeutic success or failure. Successful treatment of disease problems (biochemical derangements, thought-disordered speech, anxiety) can occur along with unsuccessful treatment of illness problems (maladaptive individual coping response, family tensions, untreated religious cause, etc.). These cultural effects on evaluations of outcome also can feed back to determine actual response to treatment since they may constrain patients to drop out of care before an adequate therapeutic trial is completed.

(6) CULTURAL INFLUENCES ON LABELING OF AND SOCIETAL REACTION TO SOCIAL DEVIANCE

"Normality" and "deviance" are as much cultural categories as are "abnormality" and "illness." Culture will affect what primary deviance (behavior originally demonstrated by the individual before labels are applied) the individual chooses to self-label or others choose to label as deviance. These labels in turn help create forms of secondary deviance that include cultural expectations about how deviants with a particular label should behave. These expectations then function, social labeling theorists assert, as a self-fulfilling prophecy. Behavior popularly labeled as social deviance need not represent psychopathology as defined by psychiatric disease categories, and the latter may not receive a label of social deviance. Perhaps one reason that homosexuality is infrequently encountered as a problem brought to psychiatric clinics in Chinese communities is that it is not labeled as illness. Similarly, as we have noted, minor psychological problems affecting Chinese may receive a moral, religious, or physical disease label, and thereby avoid the stigma associated with mental illness in Chinese society.

Almost no research has compared Chinese communities with other societies in the labeling of particular forms of social deviance. But if labeling theory is to be treated as a serious explanation of behavior, its hypotheses must be subjected to cross-cultural tests. Townsend (1978) has demonstrated that among German mental patients and psychiatrists and American mental patients and psychiatrists there is a greater degree of culturally shared beliefs about the cause and treatment of mental illness than professionally shared ones. The same kind of study needs to be conducted among Chinese to determine to what extent Chinese cultural views of mental illness and other forms of deviance supersede professional views.

Labeling theory also focuses our attention on conflicts in the negotiation of labels. There is no evidence that we are aware of from Chinese cultures that the label of mental illness is applied and resisted as a form of social control of political deviance as it is in the Soviet Union. But other kinds of labeling conflicts are common. One example is the routine conflict over the use of the highly stigmatizing label of mental illness, with members of the popular culture, traditional practitioners, and general medical practitioners unwilling to apply this label save to floridly psychotic or mentally retarded patients, and with mental health professionals extending its application to a much broader array of behaviors.

Since culture arguably has its greatest impact through the categories applied to conceptualize events, the labeling process offers an excellent opportunity to study cultural influences on behavior. Several contributors to this volume study somatization from this perspective (see Chapters 13, 17, and 18). In Chapter 3, Harrell sets out the cultural rules that guide rural Taiwanese in deciding what kinds of drinking behavior are deviant; and in Chapter 2, Hsieh and Spence show how certain kinds of suicide in traditional Chinese culture were viewed as deviant while other kinds were viewed as normative. In McGough's detailed description of deviant marriage patterns in traditional Chinese society (Chapter 10), we see how the very category of marriage is culturally constructed so that what is viewed as deviant or normative in imperial China varies from what is so labeled in contemporary Chinese communities and what was labeled as deviant by upper class literati may not have been deviant for peasants. Indeed, McGough shows that what is meant by "marriage" in Chinese culture is quite distinct from what this category "means" in the West. In Chapter 7, Wilson outlines core Chinese cultural values that play a large part in the labeling of deviant behavior, and he also compares Chinese and Western cultures in their tendencies to label behavior as deviant. Social deviance raises many other issues that fall outside the scope of this book (cf. Wilson, Greenblatt and Wilson 1977).

(7) CULTURAL INFLUENCES ON INDIGENOUS AND PROFESSIONAL SYSTEMS FOR TREATING MENTAL ILLNESS AND THE PSYCHOSOCIAL CONCOMITANTS OF PHYSICAL ILLNESS

A great deal has been written about indigenous and professional treatment systems in Chinese societies (cf. Kleinman et al. 1975; Kleinman et al. 1978), the point we wish to make here is that these institutions are components of local cultural systems of health care that manage mental illness as well as the psychosocial concomitants of physical illness. Most sickness, including psychological problems and stress responses, in Chinese societies is managed in the family context (cf. Kleinman 1979: 179–202). But indigenous healers (shamans, fortune-tellers, temple-based ritual specialists, Chinese-style physicians) and Western-style primary care physicians provide much of the treatment for mental illness and psychosocial concomitants of physical illness. Psychiatrists and other mental health professionals treat only a small fraction of these problems in Chinese society. This reinforces the Chinese cultural orientation we have previously described in which mental illness and psychosocial problems associated with physical disorders are labeled and managed as somatic rather than psychological phenomena requiring somatic rather than psychological interventions. In Chapter 17, Kleinman and Mechanic suggest that this is as true of health care in the People's Republic as it is of indigenous and Western professional treatment in Taiwan.

This particular organization of Chinese cultural systems of care means that many treatable mental health problems are often unrecognized, misdiagnosed or do not receive effective care by trained mental health professionals. What psychosocial interventions are provided come almost entirely from sacred folk healers and members of the family and social network. Neither in Taiwan nor the People's Republic of China is professional psychotherapy legitimated or available for the general population.

Among the range of problems treated by local Chinese health care systems are personal and interpersonal troubles, financial and work problems, family conflicts, educational failure, and many other kinds of life problems that receive their expression and therapy in the idiom of disease and medical care. The absence of appropriate social and mental health agencies means that in Chinese culture most forms of abnormal behavior and deviance are medicalized.

In concluding this brief outline of the various ways Chinese culture affects behavior, we wish again to emphasize that this is an enormous field and that in putting together this collection we have managed to cover only some of the issues. In reviewing the chapters that follow, however, we believe readers can derive an appreciation for key themes and problems in the study of normal and abnormal behavior among Chinese that we hope contributes both to deepening their understanding of Chinese culture and to broadening their comparative knowledge of behavior.

NOTE

1. Throughout this book, we use the Wade-Giles system of Romanizing Chinese.

REFERENCES

Carr, J. E.
1978 Ethno-behaviorism and the culture-bound syndromes: The case of *amok*. Culture, Medicine and Psychiatry 2: 269–293.
Doi, T.
1973 The Anatomy of Dependence. (Translated by John Bester). Tokyo: Kodansha.
Horowitz, M. et al.
1979 Impact of event scale: A measure of subjective stress. Psychosomatic Medicine 41: 209–218.
Hsu, F. L. K.
1971a Eros, affect and *pao*. *In* Kinship and Culture. F. L. K. Hsu, ed. Chicago: Aldine; pp. 439–475.
Hsu, F. L. K.
1971b Psychosocial homeostasis and *Jen*: Conceptual tools for advancing psychological anthropology. American Anthropologist 73: 23–44.
Hsu, J. and Tseng, W. S.
1972 Intercultural psychotherapy. Archives of General Psychiatry 27: 700–705.
Hu, H. C.
1944 The Chinese concept of face. American Anthropologist 46: 45–64.
Kleinman, A. et. al., eds.
1975 Medicine in Chinese Cultures. Washington, D.C.: U.S. Government Printing Office for the Fogarty International Center, N.I.H.
Kleinman, A. et al., eds.
1978 Culture and Healing in Asian Societies. Cambridge, Mass.: Schenkman.
Kleinman, A.
1979 Patients and Healers in the Context of Culture. Berkeley: University of California Press.
Lin, T. Y. and Lin, M. C.
1978 Service delivery issues in Asian North American Communities. American Journal of Psychiatry 135:454–456.
Sartorius, N., Jablensky, A., and Shapiro, R.
1978 Cross-cultural differences in the short-term prognosis of schizophrenic psychoses. Schizophrenia Bulletin 4(1): 102–113.
Schweder, R.
in press From chaos to cosmos: A Neo-Tylorian essay on explanation and understanding in psychological anthropology. Ethos.
Solomon, R.
1971 Mao's Revolution and the Chinese Political Culture. Berkeley: University of California Press.
Townsend, J. M.
1978 Cultural Conceptions and Mental Illness. Chicago: University of Chicago Press.
Tseng, W. S.
1975 The nature of somatic complaints among psychiatric patients: The Chinese case. Comprehensive Psychiatry 16: 237–245.
Wilson, A. A., Greenblatt, S. L., and Wilson, R. W., eds.
1977 Deviance and Social Control in Chinese Society. New York: Praeger.

HISTORICAL AND CULTURAL BACKGROUND OF BELIEFS AND NORMS GOVERNING BEHAVIOR

INTRODUCTION TO SECTION I

The articles in this section cover only a few of the many subjects that could be subsumed under this broad theme. But they do illustrate the types of questions that need to be addressed if we are to arrive at a more discriminating understanding of the historical and cultural background of beliefs and norms guiding behavior in Chinese culture. What are some examples of core norms and meanings concerning normal and abnormal behavior in traditional Chinese culture? How have they functioned at different historical periods and at present? What are the consequences of their continuity and change? The contributors to this section — historians, anthropologists, and a psychiatrist — examine these and other key issues. Because relatively little research has been conducted heretofore that specifically centers on the individual in Chinese culture, these chapters should be regarded as preliminary explorations that break new ground. They reflect distinctive disciplinary approaches, raise many more questions than answers, and point up the need for future studies that are informed, and perhaps even carried out, from an interdisciplinary perspective. As heuristics, the articles suggest concrete hypotheses for empirical research as well as more general conceptual and methodological problems. This section introduces subjects that reverberate throughout the book. It opens the curtain on a distinctive Chinese stage, a behavioral field, certain of whose culture-specific and universal features are highlighted in the sections that follow.

Metzger, an historian, assesses selfhood and authority in the Neo-Confucian tradition up to the present time as culturally constituted ideals guiding individual behavior, at least for the elite class of literati. He suggests that the Neo-Confucian tradition needs to be viewed afresh from *within* in order to dispel Western biases and capture salient indigenous categories of individual thought and action that have been overlooked or underplayed. He discusses the cultural articulation of affect in the moral code of literati values, suggesting that a different psychological approach is needed to grasp the experiential states and action forms associated with this distinctive language of the emotions. In reviewing the social consequences of these psychocultural patterns, Metzger develops a sophisticated framework for taking the individual into account in historical and political studies. His complex account should broaden and deepen readers' understanding of the clinical problems as well as the adaptive coping styles that emerge from this cultural matrix. It also should help restrain readers from stereotyping Chinese behavioral patterns into the crude dichotomy so often associated with the rural peasant and modern, Western technocratic distinctions of an overly narrow model of societal development.

Hsieh and Spence summarize their findings about suicide in pre-modern

A. Kleinman and T.-Y. Lin (eds.), Normal and Abnormal Behavior in Chinese Culture, 3–5.
Copyright © 1980 by D. Reidel Publishing Company.

China. Not only do they analyze its specific cultural determinants and social functions, but in addition they illustrate its use both as an explanatory paradigm and interpersonal strategy within the Chinese family. They discuss problems that result from the structural principles and social dynamics of the Chinese family system that introduce themes investigated anthropologically, sociologically, and psychiatrically in Section III. Problems associated with female roles and relationships in the family are especially well covered by these authors. They demonstrate that certain kinds of suicide in traditional Chinese society were neither socially deviant nor the result of psychological abnormality. Such sanctioned forms of suicide were culturally prescribed as normative in particular situations that Hsieh and Spence illustrate with paradigmatic behavioral exemplars drawn from historical sources.

In the third article in this section, Harrell, an anthropologist, draws on his ethnographic research in rural Taiwan to discuss the embedding of alcohol use in social institutions and cultural norms that control the social deviance frequently associated with it in other societies and that thereby may be a major determinant of the strikingly small amount of alcoholism among Chinese. Harrell describes several variables in the social organization of alcohol use that could be operationalized as testable hypotheses in empirical field studies in other Chinese communities and in other cultures. This is a subject of considerable cross-cultural importance, since alcohol has become a prodigious problem for Western societies and for a large number of non-Western societies (e.g., Native American groups) but Chinese culture appears to "immunize" against this problem. Hence what is learned from future studies of alcohol use and abuse among Chinese might have preventive significance where generalized cross-culturally.

Had space permitted, we would have liked to include other papers in this section dealing with culturally adaptive and maladaptive aspects of drug abuse, prostitution and sexual behavior generally, inter-ethnic stereotypes and conflicts, value change and conflict, interracial marriage, and other relevant anthropological and sociological themes. We hope, however, that the very limitations we have had to impose on the volume in order to select illustrative examples of a potentially enormous field will stimulate others to review these and other subjects, many of which are just as central to human behavior in Chinese culture as are the particular themes reviewed here. More importantly, since data on these subjects is often minimal, we wish to encourage our anthropological and sociological colleagues to advance our understanding of these important subjects, many of which heretofore have received only casual consideration.

The article that follows is by another anthropologist who works in Taiwan, Seaman, and is an interpretation of shamanistic cults that views them as providing culturally sanctioned idioms for articulating personal and interpersonal distress and thereby manipulating sources of power in rural Taiwanese society to resolve such problems. Seaman demonstrates how role reversals in folk religious rituals reduce social tensions that are associated with traditional sources of power while legitimating the social efficacy of ritual communication. He demonstrates the parallels between norms governing private relationships in Chinese families and public relationships between gods, shamans, and clients. Along the way, he also contributes to our understanding of both the role functions of and strains on social mediators in Chinese society and the vexed question of whether shamans are abnormal or socially deviant. Seaman's discussion of authority in a contemporary rural Chinese community contrasts in a number of interesting ways with Metzger's account of authority in the context of the traditional Chinese elite class.

The final two articles in this section specifically focus on mental illness in traditional China. In one Chiu, an historian, reexamines the legal response to insanity in imperial China. She describes key changes in the official legal position on the insane, demonstrating that shifts in attitudes followed the state's ability to devote resources to the problem. Insanity posed a threat to the Chinese social order that stimulated responses of social control via the legal system which were most intense during times of stability and prosperity. During periods of stress, especially during the collapse of imperial China in the late Ch'ing, legal interest in insanity faded. But throughout these fluctuations, Chiu reveals that the major responsibility for the care of the mentally ill in China resided with the family, a tradition that has continued up to the present (see the final article of the book). This article should be of interest to readers both for its review of forensic psychiatry in traditional Chinese society and for its description of the culturally constituted legal and moral codes through which insanity was socially controlled.

In the last article of Section I, Lin, a psychiatrist who has had some training in medical anthropology, briefly reviews traditional Chinese beliefs about mental illness and its treatment. He shows that these beliefs relate to core Chinese cultural themes that have developed into several distinctive therapeutic traditions: traditional Chinese medicine, secular folk healing, and religious folk healing. The relation of each of these traditions to mental illness is outlined. Lin underlines the fact that these traditional beliefs diverge considerably from modern Western concepts about mental illness because they do not reify a mind/body dualism or view illness as reducible to structural lesions, but rather take a holistic, bio-psychosocial approach that relates microcosmic and macrocosmic processes and interprets illness as problems in functioning and interrelationships between components in an integrated, functional system. Lin indicates the clinical significance of these beliefs in guiding individual and family treatment, utilization of folk healers, and response to psychiatry. He differentiates stigma associated with mental illness among Chinese from stigma in the West because the former attaches principally to the family not the individual. Many of the illness beliefs he reviews relate to clinical issues covered in the final section of this book.

THOMAS A. METZGER

1. SELFHOOD AND AUTHORITY IN NEO-CONFUCIAN POLITICAL CULTURE

I. AUTONOMY AND THE LITERATURE ON CHINESE POLITICAL CULTURE

Despite much emphasis on the interplay of class interests, many scholars continue to believe that cultural orientations have greatly influenced the development of Chinese society in premodern and modern times. There is also a considerable consensus that despite China's cultural heterogeneity, a single, tradition-rooted set of shared orientations has been extremely widespread and has played a leading if not modal role in China's cultural evolution coming down to the present. Moreover, there is some consensus about the content of this set of orientations. This can be seen from the wide range of writing represented in the following studies: Weber's classic on Chinese religion (Weber 1951); a symposium volume put out by a group of Chinese behavioral scientists in 1972 and sponsored by the Academia Sinica (Li I-yüan and Yang Kuo-shu 1972); a survey and critique of the literature on Chinese culture written by Morton H. Fried in 1976 (Fried 1976); another such critical survey put out by Wei Yung in 1976 (Wei 1976); an analysis of China's traditional political orientations written in 1977 by a Chinese historian who has specialized in the premodern history of Chinese government (Chou Tao-chi 1977); and the writings of modern humanists discussing China's traditional "cultural spirit", notably those of T'ang Chün-i (see Metzger 1977: 29–47). Leaving aside the more specific research on, say, changes in the life goals of Taiwan students during the span of a few years, we find three main points in this literature.

First, there is much agreement on the existence of a syndrome stressing both the importance of authority figures and the need of the self to merge into the group. Familism, "dependence", and particularism have often been linked to this syndrome. Scholars like Chou Tao-chi note a complementary trend in the polity, that toward unchecked autocracy, although he relates this political trend also to non-cultural factors, such as the communication difficulties inevitable in a vast, premodern country.

Second, many connect this authoritarianism to what can be summed up as "a relatively passive way of dealing with objects in [the] environment, whether inherited norms, social objects, or natural objects" (Metzger 1977: 241). Multifaceted, this passivity has been seen as including a tendency toward fatalism, toward patient acceptance of suffering, and away from the direct articulation of ego's own interests. Weber's emphasis on a lack of "tension" between ideals and reality also is close to this notion of passivity.

Third, humanists especially have pointed to an emphasis on the idea that

7

A. Kleinman and T.-Y. Lin (eds.), Normal and Abnormal Behavior in Chinese Culture, 7–27.

human nature is good and on education, achievement, and social mobility. Philosophers like T'ang Chün-i have gone further, arguing that Confucianism has focused on the individual as a morally autonomous being seeking to realize oneness with a transcendent, cosmic good. This view refers to innumerable Confucian calls for autonomy, such as Mencius' (371–289 B.C.?) claim that the moral individual "cannot be corrupted by wealth and high station, cannot be persuaded to change his views by the pressures of poverty and low station, and cannot be made to bend by fear of those who awesomely wield physical power" (Legge 1966: 651); Hsün-tzu's (ca. 298–239 B.C.) view that the moral person is "proud before those with wealth and high station . . . [and] regards kings and dukes lightly" (Liang 1969: 15); and the idea of "standing and acting on one's own" in the classic *Li-chi* (*Ju-hsing* chapter). Because it was ambiguously defined, the idea of authority was logically compatible with such autonomy. Both Mencius and Hsün-tzu used three partly conflicting criteria of hierarchical position: age, political or social position, and virtue (Legge 1966: 568; Liang 1969: 48). Elucidating this idea of autonomy, T'ang focused on the Neo-Confucian concern with the ontological basis of individual moral effort.

Yet due to a kind of disciplinary compartmentalization, the humanists have talked about autonomy, the behavioral scientists, about authoritarianism and passivity, and virtually no one has inquired into the relations between these three. To be sure, a variety of scholars have in effect tried to solve this problem by regarding the norm of autonomy as epiphenomenal, holding either that it was morally betrayed by the Confucians of the imperial age (Hsü Fu-kuan 1977), or that it had no influence on overt behavior outside a tiny elite circle. This standpoint has been very hard to surmount because while it appears as an evaluation of the tradition by modern standards, it is paradoxically rooted in an angle of vision with which traditional Confucians viewed their moral lives, and which has remained basic in modern times.

Confucians were less interested in analyzing their own sense of selfhood than in moralistically focusing on their frailties, in denouncing the frailties of others, and in dwelling on the norms of the ideal society, where there would be no need for autonomous behavior challenging those in power. With their eyes fixed on their ideal hierarchy or "the five relationships" along with its list of standard virtues, such as filial piety and loyalty, Confucians regarded their own emphasis on autonomy as referring merely to the determination to realize these standard virtues. Feeling that this determination was precisely what had been lacking since the golden age, they had no reason to think of it as a norm typical of the imperial period. Then modernizers intent on denouncing the tradition simply identified it with these standard virtues, easily ignoring what in the past had anyway been referred to only obliquely and had been regarded as an unrealized virtue. Similarly, when a Chinese political scientist recently suggested study of the "politically relevant concepts of traditional China", he referred only to this list of standard virtues (Wei 1976: 140).

Yet how can any ideal endlessly reiterated in the Confucian literature have had no behavioral impact? Take, for instance, the following famous statement of Mencius (Legge 1966: 599–600): "But Heaven does not yet wish that the empire should enjoy tranquillity and good order. If it wished this, who is there besides me to bring it about?" As Chou Tao-chi indicates (Chou Tao-chi 1977: 28–30), this passage combines a somewhat fatalistic view of history with a concept of ego's great moral responsibility for the world. How can we say that the former idea necessarily had more behavioral impact than the latter?

For overt behavior apparently linked to this ideal of the autonomous ego, we can turn to the bureaucratic system of "remonstrance", institutionalized almost continuously since the third century B.C., or to the pattern of rebellious behavior, the importance of which in the nineteenth century has recently been demonstrated statistically (Yang 1975). Clearly, in the case of many local disturbances sparked by economic grievances, the participants and even much of their gentry audience believed that the Confucian principle of "righteousness" (*i*) gave moral legitimation to violent illegal actions defying the will of official authority figures responsible for a particular injustice (*ta pu kung-tao*). A recent study contains unusually rich data about one such uprising that occurred in Ningpo in 1852 (Liu 1978: 353–361). Or take the case of early modernizers like Liang Ch'i-ch'ao (1873–1929), who felt that the course of history had thrust on him and a small elite the responsibility to save China (Chang 1969: 20, 45, 63–64, 74; Chang 1978: 17–18, 105). His sense of ego's capacities and mission was obviously a "politically relevant concept", and there is no question but that it was based on his Confucian heritage, which in fact did dominate his formative years. While the ideal of autonomy affected the behavior of many male adults in times of political crisis, it also influenced the self-image of scholars and bureaucrats dealing in normal times with a world they typically perceived as bad (Metzger 1977: 167–190).

II. METHODOLOGICAL CONSIDERATIONS

Therefore elucidation of this ideal is needed if we are to understand that central set of cultural orientations, or an important aspect of it, with which Chinese have entered the modern era. To start with, however, some methodological points should be made. First, based on Metzger (1977), my discussion here can apply only to that sector of the population to which the material used in this book refers. This material consists of some of the social science literature on modal Chinese personality patterns (chapter 1); some of the modern humanistic literature on such patterns (chapter 2); some of the central writings of the Neo-Confucian philosophical tradition, which dominated elite education during those centuries just before the modern period (chapter 3); bureaucratic documents from the Ch'ing period (1644–1912) (chapter 4, Metzger 1973); and a mix of primary and secondary sources regarding modern Chinese thought (chapter 5). Hence we are dealing with orientations widespread among the educated during a long period including the twentieth century — a minority, but a highly influential one.

A second problem is how best to describe the shared orientations of this group. Intellectual biography, as Wang Erh-min also has suggested (Wang 1977: 522–523), is not an approach well suited for this task. Intellectual historians have become preoccupied with individual idiosyncrasies, but by typically ignoring shared orientations, they have often been unable to explain the meaning of competitive doctrines or even specify what was distinctive in a particular thinker's outlook. Chinese philosophers have sometimes examined shared orientations, but the philosophical method is also not suited for our task. We are mainly interested not in selecting out ideas that can be defended as "true" but in describing what William James called a "state of mind" (James 1958), considering as comprehensively as possible all the verbalized feelings and ideas which together formed a certain mental pattern "defining the situation" of the population group investigated (to use W. I. Thomas's term). From the standpoint of this anthropological approach to ideas, clichés are more important than "true" ideas, even though the problem of the relation between the truth of an idea and its meaning for an historical actor remains a vexing one. Because it largely deals not with idiosyncratic doctrines but with clichés used in common by all the Neo-Confucian schools over some eight centuries, my account of Neo-Confucianism can plausibly claim to describe some of the shared orientations most basic to the thinking of the educated classes in late imperial times (Metzger 1977: 50–51).

To be sure, American philosophers are often skeptical about the possibility of "translating ... alien sentences" and so of empathetically penetrating an historical "state of mind" (Quine 1969: 1–20). Quine's doubts, however, are not shared by any of the modern Chinese philosophers who have worked on Neo-Confucianism, and whose methodology in effect coincides with Dilthey's theory of *Verstehen*. Following Dilthey, however, I would distinguish empathetic understanding from that hagiographic tone found in so much writing on Neo-Confucianism. We can empathize with an historical actor and yet still see beyond his self-image. As important, however, is the question of how to put ideas into context so as to discern the "state of mind" they form.

Context means juxtaposing ideas, but we have to distinguish between juxtaposition that plausibly occurred in the mind of the historical actor and juxtaposition in the mind of the modern scholar studying this historical figure. Sitting in an American library, we can try to contrast what Mao thought Kant meant with what Kant really meant. This kind of juxtaposition leads to what has been called a "hall of mirrors" (Wakeman 1973: xiii), but what Mao juxtaposed in his own mind is obviously a still more basic question.

Yet if we are interested in the pattern formed by ideas juxtaposed within the mind of an historical actor, we need, I think, some analytical framework not only facilitating comparison but also ensuring that we are to the best of our ability taking account of all those attitudes most basic to behavior. Most work on "shared vocabularies" has unfortunately lacked such a framework. My approach is to posit that all human thought shares certain features and then to use these universal features as themes around which to organize data.

First, I posit that all thought defines the self in its relations with the cosmos and the group, which includes the idea of authority. Historical time, the temporal context especially of the group, is a fourth category. Invariably these relations imply epistemological criteria, that is, the standards used by an audience to distinguish true or valuable ideas from ordinary or false ones. Second, these orientations usually involve a distinction between the ideal and the given state of the self and the group, along with a perception of the means available to close this gap. If the means are perceived as adequate for the job, we can speak of a sense of impending solution. If not, we have a "sense of predicament." Third, the competition between idiosyncratic doctrines in a particular cultural arena occurs among thinkers who largely share an agenda of problems, those associated with closing this gap, and a set of epistemological criteria or rules of the game. This obvious point has sometimes been overlooked. For instance, scholars have argued over whether Confucian philosophy had any living meaning in the twentieth century without inquiring into the agenda and the criteria of the audience to whom this philosophy was addressed. Yet if the interplay of ideas should be put within the context of such a shared "grammar" of thought, conversely shared cultural orientations cannot be understood without looking into the *Problematik* of historical actors as thinking people.

III. SELF AND COSMOS IN NEO-CONFUCIANISM

Using this framework and the materials mentioned above, we can describe Neo-Confucian orientations in terms of the way they defined the goal of life and the dyadic relation between ego and cosmos through which this goal could be reached. Aiming for "sagehood", Neo-Confucians envisaged a radical transformation (*pa-pen se-yüan*), not piece-meal improvement. It is striking, though, that they were preoccupied not with the ideal socio-political order of the "five relationships" but rather with a kind of transcendent precondition of this order. They wanted a totalistic moral state, endlessly worrying about the tiniest moment of deviation. They wanted total moral purity, meaning the absolute absence of any self-interest, but the idea of this purity was intertwined for them with that of a total cognitive understanding of all existence. This understanding, moreover, had to be obtained in a "living" way by confronting and overcoming "doubts", since the truth could not be transmitted in any obvious, mechanical way.

The nature of this cognitive understanding was determined by their perception of the cosmos as an architectonically unified and inherently moral whole, each facet linked to the next. Understanding, therefore, meant tracing out this pattern of linkage, particularly the triangular linkage between ego's "mind", the ultimate basis of the cosmos ("principle"), and the "things" of ordinary experience (*hsin, li, wu*). With this shared focus on linkage, Neo-Confucians typically criticized a philosophical formula by claiming that it "split mind and principle into two." Partly by using modern philosophical terminology, T'ang Chün-i has

shown with what subtlety and intensity Neo-Confucians thought about this
ideal, pursuing the oneness of the "inner" (thought) and the "outer" (action),
of subject and object, of the human and the purely natural, of the spatial community and the temporal, of the transcendent and the mundane (Metzger 1978).

With this moral and cognitive state came a peculiar emotional sensation of
power. One aimed to "collect one's spirit back into its point of utter oneness
with the heart of the cosmos" and then let it "expand outward without limit"
(*shou-shih, t'ui-k'uo*). In this moment one had absolute self-determination, being
one with *chu-tsai* (that in the cosmos which rules all else), and so one was filled
with a sense of power (*li-liang*), joy (*lo*) and pride (*tzu-tsun*).

To conceptualize this power Neo-Confucians used the political image of
"control" (*kuan*). Already in Chou times, the images of power and subservience
influenced the conceptualization of the moral mind. Hsün-tzu referred to the
"mind" as *shen-ming-chih chu* (that which controls through the spiritual force
of its utterly bright understanding) and as a *t'ien-chün* (natural ruler) which
"governed" the five senses, and by means of which "heaven and earth would
be governed and the ten thousand things would be made to serve" human
needs (Liang 1969: 299, 228–229). This theme of transformative power was
emphasized especially in the classic *Chung-yung*. The great Han Confucian
Tung Chung-shu (ca. 179–104 B.C.) emphasized the power of "the King" over
the cosmos. Yet as Neo-Confucians after about 1100 focused rather on the
"mind" of the scholar as the main vehicle of moral action, they implied that this
vehicle was as potent as the royal one. Taken from *The Classic of Changes*, the
vocabulary of "mastering" and "encompassing" the cosmos was commonly used
by them. The idea of "control" was implicit when Chu Hsi (1130–1200), the
greatest Neo-Confucian, referred to the sage's "great power" to "do" whatever
"heaven and earth failed to do"; when he said that "If there is something not
right in the affairs of the world, it is set right by the sage"; and when he made
the amazing statement that the result of one person's perfect moral effort would
be the total material perfection of the whole world. The idea of control was
explicit when he said: "Man is the mind of heaven and earth. When man is not
present, there is no one to *kuan* (control) heaven and earth."

The impact of this statement, it should be noted, comes less from the verb
kuan than from the suggestion that man's function is to serve as the "mind" for
the cosmos. For Chu Hsi, the mind was inherently a vehicle of "control." Thus
he took from Chang Tsai (1020–1077) the definition of the mind as "that
which controls the heaven-conferred nature and the feelings." Moreover, in a
completely unambiguous statement, he said that while "principle is found in all
the ten thousand things of heaven and earth . . . it is controlled by the mind"
(Metzger 1977: 78, 137, 98, 143). Therefore the modern authority Fung Yu-lan
was correct when he said that by and large "most Chinese philosophers" pictured
the sage as having "the capability to *chia-yü* (control) the actual, physical world"
(Fung 1961: 202). True, as Fung notes, there were doubts about this capability.
Yet because the pathos of such control was basic to the Neo-Confucians' sense

of themselves, they clung to the terminology allowing them to verbalize and visualize such control. In short, they demanded the responsibility totally to close the gap between the ideal and the real throughout the world. Said Wang Yang-ming (1472–1529), the leading Neo-Confucian after Chu Hsi's time: "If one thing fails to find its proper place, this shows that my capacity for virtue has not been fully realized in one way or another" (Metzger 1977: 79). To realize such control was to realize linkage, especially a society in which all people were as "one body" (*i-t'i*).

Perceiving this goal, Neo-Confucians, as already mentioned, also perceived ego as autonomously able to pursue this goal, despite ambiguities introduced by the idea of *t'ien-ming* (that which heaven has decreed) (Metzger 1977: 127–134). As I have argued, they in effect perceived two aspects of the mind: a phasic flow of feeling stemming ultimately from that point in ego's mind which coincided with the pure, indivisible consciousness in the cosmos (*hsü-ling ming-chüeh*); and what can be called ego's "intervening will", which could either guide these feelings toward the goal described above or let them lapse into "selfish desire." To guide them, the mind as will carried out *kung-fu* (efficacious moral efforts), which were repeatedly divided into three kinds: a partly ineffable process of spiritual nurture, a largely verbalized process of study, and action. Actually, though, we have to add a fourth capability. When Neo-Confucians were in the act of advancing a particular philosophical formula, say Wang Yang-ming's "doctrine" (*shuo*) of "the oneness of knowledge and action", they were not carrying out what they regarded as *kung-fu* but rather were doing what Mencius had apologetically called "arguing." Thus "arguing" about the guidelines of *kung-fu*, Neo-Confucians in vague terms differed over how to conceptualize the linkage between "mind" and "principle." Yet their differences become clearer to us when we see that largely they centered on the relation between the indivisible cosmic consciousness and the individual's "intervening will." Chu Hsi ignored this subjective will when conceptualizing linkage, while Wang Yang-ming had the insight that the linkage between the subjective will and this ultimate, given cosmic consciousness would have to be conceptualized.

Yet how could "efficacious moral efforts", not to mention "arguing", realize the goal of cosmic control and oneness described above? Committed to this goal, Neo-Confucians required a vocabulary which allowed them to think of their "efforts" as cosmically potent and of the cosmos as susceptible to their influence. This vocabulary, denoting the mind's phasic flow of feeling and its continuity with the structure of the cosmos as a whole, was dropped in modern times as science took over the task of describing the cosmos, and as new ways were found of translating moral feeling into "outer" action. Hence modern Chinese philosophers have neglected this Neo-Confucian perception of a vital dyadic relation between mind and cosmos, preferring just to celebrate the Neo-Confucian concept of the mind as an answer to Western existentialism.

This modern perspective has prevented many scholars from grasping the importance of this dyadic relation in Chinese thought. Even when the organismic version of this relation – the traditional theory of *yin* and *yang*, of the phases of ego's mind, and of the indivisible cosmic mind – was dropped, the broader epistemological and ontological assumptions defining this dyadic relation often remained integral to modern philosophizing about heroic action. This is illustrated equally well by Mao Tse-tung's main philosophical essays, 'On Contradiction' and 'On Practice' (written in 1937), and the philosophy of culture and history that was developed by the "cultural conservative" T'ang Chün-i in the 1950s, and that is well represented by three books of his (T'ang 1955, 1972, 1975).

First, even if the idea of a cosmic "mind" was dropped (T'ang kept it), there was more broadly the assumption that ultimate cosmic reality could be known as noumenon; our knowledge was not restricted to data appearing in the consciousness of the observer. Thus Mao referred to the "inner cause" of things (*nei-tsai-te-yüan-yin*) and used much other language similarly denoting the ultimate nature of reality (*shih-wu-te pen-chih, tzu-jan-te hsing-chih, tzu-jan-te ch'üan-t'i, shih-wu-te nei-pu, shih-wu fa-chan-te ken-pen yüan-yin, tzu-jan-te ch'üan-t'i,* etc). Second, even if the idea of *yin* and *yang* was dropped, the assumption was often accepted in modern China that the units of cosmic or historical action were essentially simple, each largely homogenous in character, following fixed laws of action, and so best understood in terms of an architectonic, systematic doctrine (*hsi-t'ung*). This assumption can be seen in the view of classes, societies, or national cultures as each dominated by a single idea or driving force. Said T'ang: "The culture and thought of a people or nation are virtually always concentrated in some important concept or revolve around certain commonly used terms" (T'ang 1955: 293). The resulting analyses of historical forces were usually simplistic, invariably filtering out complexities of cultural context, but they were psychologically significant in helping to constitute a vision of that cosmic-historical process to which the moral hero was oriented.

Third, this process was filled with a "power" (*li-liang*) that the moral hero could tap. Mao's idea of the power of revolutionary forces growing out of the contradictions of class struggle is an obvious example, but T'ang Chün-i had a similar perception, speaking of the "latent" "power" possessed by China's true cultural spirit. The job of the moral hero, T'ang held, was to "turn the power that has supported the victory of Marxism-Leninism in China into the power that will positively open up the future of Chinese culture" (T'ang 1955: 8). Many other references (T'ang 1955: 273, 126, 255, 269, 316) illustrate T'ang's absolutely basic assumption that the efficacy of the individual's moral action hinged on the fact that there was an irresistible force in the world ready to respond to him. Again, this view has been dismissed as a simplistic theory of history by scholars not prepared to note its psychological significance.

Fourth, this cosmic-historical process, if not divine, was at least teleologically meaningful and inherently indicated the difference between good and bad. Hence it was taken for granted, by both T'ang and Mao, that morality could be deduced from ontology. Humean skepticism about any such connection between "is" and "ought" has been exceedingly rare in modern China. Rather, moral norms have usually been seen as objective, universal givens, not the product merely of historically conditioned preferences. At the same time, the linked traditional feeling, perhaps expressed most vividly by Hsün-tzu (Liang 1969: 324–325), that knowledge of the good necessarily produces a decision to act in accord with the good, seems still important today. Sun Yat-sen's (1866–1925) reflections on this issue had a great impact ("knowledge is hard, action easy"). Another connected idea, the major Confucian theory holding that the main causative factor in history is the development of moral doctrine, has greatly influenced modern Chinese thought, beginning at least with Liang Ch'i-ch'ao and Sun.

Fifth, although knowledge of the good and its cosmic basis was possible and vital, it was also elusive, especially in terms of applying this knowledge to specific cases. A large cluster of Neo-Confucian and modern ideas revolve around this point. Sixth, this elusiveness meant that the moral hero existed in a perilous moral situation. In the Neo-Confucian framework, the moral hero was anxiously and totalistically seeking linkage in the sense of both a social environment free of hostility and a cognitive grasp of the cosmos as an ordered whole. Indeed the central ideal of *jen* (benevolence, oneness with the nurturing impulses of the cosmos) explicitly covered both kinds of linkage. Hence the quest for *jen* illustrates the definite psychological connection between the anxiety-ridden philosophical concern with linkage and that fear of social friction emphasized by behavioral scientists like R. H. Solomon.

Yet the Neo-Confucian subject was much aware of not only hostility but also gaps in his understanding of the structure of cosmos (*hsin, li, wu*). Neo-Confucians thus had defined for themselves an anxiously Sisyphean situation in that they took for granted the existence of their goal and of tremendous "inner" and "outer" obstacles impeding pursuit of it, while regarding with doubt all of the formulae advanced to overcome these obstacles. The diffuse, free-floating anxiety symbolized by this perception of their situation is confused by some historians with anxieties arising out of particular painful incidents, such as traumatic events at the imperial court. If we are to argue that Neo-Confucians had a "sense of predicament" equivalent to the pervasive "tension" Weber saw in the Puritan definition of the human situation, we have to try to demonstrate the existence of anxieties of the former sort. This is the point of chapter 3 in Metzger (1977). True, many modernizers around 1900 were filled with a sense of rising optimism as they perceived a new balance between their goals and the available means of action. Nevertheless, much evidence suggests that even within this new context, the syndrome of anxiety persisted. Certainly the emphasis on the elusiveness of truth is a commonplace aspect of the modern ideologies.

Seventh, as a series of perilous moral situations, history was perceived as a Manichaean moral struggle between heroes and villains. There is no need to comment on the obvious persistence of this traditional view in modern ideologies, whether radical, conservative, or liberal. Eighth, some heroes in the past had been successful and had even left behind written if philologically problematic and vaguely worded guidelines for moral action. Both the existence of these guidelines and the vagueness that was seen in them were psychologically and epistemologically crucial. Ego looked back to an omniscient alter, but because alter was dead and his transmitted words vague, ego had a charismatic mission of interpretation on which the fate of the world hung. Similarly, searching for moral truth by both using these guidelines and referring to his own experience, ego had major epistemological advantages. For all the elusiveness of truth, one could usually avoid the brink of radical skepticism. Few if any Chinese thinkers have felt a need to begin with the Socratic "All I know is that I know nothing." This reliance on a body of written, authoritative guidelines certainly did not end when Liang Ch'i-ch'ao and others rejected the Chinese classics as the basic source of these guidelines. T'ang Chün-i once suggested that the Chinese Communists were able to use "Marxism as a sacred classic" (T'ang 1955: 269), and in fact Mao repeatedly turned to Marxism as an authoritative voice setting thought on the right track. This is illustrated by a favorite phrase of his, *Ma-k'o-ssu-chu-i kao-sung wo-men* (Marxism tells us that). T'ang, in turn, explicitly saw himself as building on the wisdom of the Neo-Confucian tradition (Metzger 1977: 34).

Ninth, in this cosmological and epistemological situation, ego's relation to authority figures could take two morally legitimated forms. When this authority figure was perceived as moral, then he, ego, the cosmos, and these written guidelines formed a moral oneness. When, as was far more common, the authority figure was perceived as morally dubious, ego perceived himself as referring to cosmic truths and to these guidelines and so able to protest against the behavior of the authority figure. This stance not only was common traditionally but also was adopted by Mao when he rebelled and by dissenters in the P.R.C. such as the signers of the Li I-che poster in 1974 (Metzger 1978).

It is significant that these nine assumptions defining the interaction between moral hero and cosmic-historical process have been common to so much thought not only in premodern times but also after thought became "secularized" in China. Secularization meant that the traditional, organismic, and religious view of "Man" as directly oriented to the universals of "Heaven and Earth" was replaced by the modern vocabulary of "history", "society", and "culture", which all evolved in "stages." Indeed the Marxist version of this secular outlook became particularly fashionable, even in conservative circles, during the 1920s and 1930s, as did any variety of sociologistic, deterministic, and historicist views. In this new secularized context, however, Chinese found it easy to regard history as the vehicle of attributes previously projected onto "Heaven and Earth."

This transfer went back at least to the New Text vision of the "three ages" of history that Liang Ch'i-ch'ao shared with K'ang Yu-wei (1858–1927) during the early 1890s. In their view of history as moving progressively toward the goal of "great peace" and "the total oneness of all people", we can see the assumption that ultimate reality can be known as noumenon; that the units of historical action are essentially homogeneous and follow fixed laws; that history moves with inexorable power; that this process is inherently a source of objective, universal moral norms; that (paradoxically) a correct theory about this process is needed fully to realize it; that ego serves as a moral hero revealing and broadcasting this theory; and that ego has the moral duty to protest against the bad behavior of authority figures.

Within the broad framework of this relation between hero and cosmic-historical process, there were three lines of variation that should be noted. First, was the moral hero perceived as acting at the center of the polity, filling the role of "king" or "prime minister", or was he perceived as acting outside a morally enervated center? Classic Confucianism of the Chou period envisaged both possibilities but focused on the center, as did Tung Chung-shu, who stressed *kai-chih* (revising institutions) and *wang-chiao* (the teachings of the king). After about 1100, however, Neo-Confucianism, although still deeply attached to the ideal of action from the center, definitely regarded "the mind of the self" as the currently central vehicle of moral progress. Although the emperor was politely referred to as a "sage", this basic intellectual view definitely implied that the center was morally enervated. Despite not only imperial but also scholarly claims about the moral grandeur of the current dynasty, especially in the eighteenth century, Chu Hsi's and Wang Yang-ming's vision of political history as a process of moral decline was not challenged.

Second, whether arising inside or outside the center, moral action could be either euphorically transformative or more melancholy and accomodative. The former outlook is illustrated by Mencius' view that "If the ruler is benevolent, everyone will be." Hsü Fu-kuan's brilliant analysis of the thought of Ssu-ma Ch'ien (ca. 145–90 B.C.), China's most famous historian, suggests that his "melancholy" view of history served as a *locus classicus* for the accomodative view. Mencius and Hsün-tzu were aware that the correlation between virtue and success was often broken, but they still emphasized it. Ssu-ma Ch'ien, however, could no longer believe in it, having to confront the successful unification of the empire by the evil Ch'in dynasty and the moral deficiencies of the Han dynasty (Hsü 1977). This "melancholy" (to use Hsü's term) was linked to Ssu-ma Ch'ien's Taoist inclination and can be connected to what is regarded as China's romantic tradition, which, typified by the image of Ch'ü Yüan's (ca. 300 B.C.) suicide, has greatly influenced accomodative thinking in modern times (Hsia 1968; Lee 1973).

In Neo-Confucianism after the eleventh century, the moral hero perceived himself as acting outside the center of the polity and accommodating himself to evils in the polity for which there was no immediate remedy. As a bureaucrat, he thus accepted the authority of the emperor, the emperor's frequent denunciations of the officials as moral failures, and the need for morally dubious institutions and policies. *Chi-pi* (corrupt practices that had accumulated and piled up over time) confronted him on all sides. Yet with its emphasis on Chu Hsi orthodoxy, the Ming-Ch'ing state itself defined the bureaucrat as a potential sage.

Conscious of the classics as a moral code transcending the dynasty, officials poured out criticisms of the polity in all its aspects except for the emperor and his dynasty.

Moreover, many Neo-Confucians, especially in Ming times, took a transformative attitude toward their inner lives. The central point here is that traditionally there was great awareness of the distinction between the more and the less transformative approaches to *hsiu-shen* (character cultivation). Neo-Confucians said one had to *li-chih* (make the decision) to become a sage, and Chu Hsi had contempt for those who felt that "in cultivating one's character, it is not necessary to reach the level of Confucius or Mencius" (Metzger 1977: 133). The concept of this key moral decision was also used in modern times to criticize the traditional educational system. Liang Ch'i-ch'ao, writing around 1897, said that in this system, students "began with the goal of becoming a sage and ended up with the mentality of a clerk" (Chang 1969: 51). Thus enlarging his moral goals and moral role to the utmost, the transformative Neo-Confucian was acutely conscious of the contrast between his elitist moral stance and what Hsün-tzu had tellingly called *min-te* (the morality of ordinary people), who merely "approve of respect for custom, regard wealth as precious, and think of their physical well-being as the highest value" (Liang 1969: 84). This transformative stance, therefore, was traditionally distinguished from the moral stance of those who had resigned themselves to more modest goals, not to mention the accomodative, familistic, and economistic stance of the peasant who pursued "wealth" and "status" in the name of filial piety and through "industriousness and frugality." It can also be readily distinguished from the stance of popular millenarianism, which, as described by S. Naquin and D. L. Overmyer, involved praying for help from supernatural beings. The Neo-Confucian path to transformation brought ego into a dyadic relation with the cosmos and a quest for linkage realized not through prayer but by a mixture of individual will and intellectual effort.

Finally, apart from the transformative-accomodative dichotomy and the question of the hero's relation to the center of the polity, Confucians were aware of a range of positions between the extremes of a "sense of predicament" and a "sense of impending solution." Neo-Confucians after the eleventh century, as I have argued, had a sense of predicament, since, until the West came with its new ways, there was nothing on their intellectual horizon promising to solve the problems they had defined for themselves. Late Chou Confucians, by contrast, had a very different intellectual horizon, often perceiving the imminence of something that they thought might well solve all problems (the unification of the empire). In this sense too, the analogy that the early modernizers so often liked to draw between themselves and the Chou had a striking basis in fact that Levensonians have overlooked. There was also a sense of impending solution in the many eleventh-century Confucians who so enthusiastically implemented institutional reforms, including Wang An-shih (1021–1086).

Whether or not the moral hero asserted himself at the center of the polity and in a transformative and euphoric way, Confucian self-assertion implied a sense of self-esteem strong enough to counter the need to obey authority figures. This raises an important psychological question. Such self-esteem must have been based on ego-nurturing experiences occurring as part of the childhood socialization process. Yet behavioral scientists like R. H. Solomon and Tseng Wen-hsing, stressing dependency and authoritarianism, have described China's traditionally inherited pattern of childhood socialization as lacking or greatly restricting such ego-nurturing experiences (Metzger 1977: 21–23). Solomon says that the development of the child's "self-esteem" was "arrest[ed]" by the way that authority figures morally condemned the child's "aggressive impulses", "autonomous behavior", and "self-assertion" (Solomon 1971: 69, 80).

Martin M. C. Yang's analysis, however, suggests how Chinese children could develop feelings of self-esteem even when taught to devalue their appetitive and aggressive impulses. Self-esteem arose as children shared "morally articulated feelings" (ch'ing-ts'ao) giving them "self-respect" (tzu-tsun) as valued members of a social whole depending on the efforts of all its members to maintain its existence on a "high" and "civilized" level, and to achieve a ceremonial continuity in the face of death. Yang's point is not just that the child "identified with" the authority figure denying him appetitive gratifications and came to value the ideals legitimating this denial. Yang also indicates that while these ideals were conceptualized as independent of the authority figure, they gratifyingly defined ego as a vehicle of morality potentially equal in value to the authority figure (Li I-Yüan and Yang Kuo-shu 1972: 133; Metzger 1977: 23–27).

One can suggest that as academic success reinforced this foundation of self-esteem, the young scholar in late imperial times combined his feeling of self-esteem with the feelings of "righteous anger" (kung-fen) aroused by authority figures perceived as morally deficient. This sense of "righteous anger" was always near the surface in a society where a vast surplus of gifted young men competed for a tiny number of bureaucratic jobs while strangely believing that a moral government is economically able to appoint all worthy men as officials. It was precisely this "righteous anger" of young men which exploded in 1895 when the reformers K'ang Yu-wei and Liang Ch'i-ch'ao presented a memorial protesting the humiliating peace treaty with Japan and signed by 603 provincial graduates (chü-jen). That such younger men increasingly rejected the views of their government cannot be explained only in political terms. Ego-nurturing experiences had enabled them to see themselves playing the Mencian role of the moral hero who acts in accord with some cosmic-historical force and rejects the cues of immoral authority figures. At the same time, national humiliation facilitated this psychological act by serving as that overwhelming evidence of bad leadership needed to turn the resentment of authority figures from a private into a public cause.

IV. CONCLUSION: THE QUESTION OF CONTINUITY

The study of Chinese political culture can perhaps profit from more conceptual precision and quantitative testing of middle-range hypotheses (Wei 1976). At least as important, however, is more sensitive analysis of attitudes, including those in intellectual documents. With the right methodology, these documents can yield widely shared orientations, not only idiosyncratic doctrines. Even if these intellectual orientations belonged only to a minority, this was a crucial minority whose sub-culture can hardly be neglected. Scholars have lately been eager to escape from the supposedly familiar confines of the "Great Tradition" to examine popular culture, but if we are methodologically innovative, we will discover that much remains to be learned about the "Great Tradition" as well.

Certainly it is clear that the theory of dependence and authoritarianism cannot be easily applied to the late imperial elite. Yet neither can their sense of self-esteem and autonomy be described just in the terms of Chinese humanists, since it was typically combined with a sense of ego's inadequacy, often leading to a sense of predicament. This traditional perception of an autonomous yet inadequate ego pursuing a transcendent goal by trying to harness the power of the cosmic-historical process had complex implications.

On the one hand, since this moral goal embodied the norms of the family and the monarchy, and since ego's sense of inadequacy often justified alter's authority, this perception easily meshed with an accomodative attitude toward the status quo. This accomodative tendency can be associated with the Ming-Ch'ing failure to invent the new technological and organizational forms needed to channel the economic surplus that apparently existed (Riskin 1975) in the direction of per capita economic growth.

On the other hand, the "sense of predicament" often connected to this perception is not compatible with Weber's thesis that Confucian culture lacked "tension" between the ideal and the real. The "tension" that did exist, in turn, was basic to the general flexibility of Ming-Ch'ing bureaucracy (Metzger 1973); the extensive restructuring of property, class, and fiscal relations during the period 1500–1800 (Metzger 1977a); and the eagerness with which Confucians in late Ch'ing times greeted Western ways as new methods to solve old problems. For as Lü Shih-ch'iang has emphasized (Lü 1976), the early modernizers were virtually all men with Confucian convictions as deep as those of the traditional conservatives who resisted modernization.

We can never entirely avoid the question of whether such a worldview should be seen merely as a set of beliefs peculiar to a particular culture or whether those who shared these ideas held to them because these ideas were valid in some more general sense. T'ang Chün-i and others, selecting out some parts of this Neo-Confucian outlook, have sought to vindicate it as a phenomenological analysis of the universal moral experience more valid than any Western one, including existentialism. Another approach may be more tenable.

The assumptions discussed above regarding the nature of self, group, cosmos, and history may be more useful than other assumptions about these items in facilitating a defense of civilizational values, such as respect for others, love of learning and art, and reverence for nature. After all, no major Chinese ideology in late imperial or modern times has led to that corrosive skepticism about these values that currently is afflicting American life. Overarching doctrinal differences, this Chinese philosophy of civilization both reinforced and was supported by the affective structure of the socialization process, which, according to Martin M. C. Yang, linked self-esteem to the "morally articulated feeling" of participation in a "civilized" way of life.

Yet this philosophy of civilization admittedly rests on epistemologically unrigorous assumptions and celebrates a concept of self which, for all the stress on autonomy, departs from the liberal ideal of the skeptical, spontaneous, and idiosyncratically creative individual. Hence the Chinese tradition of philosophy and socialization raises a question that should interest Americans: whether it is possible to keep to the ideals of epistemological rigor and individual spontaneity without lapsing into a state of moral relativism undermining civilizational values. Unless we can answer that question, we cannot claim that Confucian philosophy is less viable than any philosophy of ours.

Finally, there is the question of the continuity of this political culture in modern times. Certainly major discontinuities occurred as the Chinese adopted a modernizing outlook by accepting a nationalistic, cosmopolitan, and multifocal image of the international world; by developing a secularized view of the group and its relation to a scientifically described cosmos; and by adopting a theory of progress stressing science, technology, economic growth, political participation, and somewhat less social deference. Hence the bulk of the literature has held that modernization was based on discontinuity with the tradition.

There is still no definite demonstration that the continuities were more than residual, but it can be justly said that those who hold that modernization was based on traditional orientations have made a case at least as strong as the opposite one, especially in that they have taken more care in examining the traditional base line of modernization. We are confronted with a complicated problem that requires much more study. One consideration that has been stressed especially by Wang Erh-min and Chang P'eng-yüan is that the generation of Liang Ch'i-ch'ao, which can be regarded as setting up the basic parameters of modernizing thought in China, adopted these parameters only after the childhood and teen-age years, if not the early twenties as well. Born in 1873, Liang Ch'i-ch'ao was 20 or older before he seriously questioned the Confucian tradition. How much change in his fundamental perception of selfhood and authority was possible after his most formative years? Moreover, as he turned from an explicitly Confucian to a more secularized outlook around the age of 25, he seemed to be in a strong mood of self-confidence; that kind of spiritual crisis associated with doubt about fundamental values has not been noted by any of his many biographers. Similarly, when he left China in 1898 and stayed for some years in Japan and other foreign countries, becoming ever more cosmopolitan and sophisticated about Western ways, his main concerns were in the field of political strategy, particularly his relations with Sun Yat-sen. To the extent that his thoughts turned inward toward ultimate values, he took for granted that the Neo-Confucian definition of the moral life was the valid one, as Chang Hao has made clear.

A most important linked consideration is that in the mid 1890s, when Liang actually made his most basic change in values, his ignorance of any foreign language plus the great dearth of translated Western works beyond books of a technical nature precluded anything but a gross understanding of Western values. This gross understanding then had to compete with his deep grasp, conscious and unconscious, of a vast and valuable civilizational tradition. Under these circumstances, as shown by his writings around 1897, he was able to appreciate as distinctively new and Western the idea that every individual had a "right" to "be his own master" and that a polity should be organized around respect for this "right." Yet as he developed the theme of what this "right" entailed, he brought in one traditional Chinese value after another (the idea of "being one's own master", the idea that the valuable human capacities are possessed equally by everyone, the idea that with this "right" everyone would "exhaustively carry out all he ought to do", the idea that thus "everyone would obtain those benefits to which he is entitled", the idea of *kung* [the public good], which would be served by this process, and the idea that through this process, "the whole world would be brought to a state of peace and order") (Chang 1969: 57).

It would be surprising if individuals under these conditions could greatly change inherited, partly unconscious definitions of selfhood, authority, and moral action. Thus Wang Erh-min has traced out some of the continuities in the concept of societal change (Wang 1977: 381—439); Price has done the same for the elitist sense of the heroic, revolutionary self (Price 1974: 193—212); and, as it has been argued here, much of the traditional concept of a dyadic relation between self and cosmos can be found in the newly secularized vocabulary of historical process. Similarly, the shift to a philosophy of progress by no means eliminated the traditional goal of linkage in all its material and spiritual dimensions.

The goal of linkage can be seen in the repeated modern reference to the goal of *ta-t'ung* (great oneness of all people); in the central philosophical quest for the elimination of all doctrinal "conflicts"; in the joint quest of materialists and idealists for a single ontological concept, whether mind or matter, under which all existence could be subsumed; and especially in the major concern with conceptualizing and realizing the *translation* of moral insight into "outer" action. Secularization and the end of the monarchy meant that such translation could no longer be realized through the role of the sage with access to cosmic power or the role of "the king." While the new idea of "the group" (*ch'ün*) carrying out "movements" came to serve as a new paradigm of such translation, as Chang Hao's work indicates, the disjunction often perceived between such "movements" and morality kept this problem of translation prominent.

For instance, Sun Yat-sen's great concern with journalism and propaganda was not just a way of copying Western political techniques; it was precisely his answer to this problem of translation. He said: "After thought is clarified and unified, faith arises. Once there is faith, it produces power" (T'ang Ch'eng-yeh 1977: 1). In T'ang Chün-i's slightly different view, this "latent . . . . power" was aroused as the "intellectual" published books which in turn influenced other intellectuals, the educational system, and then society. Certainly the new "intellectual" class (*chih-shih fen-tzu*) had much in common with the traditional literati, but as the nature of the "translation" problem changed, so did the intellectual point of attack, the curriculum, and the political activities of those in China who used learning to pursue prestige for themselves and progress for the country.

In Maoism, the translation problem was supposed to be solved through the coinciding of morality with the leadership of the revolution and the state. The perception of this coincidence, however, was lost among the intellectuals represented by the 1974 Li I-che manifesto, who once more emphasized the elusiveness of moral truth, though still far from the Neo-Confucian sense of predicament (they still had much faith in historical forces and constitutional reform) (Metzger 1978). With Mao himself now leaving behind after his death an extensive record of fallibility, it seems clear that increasing numbers of Mainland intellectuals will perceive that gap between moral truth and the "outer" vehicles of power which was referred to in the Li I-che manifesto, and which traditional writers commonly posited. Basic to accomodative thinking in China, a perception of "incomplete translation" seems now to be becoming dominant on the Mainland and logically should lead to a more tolerant and eclectic intellectual atmosphere, perhaps similar to Taiwan's.

Apart from such factors suggesting directly the continuity of Neo-Confucian orientations, there is the question of the extent to which the tools of modernization were actually perceived as a breakthrough in the traditional attempt to solve traditional problems. We can begin with the explicit claim of early modernizers that Western methods were valuable as offering new ways to realize the traditional ideals (Metzger 1977: 215–216). The problem, however, goes deeper. Certainly the new focus on the "outer" issues of political organization, technology, economics, international relations, international geography, and the natural world depended on Western influence. Yet it simultaneously was a shift between two strategies of moral action which both had traditional roots. It was a shift from a strategy stressing the "inner" life of a moral agent acting outside the center of the polity, emphasizing the partly ineffable means of "spiritual nurture" (*tsun te-hsing*), taking an accommodative approach to the polity, and perceiving the moral life as a predicament. It was a shift to a strategy stressing the "outer" activities of a moral agent oriented to the center of the polity, emphasizing the verbalized, cognitive learning needed to deal with "outer" specificities (*ko-chih-chih hsüeh*), often taking a transformative approach to the polity and to society, and optimistically seeing his society as moving from an era of failure to one of success.

This surge of optimism, also noted by Price and Wang Erh-min, stemmed from the perception not only of new means of "outer" action but also of a breakthrough in the field of knowledge. This automatically enhanced the prestige of the one class able to utilize this breakthrough for the benefit of a population that widely believed in doctrinal correctness as the precondition of national strength. The intellectuals now had the mission of describing the constituents of a physical universe stripped of *yin* and *yang*, of demonstrating how the principles of morality were derived from these ontological elements, and of explaining how these principles could be "translated" into "outer" action. True, needing doctrinal unity, they were alarmed by the confusing variety of doctrines, East and West, on these matters. Yet the opportunity to work on this problem was in itself exhilarating in that it revived their inherited and long-frustrated faith in the great possibilities of cognitive learning.

Noting that the early modernizers adopted a secularized theory of social evolution, Western scholars usually view this shift as a primary rather than a symptomatic change in viewpoint, or they suggest that evolutionism simply was an integral part of the vision of modernization imported from the West. Yet the peculiar speed and enthusiasm with which intellectuals jumped from the traditional, deeply rooted vision of a sacred socio-cosmic order to a secularized view cannot be so easily explained. The quickness of this jump, rather, reflected the fact that the new, secularized vocabulary facilitated conceptualization of the above "outer" strategy of moral action. Moreover, optimistically believing that this strategy could lead from an age of failure to one of moral and material success, the modernizers saw in evolutionism a theory of history that reinforced this hope. Still more, this theory appeared to them as part of the intellectual breakthrough currently exhilarating them. Thus they saw in it a particularly cogent version of the tradition-rooted vision of the cosmic-historical process as a force supporting the efforts of the moral hero. People do not just adopt historical theories. Rather theories become attractive when considered in the light of goals and hopes grounded in basic understandings about the nature of the self, the group, and the cosmos.

True, in his stimulating work Levenson held that when modernizers like Cheng Kuan-ying (1842–1923) characterized modernization as just a better way to realize the classic Chou ideals, they did not really mean what they were saying. Rather, Levenson held, they were just looking for a formula enabling them to break with their tradition without losing their nationalistic sense of pride in it and in themselves. Wang Erh-min, however, has shown that their intentions were far more varied (Wang 1976: 31–50), and in point of fact they did perceive the "outer" strategy of modernization as largely coinciding with the Chou emphasis on the "outer." Moreover, when we relate this issue to the "sense of predicament" which in fact preceded the enthusiasm for modernization, we cannot disassociate this enthusiasm from the psychological state of people anxiously looking for a way out of an agonizing situation arising precisely out of their commitment to traditional goals. Unfortunately, Levenson's thesis was formulated without any awareness of the need for an extensive inquiry into the nature of this base-line psychological state. It was, I would argue, this very Weberian "tension" between ideal and reality which made so many educated Chinese so eager to adopt Western ways promising to transform their society.

Conversely, other Third World nations presented with the same appealing inventory of Western methods and equally desirous of "wealth and power" have responded far more lethargically. Hence modernization theories neglecting the cultural basis of the Chinese response seem to be untenable.

When we relate all the above continuities, especially those defining the teleological interaction between ego and cosmic-historical process, to the rising sense of optimism and the continuing, unshaken faith in civilizational values, we have to qualify the prevalent thesis that the impact of Western views "broke the protective canopy which the traditional *Weltanschauung* . . . or . . . symbols of general orientation . . . provided to shield people from the threat of outer chaos and inner anxiety . . . . [thus plunging the Chinese] into a [state of] spiritual disorientation" (Chang 1976: 280–281). As we have seen, many of these "symbols of general orientation" remained firmly in place, and it is hard to see "disorientation" in the spirit of self-confident "struggle" with which so many Chinese intellectual leaders in our century have faced their problems. Doubts and despair did arise, but often within the context of a commitment to civilization and modernization that had traditional roots.

Sharing this commitment, Chinese intellectuals gradually split up into conservative, radical, and liberal schools, differing especially over three issues: should one modernize in a transformative or accomodative way? does the translation of moral spirit into "outer" action require respect for or opposition to the established structure of power and property? how should one interrelate the alarmingly various doctrines, East and West, old and new, scientistic and humanistic, in order to derive values from ontological principles, achieve doctrinal unification, and realize linkage? Those taking a transformative, revolutionary, and scientistic position did come to power on the Mainland. Yet their Marxism was in fact just one strand of a broader cultural pattern. Evolving dramatically today, this pattern celebrates the assumption that the life of the ego grows in meaning not only through the empathetic merging of ego and alter but also through growing access to civilizational values that transcend the cues of authority figures.

REFERENCES

Chang, Hao
    1976 New Confucianism and the intellectual crisis of contemporary China. *In* The Limits of Change. Charlotte Furth, ed. Pp. 276–302. Cambridge, Mass.: Harvard University Press.
Chang, P'eng-yüan
    1969 *Liang-ch'i-ch'ao yü Ch'ing-chi ko-ming* (Liang Ch'i-ch'ao and the Late Ch'ing Revolution). Taipei district: Academia Sinica, Institute of Modern History.
    1978 *Liang Ch'i-ch'ao yü Min-kuo cheng-chih* (Liang Ch'i-ch'ao and the Politics of the Republican Period). Taipei: *Shih-huo ch'u-pan-she yu-hsien kung-ssu*.
Chou, Tao-chi
    1977 *Wo-kuo min-pen ssu-hsiang-te fen-hsi yü chien-t'ao* (An Analysis of Our Country's Traditional Thought regarding the Primacy of the People's Needs). Taipei District: Academia Sinica, Institute of the Three Principles of the People.

Fried, Morton H.
 1976 Chinese culture, society, and personality in transition. *In* Responses to Change: Society, Culture, and Personality. George A. DeVos, ed. Pp. 45–73. N.Y.: D. Van Nostrand.
Fung, Yu-lan
 1961 *Hsin-yüan-tao* (A New Inquiry into the Development of Chinese Philosophy). Hong Kong: *Chung-kuo che-hsüeh yen-chiu-hui.*
Hsia, T. A.
 1968 The Gate of Darkness. Seattle: University of Washington Press.
Hsü, Fu-kuan
 1977 *Lun Shih-chi* (On the *Shih-chi*). *Ta-lu tsa-chih* 55:6: 1–48.
James, William
 1958 The Varieties of Religious Experience. New York: Mentor Books.
Lee, Leo Ou-fan
 1973 The Romantic Generation of Modern Chinese Writers. Cambridge, Mass.: Harvard University Press.
Legge, James, trans.
 1966 The Four Books. New York: Paragon Book Reprint Corp.
Li, I-yüan and Yang, Kuo-shu, eds.
 1972 *Chung-kuo-jen-te hsing-ko: k'o-chi tsung-ho-hsing-te t'ao-lun* (Symposium on the Character of the Chinese: An Interdisciplinary Approach). Nankang: Academia Sinica, Institute of Ethnology.
Liang, Ch'i-hsiung, ed.
 1969 *Hsün-tzu chien-shih* (*Hsün-tzu* with Selected Explanations from the Commentaries). Taipei: Taiwan Commercial Press.
Liu, Kwang-Ching
 1978 *Wan-Ch'ing ti-fang-kuan tzu-shu-chih shih-liao chia-chih – Tao-Hsien-chih chi kuan-shen kuan-min kuan-hsi ch'u-t'an* (The value of historical material in the memoirs of local officials in the late Ch'ing period – A preliminary investigation into the relations between officials and gentry and between officials and commoners around 1850). *In Chung-yang yen-chiu-yüan ch'eng-li wu-shih-chou-nien chi-nien lun-wen-chi*. Pp. 333–364. Taipei: Academia Sinica.
Lü, Shih-ch'iang
 1976 *Ju-chia ch'uan-t'ung yü wei-hsin (1839–1911)* (The Confucian Tradition and Late Ch'ing Reformism (1839–1911). Taipei: *Chiao-yü-pu she-hui chiao-yü-ssu.*
Metzger, Thomas A.
 1973 The Internal Organization of Ch'ing Bureaucracy: Legal, Normative, and Communication Aspects. Cambridge, Mass.: Harvard University Press.
 1977 Escape from Predicament: Neo-Confucianism and China's Evolving Political Culture. N.Y.: Columbia University Press.
 1977a On the historical roots of economic modernization in China: The increasing differentiation of the economy from the polity during late Ming and early Ch'ing times. *In* Conference on Modern Chinese Economic History. Pp. 33–44. Taipei: Academia Sinica, The Institute of Economics.
 1978 An historical perspective on mainland China's current ideological crisis. *In* Proceedings of the Seventh Sino-American Conference on Mainland China. Pp. IV-2-1–IV-2-17. Taipei: Institute of International Relations.
Price, Don C.
 1974 Russia and the Roots of the Chinese Revolution, 1896–1911. Cambridge, Mass.: Harvard University Press.
Quine, W. V.
 1969 Ontological Relativity and Other Essays. N.Y.: Columbia University Press.

Riskin, Carl
   1975   Surplus and stagnation in modern China. *In* China's Modern Economy in Histori-
          cal Perspective. D. H. Perkins, ed. Stanford: Stanford University Press.
Solomon, Richard H.
   1971   Mao's Revolution and the Chinese Political Culture. Berkeley: University of Cali-
          fornia Press.
T'ang, Ch'eng-yeh
   1977   *Kuo-fu-te hsüan-ch'uan chih-lüeh* (The Problem of Propagating Doctrine in Sun
          Yat-sen's Thought and Life). Taipei: Academia Sinica, Institute of the Three Prin-
          ciples of the People.
T'ang, Chün-i
   1955   *Jen-wen ching-shen-chih ch'ung-chien* (The Reconstruction of the Humanistic
          Spirit). Hong Kong: *Hsin-ya yen-chiu-so.*
   1972   *Chung-kuo wen-hua-chih ching-shen chia-chih* (The Spirit of Chinese Culture and
          its Value). Taipei: *Cheng-chung shu-chü.*
   1975   *Chung-kuo jen-wen ching-shen-chih fa-chan* (The Development of the Humanistic
          Spirit in China). Taipei: *T'ai-wan hsüeh-sheng shu-chü.*
Wakeman Jr., Frederic
   1973   History and Will. Berkeley: University of California Press.
Wang, Erh-min
   1976   *Wan-Ch'ing cheng-chih ssu-hsiang shih-lun* (Historical Essays on Late Ch'ing
          Political Thought). Taipei: *Hua-shih ch'u-pan-she.*
   1977   *Chung-kuo chin-tai ssu-hsiang shih-lun* (Historical Essays on Modern Chinese
          Thought). Taipei: *Hua-shih ch'u-pan-she.*
Weber, Max
   1951   The Religion of China. Glencoe: The Free Press.
Wei, Yung
   1976   A methodological critique of current studies on Chinese political culture. The
          Journal of Politics 38:1: 114–140.
Yang, C. K.
   1975   Some preliminary statistical patterns of mass actions in nineteenth-century China.
          In Conflict and Control in Late Imperial China. Frederic Wakeman Jr. and Carolyn
          Grant, eds. Pp. 174–210. Berkeley: University of California Press.

ANDREW C. K. HSIEH AND JONATHAN D. SPENCE

2. SUICIDE AND THE FAMILY IN PRE-MODERN CHINESE SOCIETY

If we survey the act of suicide across a broad span of pre-modern Chinese history, we find that it provides an intriguing intersection point at which so-called "normal" and "deviant" behavior patterns blur and overlap. The topic is a vast and almost totally unexplored one, and in this paper we restrict ourselves to three facets of the problem: How was it that the Chinese woman (especially the wife) was presented as a model figure when she committed suicide, and how did this presentation change over time? How did the legal sources view this behavior, and how did they try to separate out different elements of motivation or pressure within the family context? And how, in popular literature, did various Chinese writers try to elaborate on the sparse records available, so as to introduce more detailed elements of private anguish and responsibility?

1. WOMEN AND SUICIDE: HISTORICAL CATEGORIZATIONS

The idea of suicide as a moral imperative appears early in Chinese recorded history. Already, in the *Analects*, Confucius remarked that men might have to give up their lives in the name of goodness—*sha-shen ch'eng-jen* 殺身成仁 (Waley 1938: 195).[1] This ideal of behavior drawn from the political world of males was rapidly transposed into the ethical world of female behavior; so rapidly and neatly, indeed, that scholars in the People's Republic of China are now reassessing the development of the subjugation of women in the light of Confucius' role as the spokesman for a fading slave society (Croll 1977: 593).

When transposed into the woman's world, these moral imperatives were used to erect a strict standard for loyalty to one's husband. Thus Liu Hsiang 劉向 (77 B.C. – 6 B.C.), the Han dynasty author of the first collection of women's biographies, quotes this same Confucian passage approvingly of a woman who gave up her life to save her husband (O'Hara 1945: 151–152). In his *Biographies of Women (Lieh-nü chuan* 列女傳) Liu Hsiang developed seven distinct categories for his female subjects: Model Mothers (*mu-i* 母儀), The Noble and Intelligent (*hsien-ming* 賢明), The Good and Wise (*jen-chih* 仁智), The Pure and Obedient (*chen-shun* 貞順), The Chaste and Righteous (*chieh-i* 節義), The Perspicacious (*pien-t'ung* 辯通), and The Evil and Depraved (*nieh-pi* 孽嬖). In most of these categories women are presented as being resourceful and intelligent and able to live with dignity in difficult circumstances. Suicide emerges as a dominant theme in only two of the seven sections, those on the 'Pure and Obedient' and on the 'Chaste and Righteous', and it is on these that we will concentrate here.

When we analyze those cases, presented by Liu, in which women were driven to contemplate, threaten or commit suicide, we find that they can be bunched

29

A. Kleinman and T.-Y. Lin (eds.), Normal and Abnormal Behavior in Chinese Culture, 29 47.
Copyright © 1980 by D. Reidel Publishing Company.

under four headings, according to the circumstances that prompted the act of suicide. These headings represent one way of viewing ethical standards for women in early Chinese society and show how rigorous rationales were developed to encourage behavior that in other societies might be regarded as deviant.

Circumstance 1. The Husband Dies

The only widow expressly described by Liu Hsiang as committing suicide because of this circumstance was the wife of Chi-liang of Ch'i; in her case, the dominating factor is her loneliness combined with her insistence on not taking a second husband. Liu Hsiang records her words — before she drowned herself — as being these:

> Where shall I go? A wife should have someone to depend on. While her father is living, she depends on him; while her husband is living, she depends on him. Today, among the older relatives, I am without father; among those of the middle group, I am without husband; and in the next generation, I am without a son. In my husband's home I have no one to depend on in order to manifest my sincerity; in my mother's home I have no one to depend upon to establish my observance of propriety. How can I change to a second husband? It will be just as good if I also die. (O'Hara 1945: 114)

Two other widows threatened suicide so as to avoid having to remarry: one gave as her reason the desire to serve her mother-in-law, the other that remarriage would be a double error as it would violate both her integrity and that of her would-be husband who was also ruler of the state. One widow, instead of suicide, chose the path of disfigurement, cutting off her nose to keep the suitors away (O'Hara 1945: 115–116, 122–126). The only detailed case of a remarriage is put in the 'Evil and Depraved' category, where the beautiful Hsia-chi takes no less than seven husbands in sequence (O'Hara 1945: 201–204).

Circumstance 2. The wife is put in the position of inevitably breaking the laws of propriety if she stays alive

Here we find six clear cases. A young bride is offered inadequate ritual preparations by her husband's family (*fu-chia li pu-pei* 夫家禮不備), and dies in jail rather than go through with the marriage. A wife allows herself to be burnt to death in her home, because there is no chaperon to escort her from the blazing building. A wife attempts suicide because the carriage sent by her husband to bring her home after an accident does not have the proper seats and hangings. A wife allows herself to be drowned by a flood because the messenger sent to rescue her does not bring the proper credentials from her husband, A wife commits suicide because, after being captured in battle with her busband, the capturer wants to make her marry him while her husband is still alive and kept outside as a gate-keeper. (In this case, her husband also committed suicide, after his wife had done so.) And lastly, a wife drowns herself because her husband, returning from a five-year absence at the frontier, violates the laws of filial piety to his own mother and thus compromises his wife (O'Hara 1945: 102–113, 117–118, 141–143).

Circumstance 3. The wife's death is necessary to the husband's propriety

There are just two cases in this group. In the first, a consort commits suicide to prepare her husband's path to the Underworld. (She had previously refused to do so because she had found the husband lacking in the propriety that alone would have justified such an action.) In the second, a conquering ruler issues the order that if any of the conquered subjects commit suicide, their families will be punished by execution. So as to enable her husband to commit suicide without feeling guilty for her execution, the wife herself commits suicide (O'Hara 1945: 131–136).

Circumstance 4. An intolerable pressure is placed on the wife because of all her divided loyalties within the family situation

Interestingly, all three of the cases within this category involve a wife forced to choose between a husband and a brother – in some form – and feeling overwhelmed by the choice. In one case, the wife strangles herself because her husband murders her elder brother (O'Hara 1945: 150–151).

In another, the wife stabs herself to death because her younger brother kills her husband (O'Hara 1945: 138–139). In the third, a complex and poignant example, a mother is apparently driven to take her own life because she inadvertently places loyalty to her husband's (and her own?) line ahead of loyalty to her elder brother's (and hence her parents'?). The story is worth quoting in full:

The Virtuous Aunt of Liang was a woman of [the state of] Liang. When her house caught on fire, she was inside with her elder brother's child and her own child. She wished to take up her brother's child but in the rush she took her own son and did not get her brother's son. The fire was at its height and she was unable to enter again. The woman herself was about to rush into the flames. Her friends stopped her, saying, "You originally wanted to take your elder brother's child but being excited, in the end by mistake, you took your own son. A good conscience says, "Why should you do this? Why go to the extreme of rushing into the fire?' " The woman replied, 'Can I allow this report to go throughout the state of Liang? Bearing an unrighteous reputation how can I face my brother and my countryman? I would like to cast my son again into the fire but this would violate a mother's love. In such a situation I cannot go on living.' And afterwards she ran into the fire and died. (O'Hara 1945:147)

In this category of Husband/Brother tensions, there is an involved anti-example provided in the 'Evil and Depraved' section of Liu Hsiang's work. This concerns Wen-chiang, who has an incestuous relationship with her older brother. The husband knows about it but cannot prevent it. The brother has an assassin kill the husband; at which point the people of the country kill the assassin, but apparently leave the brother and sister to their own devices (O'Hara 1945: 193–194).

There is, of course, no way of knowing how many of the above examples were based on actual occurrences, or record dialogue which actually took place; and some of the examples are clearly designed to illustrate or amplify passages from the Confucian *Classics*. Nevertheless, Liu Hsiang's collection did itself become a classic, and was regularly reprinted, often with additional commentaries, throughout the next seventeen hundred years.[2] Furthermore, the compiling of women's biographies became a standard procedure in Dynastic Histories, and later in Local Gazetteers, and these biographies often began by stating that a given woman had grown up steeped in the *Lieh-nü chuan*.

The important thing, in considering this branch of the historical tradition, is to see how the shifting categories – and their content – reflect different attitudes to the role of women on the part of the compilers. The pre-T'ang Histories follow Liu Hsiang's categories fairly closely, though they do not have any section on the "Evil and Depraved." In the *Hou-Han shu* (comp. 432 A.D.) *lieh-nü* section, there are seventeen biographies of women. Eight of them showed the kinds of exemplary model behavior, short of self-disfigurement or death, that can be found in the general categories of Liu Hsiang's "Model Mothers," "Noble and Intelligent" and "Good and Wise," and do not commit suicide. One disfigures herself (by cutting off an ear and putting out an eye) so as to avoid remarriage. Two of them choose not to submit themselves to rebels, and are killed. Six of the group commit suicide in the kind of circumstances we have already seen in Liu Hsiang: one has divided family loyalties, two die after their fathers die, one helps her husband to escape from prison, one protects her mother-in-law from robbers, and one when forced to remarry after her husband's death. A similar balance can be found in the *Chin-shu, Sui-shu,* and *Hsin T'ang-shu:*

	Exemplary Behavior	Disfigure Themselves	Refuse to Submit & are Killed by Rebels	Commit Suicide	Total
Chin-shu	21	1	5	7	34
Sui-shu	9	–	1	4	14
Hsin T'ang-shu	24	4	7	8	43

It is with the compilation of the *Sung History* (comp. 1299) that we begin to find a rapid increase in the number of suicides that are listed in the women's biographies, and a proportional decrease in the other sorts of exemplary behavior that are considered deserving of record.

	Exemplary Behavior	Disfigure Themselves	Refuse to Submit & are Killed by Rebels	Commit Suicide	Total
Shung-shih	7	–	15	16	38
Chin-shih	1	–	3	16	20
Yüan-shih	24	1	11	59	95
Ming-shih	48	–	30	147	223

If we take a mid-Ch'ing Gazetteer as an example of later imperial trends, we find similar figures but to an even higher degree. Thus in the 1737 edition of the Gazetteer of Chiangnan (incorporating modern Kiangsu and Anhwei) the number of cases of exemplary behavior short of self-disfigurement or death for the whole area, for the vast time span from the Chou to the time of compilation, is given as 69 cases spread over the 16 prefectures of the two provinces (*fu*) (*Chiang-nan t'ung-chih* 1907:2923–2930); the numbers of examples in the other more violent categories, however, have become so large that we did not even have the time to compute them all. We can give some idea of the general trend by counting the cases for just one of those prefectures, the single *fu* of Nanking, which alone had 121 cases, that can be subdivided as follows (*Chiang-nan t'ung-chih* 1967: 2931–2934)

	Cutting off flesh to feed relatives	Death after refusal to submit to rebels	Commit Suicide
Sung	1	1	1
Yüan	1*	3	8
Ming	16	5	55
First 90 years of Ch'ing	15	9	15
Totals	33	9	79

* This case led to death.

Along with this jump in recorded suicides we find that one new category has grown immensely: namely, the brief listing, without further comment, of the fact that a woman had refused to remarry following her husband's death (*wan-chieh* 完節). Undoubtedly some of these women had threatened to commit suicide so as to avoid remarriage, though we have no way of calculating how many. The Nanking figures for this category run: (*Ch'iang-nan t'ung-chih* 1967: 3035–3042).

Sung	3
Yüan	5
Ming	89
First 90 years of Ch'ing	206

Some of this startling increase can be attributed to economic factors: we know, for example, that the attempts to make widows remarry were often made by male relatives of the deceased husband, who would receive the widow's original dowry and other resources if they could force her into remarriage (Spence 1978: 71–73). But it also seems a reasonable conclusion that the state was now deliberately fostering the cult of "loyalty" on the woman's part to one male, just as in the political sphere new emphasis was being placed on the need for an official's loyalty to only one dynasty. This process reached a peak in the later eighteenth century, when the Ch'ien-lung Emperor ordered the compilation of the biographies of those who had served two dynasties under the pejorative title "*erh-ch'en chuan*," (貳臣傳) while at the same time he extolled those who had given their lives at the fall of the Ming, rather than living on to serve the Ch'ing.

Early evidence for this trend can be found in the massive compilation of data on women's suicide during the Ming and early Ch'ing in the Imperial Encyclopedia *Ku-chin t'u-shu chi-ch'eng* 古今圖書集成 ts'e 398–404. (The numbers are so large that, despite obvious limitations in the criteria for selection, they might provide a basis for useful statistical analysis.) In the Ming, for example, there are 8,490 women's suicides gathered into 45 *chuan,* and drawn from a wide variety of gazetteers and biographical collections. For the first eighty years of the Ch'ing there are 2,749 cases in 20 *chuan.*

Though it is not easy to see how these various samples could be converted into meaningful statistics, they nevertheless point in certain directions. One, that the criteria for inclusion in the women's biographical categories increasingly became that of chastity (*chen-lieh* 貞烈). Two, that such chastity was increasingly interpreted as proper behavior at the time of a husband's death. Three, that disfigurement was transposed in motive from warding off suitors to literally feeding one's parents or in-laws. Four, that biographies were less and less concerned with actions that showed a woman's intelligence and independence.[3]

We can also see the growing numbers of recorded suicides (apparently reaching a peak during the Ming), and the narrowing of the definition of virtuous behavior, as being indicative of the rigorous codes of behavior and precise sense of duty that was inculcated in orthodox Neo-Confucianism. The *Ming-shih,* published in the late eighteenth century had this to say at the beginning of its *Lieh-nü chuan* section:

When Liu Hisang wrote his biographies of women, he selected examples of behavior which served as models and warnings; he didn't restrict himself to one kind. When Fan [Yeh, in the *Hou-Han shu*] emulated him, he also chose those of talent and distinction, he didn't just value those who were chaste (*chieh-lieh* 節烈). From Wei and Sui onward, the historians mainly took cases that showed people killing themselves because of some crisis so as to preserve their righteousness in death (*hsün-i* 殉義).

The *Ming-shih* compilers explained this trend in terms of an interest in the sensational — when the common country folk talked about something enough, the scholars recorded it. But as we saw in the tables above, the *Ming History* had far more examples of female suicide than any previous history. Later in the eighteenth century, Chang Hsueh-ch'eng 章學誠 (1736–1801) gave a different criticism (Chang 1962: 177). He said that Liu Hsiang's biographies of women were initially true "collections" (*lieh* 列); they did not just deal with the "virtuous" (*lieh* 烈). The women's biographies were now too restricted; why did not the women have their own categories of "The Literary" (*wen-yuan* 文苑) and "The Scholarly" (*ju-lin* 儒林) as did the men?

Chang's was a rare voice, and only a few others had been interested in the ethical problems at stake here. During the later Ming, Kuei Yu-kuang 歸有光 (1506–1571) had written an essay on the category of virtuous women ("Chen-nü lun" 貞女論) (Kuei 1935: 41) saying that many of the women's suicides were acts against propriety, a view that was echoed by Wang Chung 汪中 (1744–

1794) in the eighteenth century (Wang 1936: 1, 25—28). The most violent attack of all on the concept of the "virtuous woman" was made by Yü Cheng-hsieh 俞正燮 (1775—1840) in his essay "Chen-nü shuo" (貞女說) criticizing male complacency in the face of such suicides. Yü concluded his essay:

It is reasonable to expect that a man should [commit suicide] in the name of loyalty and righteousness; but this [death] in the name of purity and chastity (*chen lieh* 貞烈) by the women, how is that any glory for the men? (Yu 1941: 13, 493—495)

2. FAMILY SUICIDES: LEGAL CATEGORIZATIONS

The information available in the legal sources of pre-modern China is an essential supplement to the historical record. Without this information, we might have felt that there was a clear division of suicides by males — restricted to the political sphere — and the suicide of women in the family circle, or for reasons connected with that circle. But with the help of legal sources we can see that men were as entrapped in the hierarchical structures of the family as were the women, and faced many of the same problems.

The Chinese legal codes did not conceive of suicide as being an act carried out in isolation. On the contrary, in suicide cases as in homicide cases, they looked for an instigator, and the major category under which acts of suicide can be found in the Ming and Ch'ing *Codes* is that of "Pressuring a person to commit suicide" (*Wei-pi jen chih-ssu* 威逼人致死). In the category of *wei-pi* we find in its clearest form the desire of later Chinese codifiers to pin down an instigator for each act of suicide. The *wei-pi* category is mentioned in the Southern Sung Dynasty, in 1201, in a memorial concerning local law-and-order problems. The memorialist explained to the Emperor that he could not send on the suspected murderers from his locality for trial — as the regulations demanded — because they were all dead. The local neighbors (*lin-pao* 鄰保), anxious to avoid any further involvement with the law, had pressured (*wei-pi*) all the alleged murderers into committing suicide. The neighbors had also paid off the victims' families to stop them pursuing their quest for justice (Hsü Sung 1936: 6, 7).

A fuller and more careful formulation first appears in the *Ming Code,* in these words:

All those who for some reason pressure others into killing themselves, shall receive a hundred blows. Officials and clerks who pressure commoners into committing suicide (outside the range of their public duties) shall have the same penalty, and also pay ten taels toward the burial expenses. Those pressuring their own senior relations into committing suicide shall be strangled; if they pressure someone into suicide as a result of sexual assault or robbery they shall be beheaded.

The list of "reasons" for pressuring someone, adduced by the Ming compilers, included marriage problems, land disputes, and debts (Liu Wei-ch'ien 1970: 1531).

A Ming case from 1503 shows us this law in operation. Chiang Yüan-i killed his younger brother, seized his niece's dowry, and swore at his mother so violently that she strangled herself in rage. The first judge sentenced Chiang to strangulation in accordance with the laws for "swearing at a mother." But this judgment was reversed at a higher level by Wang Yü, who recommended beheading in accordance with the law on "beating parents." This seems to have been the precedent on which the new category was based, as the emperor agreed to Wang Yü's request that henceforth all cases of pressuring grandparents and parents into suicide be treated in this way (Shen Chia-pen 1964: 487).

The Ch'ing initially kept exactly the same formulation of this clause as the Ming. But in 1772 the Ch'ien-lung Emperor made a change in the wording of the second part of the clause. Whereas the earlier phrase had been "wei-pi" (威逼), which has the connotations of pressuring someone from a position of superiority, Ch'ien-lung argued that such a phrase could not meaningfully be applied to a junior abetting his senior's act — for example in the case of a son and his own father. Ch'ien-lung changed *wei-pi* into the more neutral *pi-po* (逼迫), to press someone to do something, so that the law would more accurately reflect reality (Hsüeh Yün-sheng 1970:870).

That an enormous number of cases did indeed occur in this general category during the Ch'ing dynasty can at once be seen from the number of sub-statutes (*t'iao-li* 條例) — twenty-five — that were added to the original clause. We are fortunately able to study these cases in some detail because of the remarkable compilation of cases by Chu Ch'ing-ch'i and Pao Shu-yün, entitled *Hsing-an hui-lan* 刑案滙覽 . Most of these sub-statutes concerned cases of adultery or sexual assault where shame or discovery was followed by suicide. The number of sub-statutes was partly due to the different ways in which suicide followed the occurrence: in some cases it was the party directly involved who committed suicide out of guilt or shame, but more often the statute was invoked because the shock resulting from the discovery of the act led a third party within the family (whether husband, mother-in-law or parents) to commit suicide. Most of the remaining cases sprang from robberies — usually because the person was so desperate at his loss that he chose to end his life — or from money-lending, when either failure to pay or the sudden demand for payment might cause either party to kill themselves. There are also examples of threats, abuse, false accusation, blackmail or defamation of character, and forcing a woman into an unwanted marriage. Among these cases we find the following: a woman who abused her mother-in-law, a man guilty of homosexual assault, a man ripping a woman's trousers during a fight, a creditor who took his debtor's water buffalo, a man attempting rape, a man making his father-in-law foreclose his land to pay a debt, a thief who stole his aunt's clothes, a woman who refused to give her mother-in-law cold food in case it made her sickness worse (Chu Ch'ing-ch'i 1869: *chuan* 33–36).

In the four *chuan* of the *Hsing-an hui-lan,* where the bulk of these suicide cases are presented, we find 187 suicide cases, of which 160 concern suicides arising from family interrelationships. For our purposes here it is valuable to subdivide these according to gender, and we find 47 cases with a male suicidee,

112 with a female, and one with an unspecified "relative" (ch'in-shu 親屬). Within these gender categories we can make finer subdivisions, by describing the suicidee in terms of his relationship to the person pressuring him into suicide, or otherwise responsible for the death. (Thus when a son presses his father into committing suicide, that suicidee is listed as a father.)

Male Suicidees		Female Suicidees	
Fathers	7	Grandmother	1
Husbands	24	Mothers	21
Sons	2	Wives	79
Uncles	4	Daughters	2
Brothers	9	Aunts	9
Nephew	1		
Total	47	Total	112

If we consider the relationship of the person applying the pressure to the suicidee, then we can see graphically that the married woman (fu 婦 or ch'i 妻) had to cope with the widest range of family problems. Thus the 24 husbands are pressed into suicide overwhelmingly by their own wives (23, with one case of humiliation by a father-in-law). The wives, however, present a different picture: though 69 of the cases can be laid to the fact that the wife has been shamed in her husband's eyes by an act of rape, adultery or public sexual humiliation, and in one the husband accuses the wife of being a thief, the other 9 cases present a complete array of family members pressuring the wife into the suicidal act.

Relationship to wife of person pressuring wife (other than her own husband) to commit suicide	
Father-in-law	1
Mother-in-law	2
Uncle-in-law	1
Brother-in-law	2
Uncle	2
Cousin	1
Total	9

When we look at these cases in terms of the contributing circumstances, we find sexual factors nearly always dominant — as indeed they tended to be in the Dynastic Histories and in the Ku-chin t'u-shu chi-ch'eng. But whereas in those compilations the suicides were usually committed so as *to avoid a circumstance that would bring shame on the woman*, the legal cases deal with cases where the person *had already been* shamed. Instead of the (rather theoretical) anticipation that life would be morally unbearable, the person knows that it already is.

Contributing Cricumstances of Woman Suicide in *Hsing-an hui-lan* (in the *Wei-pi* section)	
Insulted in public by obscene language	32
Rape attempt	4
Rape	5
Forced adultery (by a family member)	5
Adultery	32
Total	78

Though the majority of suicides are presented in the *Wei-pi* section of the *Hsing-an hui-lan,* family centered suicides can also be found in other sections of the same work, and a listing of these sections shows the range of circumstances in which the family might get involved:

Chuan 4.	Crimes committed by the aged, by minors, the ill and the disabled	1 case
Ch. 7.	Marriage while in mourning	4 cases
Ch. 9.	Forcibly abducting wives or daughters	9 cases
Ch. 18.	Theft among relatives	2 cases
Ch. 22.	Homicide	1 case
Ch. 26 & 27.	Husband avenging adultery	3 cases
Ch. 33.	Killing a junior member of the family, or a servant, and falsely accusing another	1 case
Ch. 39.	Affray between master and subordinates	1 case
Ch. 39.	Servants beating a master	4 cases
Ch. 40.	Wife or concubine beating a husband	2 cases
Ch. 45.	One's family senior beaten by an outsider	1 case
Ch. 48.	Ritual impropriety	1 case
Ch. 49.	Son or grandson disobeying a family order	23 cases
Ch. 50.	Unreasonable demands by a household servant	1 case
Ch. 52.	Adultery (treated as a separate category here, because no one brought pressure)	13 cases

But a preliminary examination of these cases shows that the suicidee was generally motivated by fears of legal sanctions resulting from an act performed by a family member; and if we are to gauge the male's response to social pressures and his susceptibility to family tensions, the *Wei-pi* Section still probably remains our best source.

Derk Bodde, in *Law in Imperial China*, has translated two cases which illustrate male responses within the family; Case A shows two examples of husbands who commit suicide after initially condoning their wives' adultery. Case B shows a father's suicide out of chagrin at his daughter's behavior.

Case A: We have examined a case reported from Mukden in 1813, in which Ma Huan-lung tolerated an adulterous relationship between his wife and Ch'i Ta. Later, when Ch'i saw Ma stealing hemp stalks from Ma's landlord for fuel, he (Ch'i) reproved Ma and injured him by striking him on the left temple. On top of this, Ch'i also ran away with Ma's wife. After searching for them in vain, Ma, afflicted by shame, committed suicide. Ch'i was then sentenced under the sub-statute on seduction.

The present case is one which Lin K'o-chin, because of greed tolerated the adulterous relationship between his wife and Wang Fu, in return for which he repeatedly received money from Wang. Finally, however, Wang was unable to meet Lin's numerous demands, whereupon Lin forbade Wang to sleep with Mrs. Lin. At this, Wang demanded restoration of the money he had previously given Lin. Lin berated Wang in return, and Wang then struck Lin with his fists, injuring him on the left eye and elsewhere. Lin, after proclaiming the fact that Wang had not only been unwilling to give him money, but had also struck him, fell into such a state of uncontrollable passion that he hanged himself. (Bodde 1967: 358)

Case B: The governor of Honan has memorialized concerning a case in which Mrs. Ch'en nee Chang committed adultery with Wang Chieh and was abducted by him. The result was such shame and indignation on the part of her father that he killed himself. The governor has recommended strangulation after the assizes for Mrs. Ch'en, under the sub-statue providing this penalty for a married daughter (*fu*) or an unmarried daughter (nü) whose parents, after learning that she has entered into an illicit sexual relationship unsanctioned by themselves and after trying in vain to kill her seducer, commit suicide out of shame and indignation. (Bodde 1967: 359–360)

Both of these cases have a dramatic content of sexual activity and shame. We should not take them as typical examples without also adding cases that swung on smaller humiliations, involving men who themselves lived on the edge of subsistence and found an additional family humiliation to be intolerable.

Case C: Ch'eng Yu-lin borrowed and used his elder brother Ch'eng Yu-hsiu's farm tools, and damaged them. Ch'eng Yu-hsiu wouldn't let it be [without recompense], and swore at him. [The younger brother] tried to calm him with kind words, but Ch'eng Yu-hsiu picked up a rock and tried to hit [Yu-lin] with it. [Yu-lin] was afraid, and ran away to avoid him. Ch'eng Yu-hsiu chased him but could not catch him, and hurt his own forehead. After some people persuaded them to end [the episode], Ch'eng Yu-hsiu was angry and committed suicide. (Chu Ch'ing-ch'i 1869: 34, 31)

Case D: Because Yen Chin-kung's paternal uncle Yen Shou-yu owed him wheat and beans, and didn't pay him back, [Yen Chin-kung] demanded that Shou-yu take off his leather jacket and give it to him in payment. Because the weather grew cold, [Shou-yu] demanded it back. Yen Chin-kung wouldn't give it back. Because Yen Shou-yu had no leather jacket to get through the winter, he was in great distress and strangled himself. (Chu Ch'ing-ch'i 1869: 34, 33)

The challenge here — though it is beyond the scope of this essay — is to try to assess, in these and many other parallel cases, the extent to which the family relationship affected the outcome; and to what extent the closeness of a family, and the rigid insistence on maintenance of generational dignity within that family (on which so much weight was placed in Confucian writings) led to the constant recurrence of such tragedies. And in the case of women — perhaps especially for young brides — we need to know how much the everyday unremitting labor within the family circle pushed them towards suicide, such suicide being either a sole means of escape, or a sole means of striking back at those who oppressed them.

3. LITERARY EMBELLISHMENTS

In most cases neither the historical nor the legal sources present us with the nuances and shadings that would fill in the subtler sides of the pressures implicit in family relationships. For these we must turn to literary sources and in this area — as even a brief survey we hope will show — there is a wealth of absorbing detail.

One of the earliest such treatments is an anonymous poem from the first century B.C. Here the theme is the yearning for suicide by an orphan, living with his elder brother and sister-in-law. The poem (translated by Arthur Waley) is both bitter and haunting.

> My tears fell and fell
> And I went on sobbing and sobbing.
> In winter I have no great-coat;
> Nor in summer, thin clothes.
> It is no pleasure to be alive.
> I had rather quickly leave the earth
> And go beneath the Yellow Springs.
> The April winds blow
> And the grass is growing green.
> In the third month — silkworms and mulberries,
> In the sixth month — the melon-harvest.
> I went out with the melon-cart
> And just as I was coming home
> The melon-cart turned over.
> The people who came to help me were few,
> But the people who ate the melons were many,
> All they left me was the stalks —
> To take home as fast as I could.
> My brother and sister-in-law were harsh,
> They asked me all sorts of awful questions.
> Why does everyone in the village hate me?
> I want to write a letter and send it
> To my mother and father under the earth,
> And tell them I can't go on any longer
> Living with my brother and sister-in-law. (Waley 1920: 28–29).

The poem does not say if he did, in fact, kill himself, and perhaps we do not need to know, since the misery of the boy's life and his desire to die are already so strongly expressed.

But in another early *yüeh-fu*, "Southeast Fly the Peacocks," a double suicide springing from the family situation is meticulously documented. The young wife of a clerk, driven away from her loving husband by a cruel mother-in-law, returns home only to be bullied into remarrying by her own elder brother. From this point, the tragedy of the suicide is led up to in three stages. First, the separated couple, after a brief moment of anger, agree that both must end their lives:

> Said the prefectual clerk to the young wife:
> 'Congratulations on your lofty advancement!

The flat rock is still firm,
It can last a thousand years.
The reed was tough and pliable for a while,
From dawn until evening.
You'll prosper and move up from day to day,
I just go alone to the Yellow Springs.'
Said the young wife to the prefectural clerk:
'I'd never have thought you'd say such things.
We were both coerced,
It happened to you and also to me.
Below the Yellow Springs we'll see each other,
Let's not go against what we say today.'
They shook hands and went their separate ways,
Each returned to his house. (Frankel 1974: 256–257)

The clerk then tells his mother of his intention through the way in which he bids her farewell:

The prefectural clerk returned to his home,
Went up to the hall, and made obeisance to Mother.
'Today the great wind is cold,
The cold wind breaks the trees,
Severe frost forms on the orchids in the courtyard.
Your son's day is now darkening.
I'm causing Mother to stay behind alone,
This is my own evil design,
Do not blame ghosts and spirits.
May your life last like the rocks of South Mountain,
May your four limbs be strong and straight.' (Frankel 1974: 257)

The mother tries to dissuade him — "you must not die for the sake of your wife" — but the clerk had "made his plan and determined to carry it out;" he rejects his mother's pleas, and both lovers die as the celebration for the new wedding reach their climax.

On that day, cows lowed and horses whinnied.
The young wife entered the green wedding tent.
Gloomy, gloomy, after dusk,
Quiet, quiet, when every one had settled down.
My life will be cut off today,
My soul will depart, only my corpse will remain.
She grasped her skirt, took off her silk slippers,
Raised her body, and plunged into the clear pond.
When the prefectural clerk heard of this event
He knew in his heart the eternal parting was at hand.
Back and forth he walked under the trees of the courtyard,
Then hanged himself from the southeastern branch of a tree.
(Frankel 1974: 258)

The contrast with the Confucian morality of the virtuous woman (*lieh-nü chuan*) tradition, or of the conventional imagery of filial piety — both of which were developing strongly at the same time as this poem — is of course immediate and total. The two acts of obedience in accordance with the requirements of proper behavior, namely the son's letting his mother evict his wife, and the wife letting her elder brother arrange another marriage, are both rendered hollow by the final act of defiance. Here popular literature provides a totally different slant on conventional morality, though it should be emphasized that the need to express the protest by suicide also reemphasizes the force of the prevailing conventions.

A strong-willed mother again plays the dominant role in the famous tragedy 'Prince Huo's daughter,' Chiang Fang's ninth century short story. (Chiang Fang 1962: 32–43). The idyllic passion between the young scholar Li Yi and the courtesan Jade is wrecked by the insistence of Li's mother that he get married. The mother was "so strict that Li, though hesitating, dared not decline," and he ends up abandoning Jade. Various supernatural elements then enter the story, but they do not blur the basic point, that Jade, in her anger at being betrayed, vows to end her life so that she can become "an avenging spirit" and ruin the lives of Li Yi's later wives and concubines. The last page of the story is bleakly realistic as Li Yi's life becomes a misery after Jade's death; not because Li himself suffers physically in any way, but because he becomes convinced of the fickleness of all women (in a cruel inversion of his own guilty conscience) and beats up and divorces his own wife and treats even his most beloved concubines with sadistic paranoia.

Subtlety is added to Jade's story by the fact that her own mother — Prince Huo's former concubine — is depicted as a very warm and supportive person, "a slender, attractive woman with charming manners" to whom Jade feels free to confide her dreams.

Equally complex is the relationship between the young widow Tou Ngo and her mother-in-law, recorded in the Yuan play *The Injustice Done to Tou Ngo:* Tou Ngo is contemptuous of her mother-in-law, when the old lady is browbeaten into marrying again —

> You say he is full of joy,
> But I fear endless shame will be yours,
> Shame that you cannot bring yourself to swallow the nuptial wine,
> Shame that with your poor eyesight you cannot fasten the
> One-Heart button.   (Liu Jungen 1972: 127)

And yet she confesses to a murder she did not commit in order to save her mother-in-law from being beaten. Further irony is provided by the fact that Tou Ngo's frustrated suitor — who was in fact responsible for the murder — is never even suspected because he vociferously invokes the tradition of filial piety which would make it unthinkable for a son to kill his father. Tou Ngo's great poem of outrage has been seen as a Han Chinese protest against Yuan rule; it makes admirable sense, however, as the anguished cry of a young woman trapped in a family situation that admits of no solution.

Without knowing I have violated the laws of the land,
Without any defence I am to meet with this punishment.
I cry Injustice! let Earth be moved, let Heaven quake!
Soon my spirit will descend to the deep all-embracing Palace of Death.
How can Heaven and Earth not make complaint!
There the sun and moon hang by day and night,
There the spirits and gods dispense life and death.
Heaven and Earth!
It is for you to distinguish between right and wrong,
What confusion makes you mistake a villain for a saint?
The good suffer poverty and want, and their lives are cut short;
The wicked enjoy wealth and honour, and always live long.
Heaven and Earth!
You do but fear the strong and cheat the weak,
You too take the boat the current favours.
Earth! You cannot distinguish good and evil, can you yet be Earth!
Heaven! who mistake the fool for the sage, you are Heaven in vain!
Oh, nothing is left to me now but two streams of flowing tears.

(Liu Jungen 1972; 139—140)

Numerous other examples of suicides exist in both the Yuan, Ming and Ch'ing: in the dramas *Ch'iu Hu Hsi Ch'i* 秋胡戲妻, *Tzu-ch'ai chi* 紫釵記, *Hsi-hsiang chi* 西廂記, in the story "*Tu Shih-niang nu-ch'en pa-pao-hsiang*" 杜十娘怒沉八寶箱 and others in Feng Meng-lung's collections, as well as in the novels *Chin-p'ing mei* 金瓶梅 and *Ju-lin wai-shih* 儒林外史. But the greatest concentration on suicide is perhaps in the novel *Hung-lou meng,* where we find at least ten cases, all arising in different contexts. Two are double suicides, involving both men and women: Chin-ko and her fiance take their lives after Hsi-feng's meddling leads to the cancelling of their engagement (Ts'ao Hsüeh-ch'in 1957: 148); and Ssu-ch'i's lover — who had abandoned her — commits suicide after learning that she has taken her own life in despair (Ts'ao 1957: 1033—1034). Two maids kill themselves to accompany their dead mistresses to the underworld (Ts'ao 1957: 111, 1228—1229), and one jumps into the well after being scolded by her mistress (Ts'ao 1957: 335—337). On at least one occasion the novelist Ts'ao Hsüeh-ch'in intended a character to commit suicide but then changed his mind, thus Ch'in-shih dies a natural death, though Pao-yu in his dream had seen a picture of "an upper room in a tall building in which a beautiful girl was hanging by her neck from a beam, having apparently taken her own life" (Hawkes 1973: 135). This suicide was the result of her too great lust, which led her into incestuous relations with her father-in-law Chen. Ts'ao Hsüeh-ch'in has a beautiful echo of this in the twelfth of the poems which Pao-yu reads in "The Dream of Golden Days".

Perfumed was the dust that fell
From painted beams where springtime ended.
Her sportive heart

> And amorous looks
> The ruin of a mighty house portended.   (Hawkes 1973:144)

This (projected) suicide out of remorse, with its inter-connections with the fate of the novel's main characters, is supplemented by the two suicides of the Yu sisters, one out of anger at being rejected by her fiance, and one out of misery (Ts'ao 1957: 737–738, 772). It is Yu Erh-chieh's death, out of misery and humiliation following her miscarriage and her mistreatment on the orders of Hsi-feng that is undoubtedly the most poignant. Here we see clearly how the leisurely format of a novel allowed Ts'ao Hsüeh-ch'in to elaborate on character and context in a way that had been denied to the poet or dramatist. (In this vivid translation by Cyril Birch, "Second Sister" is Yu Erh-chieh and "Violet" is Ch'iu-t'ung, the maid who had been gaining Chia Lien's favor.) Even out of context this passage gives testimony to the range of misery to which a mistrusted woman could be subjected by other women in her own household.

The Matriarch's displeasure was the signal for the servants to trample on Second Sister in their efforts to curry favor with their superiors. She could have wished for death, so impossible had her life now become. And still it was to Equity's credit that behind the back of Phoenix she did what little things she could for the girl.

Now Second Sister was one of those people with 'guts made of petals, flesh like snow' – she was in no way fitted to stand up to this kind of maltreatment, and after less than a month of such veiled malice exhaustion developed into sickness. Her limbs were overcome with lassitude, she could take neither food nor even tea, and gradually her features took on a pallid and wasted look. . . .

The vinegar of jealousy had already begun to collect in Violet's bosom as she watched Chia Lien sending for doctors and beating and cursing the servants in his concern for Second Sister. Now, when the blame was put on her and Phoenix herself came to urge her to go away for a few days, Violet burst out in tears and imprecations: "You've been listening to that pack of mangy mongrels flapping their vicious tongues! 'Both are water, but the well-spring doesn't interfere with the river' – how have I ever injured her? Such a darling creature – I suppose she had no contact with anyone outside, but as soon as she comes here somebody does something to 'injure' her! And what sort of little monster was it anyway – red eyes and white brows? She's only been trying to make a fool out of our master with his big, soft, cottony ears! Suppose there *is* a baby – who's to say whether its surname should be Chang or Wang or what? First Mistress may treasure a bastard brat of that sort, but not me! What's so special about a baby? Anyone can have one – takes a year or thereabouts, and there's no need for any hanky-panky to get it, either! . . . .

Now Second Sister searched her thoughts: 'My sickness has taken full hold, I grow worse instead of better as the days pass. Surely there can be no recovery for me. And now I have lost my baby and have nothing to hope for – why should I put up with this rage against me? Better to die and have done. I've often heard that a person can suffocate by swallowing gold, and surely that's a cleaner way than hanging or cutting one's throat.'

Her resolution made, she struggled to her feet and from one of her cases searched out a piece of gold of a certain weight. She placed the gold in her mouth and gritted her teeth to force it down her throat. She had to stretch her neck back several times before she could swallow it down. Then she hastened to dress herself and ornament her hair as neatly as she could before she lay down on the bed again. And neither man nor demon knew of this. (Birch 1972: 252, 254–255)

Ts'ao Hsüeh-ch'in's concluding observation here reminds us of the layers of evasion and privacy that cover most suicide acts. There is a point, he seems to be saying, where only empathy and imagination can serve to supplement the more accessible record of rhetoric and institutional response. Whether one can move such literary insights out of the realm of embellishment and truly incorporate them into the historical and legal bodies of data is a challenge that demands the most serious consideration.

CONCLUSION

The cases that we have examined in this paper suggest that for long periods of China's pre-modern history the act of suicide was not regarded as deviant. Indeed, the build-up of historiographical evidence shows that from the beginning of the Ming dynasty or earlier, and at least through the Ch'ien-lung reign in the eighteenth century, the act of suicide was encouraged by the state and openly praised. At the same time in all the realms surveyed here – whether in histories, legal cases, or literature – there was a strong sense that it was wrong to pressure people into suicide against their will, and that lurking in the background of most suicide cases one would find a specific human culprit who should be held responsible and punished. One might summarize the situation, then, by saying that what was deviant was not the suicide act, but the pressuring of a person into suicide.

This had certain implications. Firstly, it largely exonerated Chinese "society," in any form, from being responsible. A widow killing herself after her husband's death was seen as acting both correctly and freely, and few people spoke out against this practice until the early twentieth century: one of the pioneers here was Mao Tse-tung, who in one of his earliest essays took the step of blaming the townspeople of Changsha and their social ethos for "causing" the suicide of Miss Chao (Schram 1969: 334–337).

Secondly, by emphasizing either individual rectitude or outside harassment, the focus turned away from considerations of personal misery or intense depression – unless such emotions were aroused by the death of a husband or the fall of a dynasty. The woman in the family thus was presented as acting in a way that corresponded to the actions of the man in the realm of the state: both were shown as committing suicide out of a sense of loyalty or duty, though in the man's case the object of that loyalty was presented as a deceased or defeated emperor. Death, for either woman or man, was seen as preferable to a transference of loyalties, and was praised accordingly, whereas men or women who committed suicide out of misery or unhappiness with the general state of society could be vigorously censured by the authorities (Spence 1978: 14–15).

Thirdly, there is a strong implication in many cases that purposeful suicide was seen as being effective; it could either be a way of pressuring the survivors – whether family or emperor – to pursue a better line of conduct (sometimes, here, the threat to commit suicide might be enough); or it could contain an element of vengeance, as the restless spirit of the deceased returned to haunt the living.

Lastly, suicide was presented as a swift and clean act. Though there are early cases of suicide by sword or dagger and of self-immolation by religious fanatics, the most common methods were those that were literally bloodless; death was found either through poison, by drowning, by self-strangulation or (in the nineteenth century) by swallowing raw opium. The emphasis in so many Chinese sources, across such a great stretch of time, that suicide could be tidy and painless may ultimately be the most important index we have of the pervasiveness of the idea that suicide, as an act, was truly exemplary.

ACKNOWLEDGMENTS

We would like to thank the members of the "core group" of our faculty seminar on suicide in China, that met at intervals during the academic year 1973–1974 at Yale: Emily Ahern, Hilary Beattie, Hans Frankel, Jerry Guben, and Steven Owen. We would also like to thank visitors to the seminar who offered valuable critiques of our earlier draft presentations on law, family and literature: Randle Edwards, C. T. Hsia, Olga Lang, Leo Ou-fan Lee, and C. K. Yang. Their discussions were ably summarized by our valiant rapporteur William Alford. We are also grateful to the Ford Foundation, which through a grant to Yale's Concilium on International and Area Studies provided us with the initial resources to launch this enterprise.

NOTES

1. The authors are preparing a separate paper that will concentrate on the problem of suicide as a political act in Chinese history.
2. See for example *Ssu-k'u ch'üan-shu tsung-mu t'i-yao* 四庫全書總目提要, *History*, section on *Biography*, the discussion of Liu Hsuang's *Lieh-nü chuan*, and the List in *Chung-kuo ts'ung-shu tsung-lu* 中國叢書綜目: pp. 437–441.
3. It should be noted that the high figure in Nanking-fu of those who refused to remarry could be explained by a number of factors: that local historians had better knowledge of such persons than compilers of dynastic histories; that they had more space to include them; that the Ch'ing practice of displaying the names of virtuous widows in their own locality had a considerable propaganda effect. (Tseng T'ieh-ch'en 1935: 42–59)

BIBLIOGRAPHY

Birch, Cyril
    trans 1972
        Red chamber dream. As printed *in* his Anthology of Chinese Literature. New York: Grove Press.
Bodde, Derk and Morris, Clarence
    1967 Law in Imperial China. Cambridge: Harvard University Press.
Chang, Hsüeh-cheng 章學誠
    1962 *Wen-shih t'ung-i* 文史通義. Taipei: Shih-chieh shu-chu.

Chiang, Fang 蔣防
 1962 Huo Hsiao-yu chuan, 霍小玉傳 as printed in Yang, Hsien-i and Yang, Gladys, trans The Dragon King's Daughter – Ten T'ang Dynasty Stories. Peking: Foreign Languages Press.
Chiang-nan t'ung-chih 江南通志
 1967 Reprint of 1737 Gazetteer of Chiang-nan. Taipei: Hua-wen shu-chu.
Chu, Ch'ing-ch'i 祝慶麒 and Pao, Shu-yün 鮑書芸
 1869 *Hsing-an hui-lan* 刑案滙覽. no publisher.
Croll, Elisabeth
 1977 A recent movement to redefine the role and status of women. China Quarterly 71: 591–597.
Frankel, Hans
 1974 The Chinese ballad "Southeast Fly the Peacocks." Harvard Journal of Asiatic Studies 34: 248–271.
Hawkes, David
 trans 1973
  The Story of the Stone. London: Penguin Books.
Hsü, Sung 徐松
 ed 1936
  Sung hui-yao kao 宋會要稿. Peiping: National Peiping Library.
Hsüeh, Yun-sheng 薛允升
 1970 *Tu-li ts'un-i* 讀例存疑. Taipei: Chinese Materials and Research Aids Service Center.
Kuei, Yu-kuang 歸有光
 1935 *Chen-ch'uan hsien-sheng ch'uan-chi* 震川先生全集. Shanghai: Commercial Press.
Liu, Jung-en
 trans 1972
  Six Yüan Plays. London: Penguin Books.
Liu, Wei-ch'ien 劉惟謙
 1970 *Ta-Ming-lü chi-chieh fu-li* 大明律集解附例. Taipei: Hsüeh-sheng shu-chu.
O'Hara, Albert
 trans 1945
  The Position of Woman in Early China (Liu Hsiang's Lieh-nü chuan 列女傳. Washington, D. C.: The Catholic University of America Press.
Schram, Stuart
 1969 The Political Thought of Mao Tse-tung, revised edition, New York, Praeger.
Shen, Chia-pen 沈家本
 1964 *Shen chi-i hsien-sheng i-shu* 沈寄簃先生遺書. Taipei: Wen-hai chu-pan she.
Spence, Jonathan
 1978 The Death of Woman Wang. New York: The Viking Press.
Ts'ao Hsüeh-ch' 曹雪芹
 1957 *Hung-lou-meng* 紅樓夢. Peking: Tsou-chia ch'u-pan she.
Tseng, T'ieh-ch'en 曾鐵忱
 1935 Ch'ing-t'ai chih ching-piao chih-tu 清代之旌表制度. *Chung-kuo she-hui* 中國社會 1(5): 42–59.
Waley, Arthur
 trans. 1920
  170 Chinese Poems. London: Constable and Company.
Waley, Arthur
 1938 The Analects of Confucius. Paperback ed. New York: Random House.
Wang, Chung 汪中
 1936 *Shu-hsüeh* 述學. Shanghai: Chung-hua shu-chu.
Yü, Cheng-hsieh 俞正燮
 1941 *Kuei-szu lei-kao* 癸巳類稿. Hong Kong: Commercial Press.

STEVAN HARRELL

3. NORMAL AND DEVIANT DRINKING IN RURAL TAIWAN[1]

Ou-yang Hsiu, the most famous of the Neo-Confucian scholars of the early Sung, once wrote a poem entitled The Drunken Old Man's Pavilion. In it, he described the joys of watching the daily and seasonal changes in a misty pavilion on a mountain top, joys realized through the medium of large amounts of wine (Ou-yang 1963). Other poets as well extolled the pleasures of drink, poetry, and friendship. Not only in the sensuous lines of Li Pai but even in the restrained and correct verse of Tu Fu, wine and human warmth go together (T'ang-shih san-pai-shou 1968).

R. F. Johnston, British vice-magistrate at Weihaiwei in the first decade of this century, prized the Chinese of humbler social class for their temperance in matters of alcohol. He stated: "I have been obliged to punish only six Chinese for drunkenness in five years" (1910:145). Other contemporary accounts rarely mention alcohol, even when they spend many pages talking of the dangers of opium.

These two very separate vignettes suggest something about the place of alcohol in Chinese society. It has nearly always been accepted as an accompaniment to meals or even to poetry, and has always been widely available, even to the poorest classes, everywhere. Yet there is a strong suggestion that this very dangerous drug has been quite successfully tamed in Chinese society, that alcoholism and drunkenness are minor problems, especially in comparison to the scourge that was opium. Why should it be that the substance usually considered to be the most potentially harmful of all common psychotropic agents should hold such a benign, even honored place in Chinese civilization, and should create, seemingly, so little of the devastating effects usually associated with drinking in Western societies? This paper, based on ten months of participant observation in society, hence in drinking also, in rural Taiwanese villages, will try to suggest some answers, based on experience in that small corner of Chinese society.

It is clear to begin with that the answer is not, as some have suggested, physiological. It is true as reported by Wolff (1972) that some Chinese, after drinking very little alcohol, experience a "flush response" in which the skin becomes very red and which is reported by some subjects to be quite uncomfortable. But most Chinese males I have known do not experience this response, and even those who do often drink quite heavily in spite of it. I have often seen young men with faces quite red participating boisterously in drinking and even in drinking games.

The fact that drinking has not been recognized as a major problem cannot be attributed to moderation, either. It is possible to drink a little bit, if one is in the

49

company of very good friends at times other than festivals. Otherwise, a decision to drink generally means a decision to drink until inebriated, because drinking involves reciprocity, and one must not only drink the specified amounts in toasts proposed by others, but also counter with toasts of one's own. This means that it is extremely difficult to get away from a festive meal without at least a light head. Some people go much further and have to be helped home.

The facts are, then, that most Chinese adult males, at least in rural areas of Taiwan, do drink and that when they do, they drink until at least tipsy if not downright drunk. If drinking is not a major social problem, then, the reasons must be sought in the ability of the society to put drinking in its place, to define the social context of alcohol consumption so that it becomes, not an antisocial activity, but a social activity, one that is integrated into and even contributes to the ordinary activities of social relations. This becomes clear when we take a broader look at drinking in rural Taiwan and realize that not all drinkers do conform to social rules, that there are deviant as well as normal drinkers, and that such deviant drinkers, or *ciu-kui* (Hokkien, alcohol ghosts) are scorned and disregarded like any other social deviants. Drinking itself is not a problem, but wrong drinking is. Let us examine the nature and context of normal and deviant drinking, which will give us a better idea of how Chinese society has been moderately successful in controlling alcohol, and of what happens where it has failed.

NORMAL DRINKING

Normal drinking is drinking that is accepted by most members of society. It is accepted because it is part of social relations and because it can be justified in terms of popular beliefs about diet and preventive medicine. For one's drinking to be considered normal, it must meet three absolute criteria: one should never drink alone, one should never drink without eating at the same time, and one should not drink so often that one cannot continue one's contribution to family and community. Drinking with others over meals or snacks on appropriate occasions is normal, for adult males at least, no matter how long a drinking session lasts, no matter how much is drunk, and no matter how inebriated the participants become. In order to understand this, we must take a closer look at the contexts in which men in rural Taiwan drink, and at the social relations and customary behaviors of drinking in such contexts.

The archetypical context in which drinking is allowed, or even expected, is that of a banquet for a wedding, moving into a new house, or killing a pig in honor of the local god during the first month of the Chinese lunar calendar. On all these occasions, people hold enormous feasts, providing neighbors, relatives, and friends with ten to fourteen catered dishes and liberal amounts of alcohol. Just by bringing so many people together to honor a particular occasion, such a banquet is already an important aspect of social relationships. And the drinking which goes on, by following certain rules, conforms to and reinforces the social relationships which are being affirmed on such an occasion.

Typically, the guests at a banquet will be seated at a number of large round tables, each accommodating about ten people. Although men tend to sit at separate tables from women and children, there is no hard and fast rule about this, and some tables are mixed. When guests arrive, bottles are already on the table, but they are not opened while people are eating roasted watermelon seeds and waiting for the first dishes to arrive. When the food comes, the liquor can be opened and the drinking begins. For a male sitting at a table with other men, there is already a decision to make: alcohol or a carbonated soft drink. One cannot choose the latter easily, because it is much more difficult to participate in the important social relationships of drinking when one is ingesting something with no alcohol and hence no drug effect in it. Drinking is reciprocal, and sugar does not reciprocate alcohol, so a man who chooses Coke, for example, will be pressured to drink, even if just a little, in order to be part of those social relationships. He must, through the first few dishes of the meal anyway, keep his glass full of Coke and guard against others' attempts to fill it with liquor. If he really means it, people will stop trying to get him to drink after a few rounds, and toast him, liquor to pop. This may be a disappointment to others at the table who were looking for a rousing time drinking, but it is no social stigma to the man who refused. There are perfectly good reasons for not drinking, such as taking medicine, feeling sick, or simply having something important to do after the banquet. But to be a full participant, a man must drink, and others will try to get him to do so. If he does give in and drink a little, he is in the game, and will have to participate fully or else be even more skillful at fending off others' attempting to fill his glass and to toast him.

Once the drinking itself begins, those who are participating must do so in a particular way: They must toast each other, and must do so in equal amounts, unless agreed upon otherwise. A man can toast the whole table, for example, and often the first toast is made in this way. If the host is present at the table, he is expected to make the first toast, and to toast the whole table. To do so, he lifts a full glass in the fingers of his right hand, with the left hand held out flat, palm up, with the little finger against the side of the glass. He will describe an arc in front of everyone at the table, and they will all raise their glasses in a similar manner. Then the person proposing the toast declares how much is to be drunk. Usually it will be the entire shot-glass, in the case of rice wine (about 20% alcohol) or an entire tumbler, in the case of beer. If all agree, then all drink. If not, someone may object, out of fear of becoming drunk or protest of inability to drink, and state that we should just drink half, or even just drink "according to our wishes (Hokkien, *sui-i*)" which means just touch the glass to our lips or at most take a small sip. The proposer of the toast may or may not agree to this; if he does, people will drink; if not the negotiations go on until a consensus is reached, and then everyone drinks. After drinking people hold up their glasses in the same position, to show how much, either the whole glass or half of it, they have actually drunk. To propose a toast to a single person, rather than to the whole table, one simply holds up one's glass in the direction of that person, and says "invite you to drink," or "thank you for the meal," or "thank you for coming" or some such sentiment, and the two then proceed as before in the matters of negotiating how much to drink and holding up the glass in demonstration afterwards. When people have drunk, whoever is managing the bottle then refills their glasses, ready for the next round.

A very important aspect of this toasting is that it is reciprocal, in two senses. First, two men who are parties to a toast must drink the same amounts. Second, if one man toasts another, the other must toast him back after not too long. This second rule is not observed rigorously, as long as there is a rough equivalence between the toasts initiated by each partner. This insures a kind of equality in social relations, or at least a reaffirmation that an unequal relationship is proceeding on a normal and expected basis, but it does not insure that all participants in drinking at a particular table are drinking the same amount. It is perfectly possible to gang up on someone, just to test his capacity for liquor, and this has happened more than once to visiting anthropologists.

As the meal progresses through its various courses, the drinking at a particular table may follow one of two sequences. At some tables, polite and reciprocal toasting continues to the end, when only slightly tipsy men leave and return to whatever they need to do. At other tables, however, where some men may be really interested in drinking, their drinking may take over the table. In this case, others will tend to withdraw and the real drinkers will toast only each other. As they become more and more drunk, they will begin to consume larger and larger amounts, and to have longer arguments over who is really consuming how much. Often, if they have been drinking rice wine out of shot glasses, they will switch to small tumblers to avoid having to pour so often. They may become quite boisterous and begin to sing songs. They may very well ignore the food which continues to be brought, and those who are having a really good time may progress to the stage of finger-games. In the most common of these, two men begin with full glasses of liquor, and simultaneously thrust their right hands downward into the space between them, holding out any number of fingers from none to five, and each shouting any number from zero to ten. When either one shouts a number which equals the sum of the fingers both of them are holding out, the other has to drink a specified amount. This can go on for hours until one or both get too drunk to be able to count fingers. By this time, usually most guests, including those who have drunk moderately, have already left the banquet house or hall, while the "serious drinkers" continue their games.

I have dwelt so long on drinking behavior of men at large banquets because it illustrates nearly all the important points about normal drinking. First, it always accompanies food, and always is done together with others. Second, it proceeds according to quite rigid rules — one cannot, just because one is attending a banquet, pick up one's glass when one is thirsty and just take a drink. To do so would be to violate the basic rule that drinking helps to establish and affirm social relationships between drinkers. Because of this, drinking is not just tolerated but expected on such occasions, and those who refuse to drink must be both strong willed and ready with acceptable excuses. Finally, drunkeness is tolerated at such times. People nearly always take the whole day off on occasions which call for a banquet, and their drinking thus will not only be sociable, but will not interfere with work or other serious pursuits. When I once apologized for some silly remarks made while drunk at a wedding feast, people seemed surprised that I had bothered. One is expected to get drunk on such occasions.

Another important context in which drinking is tolerated and expected of adult males is during religious festivals. These are usually scheduled on different days in different neighboring communities, so that people from one village or section of town can visit while friends or relatives in another celebrate their festival, and have these same friends or relatives visit them when their own turn comes around. On such occasions every family makes offerings to the god whose birthday the festival commemorates, and then prepares a fancy meal, accompanied by alcoholic drink. Visitors who know several people in a community are expected to visit as many of them as possible, to eat and, in the case of men, to drink as well. Taking food from someone or offering it to a guest reaffirms a social relationship between the guest and the host, and the same goes for drink. The same rules of reciprocal toasting apply, though a guest who is expected to put in appearances at several households must not stay too long at any one. The extreme of such mobile drinking is reached by political figures who will attempt to take literally a bite of food and a sip of liquor at tens of households or even a hundred a night for several weeks. As a consequence of all this visiting, the streets are full of drunk and semi-drunk people on festival nights. But again, such drinking behavior is expected, controlled, and normal for most men. Festivals are days that everyone takes off, and drinking gets in the way of very little, especially since what there is to do mainly consists of more drinking. Restricted to a particular occasion with others, with food, and obeying the social rules of toasting and reciprocity, such drinking is normal and expected. In other, similar contexts, such as guest meals at another's house or trips to restaurants, as long as they are not too frequent, drinking is controlled in the same way, and is tolerated and considered normal. It is a part of social relations, in the same way that eating is.

If certain kinds of drinking are socially normal, because they fit in with other activities, they are also normal in the sense of beliefs about health and the body. Chinese beliefs about preventive medicine contain a strong notion that most substances which are ingested are either hot or cold, and affect the body by "heating" or "cooling" it. Alcohol is subsumed into the same system – beer, which is cold, is the drink of choice at all occasions during the hot summer months, while rice wine (Hokkien, *siou-chiu*, "hot wine"), which is considered hot, is drunk exclusively in the winter (see also Anderson and Anderson 1975: 146–148). In addition, certain kinds of alcoholic beverages, particularly those made from medicinal herbs, are themselves thought to have medicinal value, and

can be consumed in small amounts by anybody, anytime, because of their presumably prophylactic physiological effects. Wine as a biologically active substance is included in the folk culture of physiology and medicine in the same
way that wine as a social drink is included in the system of social relations.

Just as certain kinds of social drinking are considered normal and acceptable,
those who engage in drinking, even quite heavy drinking, on such occasions can
be fully acceptable, respected, even prominent members of the community.
Political figures, as mentioned before, often find it difficult to avoid drinking
large amounts on ceremonial occasions, and some men who are otherwise
prominent as community leaders are also renowned for their drinking ability.
One good acquaintance of mine who was a section head in the local government
was also widely known for his ability to hold liquor, and indeed was able to do a
whirlwind job of getting a visiting young anthropologist drunk by reciprocal
toasting while remaining very much in control of the situation himself. Since
he drank according to accepted rules on accepted occasions, he was not censured
for his drinking behavior, even though he often drank quite heavily on those
occasions.

Such, briefly, is a way in which a society can allow drinking, even heavy
drinking, and keep it in control. But it must not be imagined that even such
normal and accepted drinking is without at last minor deleterious consequences,
or that people see such drinking as having no bad effects on themselves or their
communities. A man who does not drink at all (and there are a few) can be
respected for it, especially if he works hard and keeps up all other aspects of
social relationships. And people recognize that even normal drinking has its
costs, especially when heavy banquet drinking leads to suppressed quarrels being
brought out into the open. Members of two of the most prominent families of
the village in which I lived actually came to blows one night after a rousing bout
at a banquet, and many people blamed their indiscretion on the fact that they
were drunk. On the whole, however, normal drinking does not lead to antisocial
behavior.

DEVIANT DRINKING

If drinking by adult men, over food, with friends or acquaintances, at festivals,
banquets, or other special occasions, is considered normal and has relatively
minor deleterious consequences either for the society or for the position of the
drinkers in that society, any drinking which occurs outside that context is
abnormal, because it is perceived as having deleterious effects on the drinkers
and on the community. And those who drink outside the normal, accepted
context are deviant drinkers, and are less well regarded by society for that and
subject to social control. There are several kinds of drinking and drinkers that
violate these rules of social context, and I will describe each of them briefly
here.

First, there are women who drink. Most women do not, or at least not to any appreciable extent.[2] When a woman, from a bride to a mother-in-law, is called upon to share a toast with a man, she may acceptably drink *sui-i* (just touching the glass to her lips) if it contains something alcoholic, or alternatively may drink soda pop to the man's alcohol. Some women will actually drink a glass of beer or rice wine, especially at a family festival, but only one. Men often attempt to get women to participate in the ordinary round of toasting and counter-toasting, but usually without success. It is easy for a woman to refuse to drink, and most women do so.

Those who drink in the same way men drink, that is, until they are drunk, are looked upon as somewhat deviant. I only knew one woman who habitually got drunk – she was a widow with a slightly usavory reputation otherwise, and could occasionally be seen being helped up the street by a friend, unable to walk by herself. This behavior was looked on with mild disapproval. Since she functioned reasonably normally in the community otherwise, however, her drinking was a target of only moderate criticism. It was, however criticized, and probably would not have been, had she been a man.

A second and more serious breach of proper context for drinking comes when men drink on inappropriate occasions, or drink too often. It is certainly permissible to drink quite a bit of alcohol on occasions other than festivals, especially if it is done with friends over meals in restaurants. But men who do this habitually have a difficult time being taken seriously. In the community where I lived, for example, there were five or six men who spent large amounts of time either after work or on days off drinking. They would meet at each other's houses, or more frequently in the local noodle shop, and consume bottle after bottle of the cheapest liquor, usually mixed with soda pop, over plates of small snacks such as peanuts or dried watermelon seeds. Not all of them did it all the time, but each of them did it often enough that they were considered *ciu-kui*[3] (alcohol ghosts), men who drank inappropriately. They all held jobs, but most, significantly, were poor, and none of them was respected in the community. When one would show up in someone else's house, drunk after a session with the others, it was something of an embarrassment. People would whisper to me not to pay any attention to so and so, because he was drunk, and it seemed to me they were always waiting for the fellow to leave. Once I was sitting in the local noodle shop, where I took my meals, and noticed a young man of my acquaintance, and started to talk to him. As I did, two of these *ciu-kui,* both of whom I knew well, came over to my table, took my hand, tried over my eventually successful protests to pour me a glass and began to swear eternal friendship. The other young man moved away quietly. I ultimately managed to walk out, leaving the drinkers to their next bottle, but by that time the slightly disgusted young man was long gone. He, like most respectable people, wanted as little to do with the drunks as I did.

A further departure from normal drinking behavior comes when someone drinks either alone or without food, or both. Someone who indulges in alcohol outside any kind of social activity is engaging in an anti-social activity, and someone who drinks without food has not even a pretense of using alcohol as part of a normal activity such as eating. Those who drink alone or without food are the real wine ghosts. One of the less serious offenders in this category was a man called "Big Dumb Ciu", a retired coal miner. He usually seemed mildly inebriated, and once answered my greeting of "Have you eaten yet?" with "Half eaten — wine!" He was a ne'er-do-well and was the open target for kidding, more for his stupidity than for his drunkenness, by young and old alike. But he rarely caused any harm, and was tolerated if not respected. More serious problem drinkers are those whose behavior is anti-social in other ways. A prime example of a wine ghost of this sort was a man named Peq, who cohabited with a widow in a house behind the one I lived in while I resided in the village. Every evening in the summer, the woman he lived with would set a chair and a bench in the courtyard between the two houses, and place an opened bottle of cheap wine on the bench, sometimes accompanied by seeds or peanuts. Peq would manage to drink this much in an hour or less, and would often then go out to start some trouble. When drunk, he would insult people, provoke others to fight with each other, or simply act "drunk and disorderly" out on the street. To provoke fights, especially where one has no personal interest of one's own, is the height of anti-social behavior in a society which holds harmony to be one of the highest virtues, and Peq was thoroughly despised for this habit. People connected it directly with his drinking, because he only did it when drunk. Even though he was probably not drunk as much of the time as some of the other habitual wine ghosts, his behavior was much more deviant. The others did not really hurt anything, they were merely occasional pests who could be tolerated if never respected. But Peq drank alone, and drank even though he knew perfectly well that it would lead to antisocial behavior. It is as if he were deliberately ignoring the importance of social relations generally — his drinking was antisocial in the sense of the direct opposite of social; done without companionship, it caused conflict.

Having described deviant and anti-social drinking and drinkers, it might be worthwhile to speculate on the causes of such drinking. Most but not all wine ghosts are poor, and the question arises whether they are poor because they drink or drink because they are poor. I suspect it is the latter, because in no case did even the most anti-social drinking prevent anyone I knew from earning a living. A few of the drinkers were retired, anyway, but most of them held down regular jobs and drank only after work or on days off. Even Peq went every day to one of the Taipei city markets, where he was a custodian. So it was not their drinking which caused their economic plight. Their social plight, on the other hand, was somewhat different. Not knowing the history of how they became problem drinkers, I cannot determine for sure if they were disrespected because they drank or if they drank because they were disrespected. But whatever the initial cause of disrespect, it was certainly intensified by drinking. Again, the worst case, that of Peq, serves to illustrate the point. He came from a distant part of Taiwan and was only cohabiting with a village woman, and thus had no formal ties to the community. This already was a handicap, though other men who had married into the village or who had simply moved in with their families, at least, by hard work and skillful social relations managed to become accepted after a few years. Peq was not, and his drinking, together with its consequences, made the situation a lot worse. One village woman told me I could tell right away that Peq was not one of the locals, for he caused trouble among people, something anybody with real ties in the community would never do. Drinking alone was in one sense a symptom of his isolation, but by continuing the behavior, Peq assured that the isolation itself could never be broken. He eventually moved out of the village and left his woman friend to be cared for by her sons.

CONCLUSION

We can see from this brief account that the rules which define drinking in this Chinese community as normal or deviant fit in with two important aspects of Chinese culture: the system of folk biomedical beliefs and, more importantly, the system of social relations. As part of an accepted social activity — eating, especially ceremonial eating — drinking is normal, even desirable. Outside the context of such a social activity, it is undesirable and deviant. But while these associations have a symbolic content, they are more than simply symbolic. Drinking in accepted social contexts can be controlled, so that the potentially dangerous drug consumed does as little damage as possible. Outside the accepted social contexts, however, drinking becomes dangerous. People who simply drink too often are dangerous mainly to themselves — they can make little contribution, but are relatively seldom directly harmful to others. The most deviant drinkers of all, those who drink alone, are posing a direct social danger, and their behavior is strongly condemned. Drinking behavior, like any other behavior, is ultimately judged normal or deviant by its effect on social relations.

But a further question arises. Even if Chinese communities in rural Taiwan are able to control drinking behavior and render it socially harmless most of the time, we see that they cannot always do so, and thus we must ask what is done to try to control problem drinkers when they do emerge. The answer is that very little is done in most situations. If a drinker becomes violent or threatens to do so, people will restrain him physically, and even threatened to call the police on one occasion when the wine ghost Peq was making convincing threats. But otherwise, criticism and the realization that a problem drinker would never be respected serve in themselves to control most deviant drinking behavior. As long as it does not directly threaten the livelihood of others, people in this area are very tolerant of drinking behavior. Because it destroys a man's opportunities for economic advancement and social respect, most men will never engage in this kind of drinking, which will thus not become a large-scale social problem, as long as there are economic gains to be made and social respect to be had. The few men who succumb to drink, either as a result or as a partial cause of losing respect and economic standing, can be left to do so, perhaps criticized because they are deviant, but not directly sanctioned in any way. They serve as a negative example which, along with socialization into proper social behavior, including proper drinking, keeps most men from ever becoming problem drinkers.

This description applies to drinking behavior only in one section of rural Taiwan; it might be profitable to speculate on how applicable it might be to other sectors of Chinese society. I have very little experience with drinking in other Chinese contexts, but when I have attended banquets with Chinese academics, their behavior has been quite similar, with only a few famous drinkers really consuming much, and perhaps with less pressure on the non-drinker to participate in drinking. And with little evidence, I would expect similar behavior in most Chinese communities, because the assumptions about eating as an aspect of social relations, assumptions which include drinking behavior, seem to be the same everywhere. In any Chinese context, creating and maintaining social relationships is crucial to maintaining or advancing one's social and economic status. And drinking is one way to maintain or even create social relationships. As such, it can be abused only at the drinker's peril. There are sure to be more problem drinkers in communities where other kinds of socially deviant behavior are common or even expected within the community, but in most contexts the cultural values of work, striving to get ahead, and social cooperation are probably enough to keep real problem drinking under control. I have no evidence that this is the case, but it makes logical sense. I would hope that further research could test this hypothesis, and allow us to discover whether indeed Chinese culture has managed to tame alcohol to the dimensions of a minor social problem.

NOTES

1. This paper is a sidelight of ten months' field work in 1972–73, and two months' further research in 1978, in rural northern Taiwan. The support of the National Institute of Mental Health and the Social Science Research Council is gratefully acknowledged, as is the intellectual and institutional assistance of the Institute of Ethnology, Academica Sinica, Taipei.
2. A woman in the first month after childbirth is expected to each mainly *kei-chiu* (Hokkien, chicken wine), a dish of chicken stir-fried in sesame oil and then simmered in wine. This dish does not really have the alcohol simmered out of it, and I imagine that eating large amounts might cause slight inebriation. But it would be hard to get drunk on it and anyway consumption of *kei-chiu* is justified in dietary terms (chicken, wine and sesame oil are all classified as hot and thus restorative), and is thus considered normal.
3. (p. 11) The term *"kui"* (Hokkien, ghost) is suffixed to various words to indicate someone with a particular undesirable behavior. A *la-sap-kui*, or dirt ghost, for example, is a slovenly person, as a *ciu-kui* is a problem drinker.

REFERENCES

Anderson, E. N., and Anderson, Marja L.
   1975 Folk dietetics in two Chinese communities and its implications for the study of Chinese medicine. In Kleinman, A., *et al.* (eds.): Medicine in Chinese Culture. Washington, D.C.: Fogarty International Center.

Johnston, R. F.
    1910 Lion and Dragon in Northern China. New York: E. P. Dutton.
Ou-yang Hsiu (Ouyang Xiu)
    1963 *Zui-weng Ting-ji. In Gudai Hanyu,* Volume 2, Part 1. Peking.
           Zhong-hua Publishers.
T'ang-shih san-pai-shou
    1968 Taipei: *Chung-hua shu-chü.*
Wolff, P. H.
    1972 Ethnic differences in alcoholic sensitivity. Science 175: 449–450.

GARY SEAMAN

4. IN THE PRESENCE OF AUTHORITY: HIERARCHICAL ROLES IN CHINESE SPIRIT MEDIUM CULTS

A review of the literature relating to shamanism and similar altered states of consciousness reveals at least two main approaches to the phenomena. One approach defines the subject by examining the state of mind of shamans, mediums, hysterics, etc. and, by reviewing the life history of such individuals, seeks to determine what aspects of their personality are involved (e.g., Yap 1954; Silverman 1967). The other approach concentrates more on social structures and seeks an explanation of the phenomena through an analysis of the web of social relations surrounding the shamans, witches, spirit mediums, etc. who are under study. The question asked in the former approach is likely to be "Who becomes a shaman?" The question framed by the latter approach is most likely to be some variation on "What kind of society produces shamans, or witchcraft, or spirit possession and where is it most likely to occur?" The latter view is perhaps best represented by Lewis, who holds the opinion that "it is overall instability in the socioeconomic circumstances which provides the necessary, if perhaps not always sufficient condition for the existence of the possession response" (1971:203).

The logic of both approaches tends to produce differing opinions of the "normality" or "abnormality" of the behavior under consideration. Proponents of the first approach, with their focus on the syndromes exhibited by individuals who act in ways far removed from the ordinary rules of behavior, and who may be so alienated from their ordinary social networks as to require hospitalization (e.g., Yap 1960), are almost sure to pronounce the shaman or other individual exhibiting a possession syndrome as abnormal. On the other hand, the social anthropologist, whose stock in trade is whole societies and their patterns of behavior and belief, is loathe to pronounce the verdict of abnormal upon behavior which he sees as the predictable effects of the social structure. This is particularly so when he views the role of shaman or medium as having a social function, as for example in "defusing" potentially explosive social conflict (Lewis 1971; Kilson 1972).

The approach used in this paper conforms to the social anthropologist's structural/functional analysis. In particular, my concern will be the roles, statuses and behavioral sequences observed within shamanistic cults in Taiwan, and the (hypothetical) ways in which these can be related to conflict within the traditional Chinese social hierarchy. The focus for my discussion is the change in role relationships during séances, when the shaman (or spirit medium) undergoes a radical shift in behavior and personality. This shift is accompanied by a corresponding change of attitude and behavior of other cult members within the the context of a continuing relationship. Before beginning the discussion of

A. Kleinman and T.-Y. Lin (eds.), Normal and Abnormal Behavior in Chinese Culture, 61–74.
Copyright © 1980 by D. Reidel Publishing Company.

roles, however, I will first consider the more general aspects of Chinese social structure in which shamanistic cults are embedded.

China, as neatly as most peasant cultures, has a structural divide running between the localized, face-to-face, multiplex, primary socializing and production group of the rural village, and the absolutist, elitist, literate and refined (and often alien) ruling class (Stover 1974). Studies of social mobility, seeking to prove that recruitment into the ruling class was broad-based, have also shown how great the gap and, consequently, how great the reward for crossing it (Chang 1967; Fei 1968). In the sociological literature, China has thus been characterized as lacking vertical solidarity. Likewise, the basic social groupings, residential units or kinship groups, have little sense of mutual solidarity or interest; consequently, exchanges and relationships between these groups are often marked with hostility and distrust (Freedman 1966:44–48; cf. Nakane 1970). If such a view of Chinese society has any validity, it is not surprising that a crucial role has been allotted to the "middleman" or "go-between," who mediates relationships both vertically and horizontally.

As Fei points out, the combination of the functions of administrator and mediator in the same office and person leads to direct conflict of local interests versus central authority (Fei 1968:88–90). The holders of such offices are personally subject to much stress and tension, and this in turn leads to aberrent and self-destructive behavior. For example, this is what E. Grey Dimond has to say about middle-level bureaucrats and cadres in People's Republic of China:

All of the accomplishments of these past twenty years attributed to Mao Tse-tung had to be carried out by the loyal, committed Party members and cadres. It is this group of people, as well as the managers in industry, in the communes, in the military, in the bureaus, which has carried the actual day-to-day responsibility for results. This is the group where tension and stress come to rest . . . . Combining high responsibility with relatively little policy authority generates tension (1975:145).

Dimond goes on to describe a high incidence of hypertension, compulsive behavioral patterns, and cardiovascular disease among this group. The key phrase is "combining high responsibility with relatively little policy authority." Traditionally, the low-level mediators of high-level fiat were members of a group having a despised, almost outcaste, status:

Those who made the actual contact between the yamen and the people, the ruler and the ruled, were the servants of the officials. These official servants (ya-i) occupied one of the lowest positions in the Chinese social scale; they were deprived of most of their civil rights and their sons were not allowed to take the examinations. It is a significant point in the Chinese power structure that these men who were in the position of most easily abused power should have been so low. If society had not suppressed them by despising them and depriving them of a decent social position, they might have become as fearful as wolves (Fei 1968:80).

In traditional China, direct appeal to central authority on the part of competing individuals at the local level was thought to be an invitation to ruin for everyone concerned, since it resulted in falling into the hands of these very yamen servants. And yet, in the mature sections of Chinese peasant society, where access to the means of production (largely land) was severely competitive, there existed a strong tendency to seek advantage by appeal to political resources outside the purely local arena. For any given individual, the question he had to solve was how to attain access to outside sources of authority without attracting the negative opinion attached to yamen servants, "running dogs," and other power brokers. One solution to this problem was that of the Chinese gentry, who exercised influence indirectly through education, personal contacts, and elitist civil rights available only to members of this status group.

Another way of solving the problem of the power broker is found among some of the religious cults of China. These cults have developed a unique way of dealing with the tensions and pressures that are focused on local leadership when they must translate high-level policy statements (or moral principles) into action. The solution which these cults have evolved is to employ a "spirit medium." Such a cult is characterized by predictable episodes of possession among its members. During a possession the role hierarchies among the members of the cult are radically transformed: it is not too much to speak of role reversals. A key feature of a possession is that the behavior of a medium when he is possessed does not reflect on his status or reputation when not possessed.

The strategy which I will use in exploring this aspect of shamanism in China is a simple one. I will accept the ideological position of the cult about what happens during a séance, i.e., that possession is the displacement of one personality by another, and that the displacing personality is a discrete and separate identity, a free soul making temporary use of the spirit medium's body. I will first consider the behavioral, structural and organizational aspects of a séance in a particular cult, to provide a framework within which to view changes in hierarchical role relationships. These changes in role relationships will then be related to the character of possessing spirits and the way in which they reflect Chinese ideas about power and authority.

Authority, as I will use the term in this paper, is an attribute of social power, or the ability of one individual or social entity to influence the behavior of another, ultimately derived from the ability to punish and reward. It is closely linked to the idea of *legitimacy*, that is, the acquiescence, usually approbriative, of those whose behavior is influenced or controlled (cf., the discussion in Adams 1975:30–36). The legitimate locus of authority in Chinese peasant households has been, par excellence, the pater familias. The cultural ideal sees the father as having absolute power over the resources of his family, not only over the land, but the labor and even the lives of his children. The developmental process of the Chinese family is characterized by two opposing features which impart an expansionist dynamic to the Chinese family system. First, the accumulation of a family estate is strongly supported by the authoritarian position of the pater familias and the husband's and wife's joint interest in raising a large family to create a common estate. In the interests of everyone, submission to the authority of the father is required in order to coordinate the family's efforts to enlarge the economic base of the household. But working against this spirit of cooperation and internal cohesion is the rule of equal inheritance among brothers, which demands that as a family group matures, and as each brother in a sibling set becomes differentiated by taking a wife and producing children, his interests become more and more opposed to those of his siblings. As a result, at some point (according to the cultural ideal upon death or retirement of the father) brothers will divide their common estate.

The divisive forces in the developmental process of the domestic household are paralleled by similar pressures in the development of cult groups. As the economic base of the cult grows, as the process of differentiation among cult members advances and as the problems of succession within the hierarchy of cult statuses proliferate, then the cult becomes more and more susceptible to friction and backbiting. Ultimately, charges against those responsible for the cult's economic resources will be made — charges of manipulating the cult in their own economic interest (cf., Baity 1975:129—130). Thus the developmental cycles of both the Chinese family and the religious cult have parallel centrifugal tendencies as they grow and become more complex.

The authority of the Chinese father is based on the principle of descent, and the power he exercises in the deployment of the family's resources, both material and labor, is derived from the maintenance of the ancestral cult. The authority of the executive of a religious cult, however, is not similarly hallowed by descent, or only rarely so. In enforcing his authority, the father has no need to refer to sources of power outside his intrinsic rights as father. The basic support for his authority lies within the family structure, not outside it. But those who manage the activities of cults do so on behalf of spirits who are in the relationship of guests, not ancestors. Cult leaders are thus in the position of the "yamen servants" described by Fei in the quotation above. The problem they have in legitimizing their power over the cult's resources becomes more acute as the cult grows more powerful and attracts more and more members. The cult leadership becomes more and more vulnerable to allegations of abusing their position precisely because they must both administer and mediate. The problem which the cult leadership faces is, then, how to avoid the harsh judgment which their functional roles entail, and keep from attracting a negative status similar to "yamen servants". As indicated above, the solution has been to develop the institution of the spirit medium or shaman as an alternative to an ideology of descent.

It is convenient to analyze the structure of Chinese religious cults in terms of two main functions. The first of these functions is domestic and economic and is best conceived of as the "household economy" of the cult. The second function is dramatic and informational, consisting of the "communication system" between living cult members and the spirits which the "household economy" of the cult supports.

The focus of every Chinese religious cult is an incense pot. The daily burning of incense in the pot is the minimal form of interaction with and symbolic recognition of the existence of the spirits. In an organizational sense, a cult focused on daily, repeated offerings of burning incense requires the same basic activities as that of any familial household, providing shelter, feeding, nurturing and a daily round of communal intercourse. The ancestral cult offers a good example, being an extension of the household economy to share shelter, food, incense, etc., with the souls of the dead members of the family. In cults which are intended to include the spirits of souls not belonging to the descent group, the simplest way in which to organize the extension is to locate these spirits on the family altar as "guests." The locus of representations of these guest spirits is always on the left hand of the ancestral tablets, the place of seniority and honor. The ritual associated with such cults is essentially dumb, in the sense that the interaction between humans and spirits (ancestral or other), requires only the performance of maintenance activities, not the production of encoded linguistic intercourse. Thus the performance of prescribed "customary rites" is a sufficient condition for the perpetuation of the cult organization.

In most cults, however, the communication system between living individuals and the souls of the dead is well developed. The minimal form of such a communication system may be a device such as "moonstones," or even coins, which are cast to determine the opinions, desires or other attitudes of the spirits. In more elaborated forms, the medium is a person whose body is "borrowed" by the spirit which then is able to speak "in the clear" to the living. It is a given of the ideology of spirit medium cults that the spirits of the dead have access to information and social networks in the form of otherworldly social hierarchies, which allow them to influence the fate of the living. Simply put, the spirits of the dead have power over the living. The social hierarchies of the dead are conceived of as essentially the same as that of the living, thus those spirits who have most power are precisely those souls that have the status of warrior, scholar, statesman, judge, bureaucrat, emperor or just a plain, powerful "local bully." They occupy statuses which reach outside the village arena to levels of national, international and even cosmic extent. These supernatural authority figures are mediated by shamans who perform miraculous feats of physical dexterity and self-mutilation. They also compose extemporaneous poetry and prose: messages derived from the communal worldview, full of the power of affective content.

In the cult group which focuses on the altar in Mr. Lim's house (located in central Taiwan), Mr. Lim himself fills all of the roles required for the household economy function (Seaman 1977a). He "invites" images from a local temple to "visit" his home for extended periods of time, where they reside on the altar table next to his ancestral tablets. It is Mr. Lim who sets out fresh brewed tea every morning and evening. He is the one who provides a candle when night draws near, and who buys the bouquet of flowers, the fish and the fowl, the rice and the cakes, that are offered to the gods before he or his family partake of them. Most important, Mr. Lim is the one who never allows the fragrant incense to go out. Every morning and every evening, Mr. Lim arranges several kinds of incense to provide his "guests" with an atmosphere most pleasing to their kind of being, and he thus induces them to remain with him.

Very few cults are merely chance expressions of piety. The incense pot burns with a fire that has a definite source in the pot of another cult, usually referred to as the "incense source." Mr. Lim periodically "cuts incense" at a nearby temple which is the source for thousands of similar cults throughout the island, and whose source in turn is a temple on the Mainland. Pilgrimage routes in Taiwan and the Mainland tend to reproduce the hierarchies of such "incense sources." On feast days, these linkages are renewed by the physical transportation of new "cuttings" of burning incense from the "sources" to the local pots. Thus the maintenance of the incense pot provides a focus for the economic and social structure of the cult. The power of central places is never more explicit than in the pilgrimages to nowadays far out-of-the-way places, which still call back the descendants of long ago immigrants to their origins (cf., Baity 1975: 125). (In this paper I use as my example a cult group which exhibits the minimal organizational form necessary for the functioning of the cult. For those interested in a more lengthy examination of the developmental process of a spirit medium cult and the complex interaction of village politics with temple cult, I refer the reader to Seaman (1978).)

Mr. Lim is the organizational head of his cult. It is his function to "stick his neck out", i.e., serve as the public front for the cult. His reputation and that of his cult are very closely intertwined. Whatever events happen in his house which involve questions of law and morals are his responsibility. He must answer to public opinion and to the legal authorities of this world. His position in the cult vis-à-vis others who frequent his home and thus may be considered members is, by the same token, that of authority. It is Mr. Lim who chooses whether to remain at home and keep his doors open to those who come visiting, or whether to lock up the hall and go elsewhere that night. It is Mr. Lim who decides the amount and splendor of the offerings, the trappings, the kinds of incense, etc. It is he who decides whether the images of the gods will make public pilgrimages often or never. Mr. Lim's cult is also atypical, in that he himself is a skilled craftsman who manufactures the ritual weapons and other paraphernalia used by shamans in their séances. As a result, the number of shamans who frequent Mr. Lim's hall is rather great. The high probability of a shaman's being possessed is, in turn, a great part of the attractiveness of Mr. Lim's cult to other villagers. Mr. Lim's social network, which contains dozens, perhaps hundreds of active shamans, is another inducement for villagers (and outsiders) to contact Mr. Lim when they wish to invite a shaman to spend an evening at their homes in order to "take care of business," i.e., deal with some spiritual problem or handle a matter of serious concern.

Mr. Lim and the shamans attached to his cult are professionals and the majority of their séances are in the form of "house-calls," performed at the invitation of some supplicant in his home. The basic roles in such a séance consist of Mr. Lim, who serves as contact man and general organizer of the event, the shaman (sometimes several) who serves as spirit medium, and the supplicant, who desires the intervention of a god of high status and authority in some personal or familial problem. It should be clear to the reader that both Mr. Lim and the shamans undertake a séance for money. They are hired to perform a service and they get paid for it (although they are paid by *ang-pao* (Hokkien, red envelope) which makes the transaction a little less "commercial"). On the face of it, then, there would seem to be little functional difference between Mr. Lim and the shaman as compared to the "yamen servants". There is a difference, though, and it lies in the idiom of authority which links the god, the shaman, and the supplicant. It is through the "domestication" of outside authority (the gods and their universalist laws of morality) by means of affective idioms of "guestship" and "fatherhood", that the cult exercises its influence without necessarily incurring the negative sentiment attaching to this-worldly power brokers. First, the cult establishes a direct relationship with what is basically a very distant force, that of the heavenly bureaucracy, by use of a concept of "guestship". Gods are induced to take up residence on the cult altar by means of "incense cutting" and the setting up of idolic representations, and especially by incorporating them into the commensality of the household economy. They are provided with subsistence payments of "spirit money" on a regular basis. The reciprocal obligation of the god for this support is to tap the spirit hierarchies to which he has access on behalf of the cult members. In this way, the administrator of a cult has a great deal of power in influencing the gods, since he is the one who normally makes the decisions concerning where the images of the gods and their incense pots will relocate, if they are to move at all.

The power of the administrator of a cult comes, then, from the host relationship that he has with the gods. The position of the shaman in Mr. Lim's cult is somewhat ambivalent as regards to the household economy of the cult. The shaman is often in the position of being a client of Mr. Lim. Everyone recognizes this, and it is perceptible in the attitudes of deference which shamans exhibit towards Mr. Lim. Since it is the function of the shaman, while possessed, to act out the role of ultimate authority, that of the gods themselves, it might be thought that the shaman would be especially vulnerable to charges of pecuniary self-interest, particularly since Mr. Lim will often decline proffered payment, while shamans nearly always accept such payment. In a way this is true, and one often hears such charges made in casual conversation. What normally rescues the shaman from such charges, however, is his particularly intimate relationship with the god which possesses him: he is the ritually adopted child of the deity. As such, the relation between shaman and god is that of father-child, and the relationship is thus legitimized. The shaman is no mere go-between, but stands in the relation of son to divine father. Early in a shaman's career, when he is first possessed by a deity, it is necessary for the god to "buy" the body of the shaman from his parents (Seaman 1977b and n.d.). This amounts to the parents giving up their son to be the child of the god (thus providing one possible etymology of the term *tâng-ki*[1], or shaman). It must be understood that this is an extremely serious step. Not only is the son lost to his parents, but his entire "spirit line" of ancestors loses one of its descendants. In any possession by the god, the shaman functions not merely as a casual representative, but as the legitimate lineal *descendant* of the god. The shaman's behavior is thus not merely that of a member of another village household, but of someone who has the high reputation of his divine father to consider. The shaman is not merely performing the normal role of a go-between, but also operates within the constraints of fatherly authority. As such, unseemly, self-interested behavior on his part would bring upon him the wrath of his divine father.

In the actual behavior of participants in a séance, the role relationships undergo a fascinating evolution. A séance of Mr. Lim's cult begins in a manner which is hard to distinguish from any casual social visit. Most house-calls occur at night, since most supplicants do not have the leisure to deal with their problems during the day. Mr. Lim may or may not bring the various paraphernalia necessary for a séance with him, although he likely has made the arrangements for its presence. Oftentimes, a divining chair is used to provide the rhythmic movement and general atmosphere which may serve to induce possession (Seaman 1977b). Posession when it comes, is not unexpected. Hours of breathing the heavy fumes pouring from the incense pot, of hearing the rhythmic clack-clacking of the divining chair, of emotionally-charged, expectant waiting, have their desired effect. For each shaman, the change of role identity has a different, individual expression. This one breaks off in the middle of cracking a joke, and his smiling face is transformed in an instant into a somber mask. Another shaman will sit quietly in a corner for minutes on end, slowly tapping his foot, regulating his breathing, and sliding slowly, imperceptibly into another world. Shamans as men are fellow villagers, not strangers, and only "guests" in the most informal fashion. But then, when they are taken and seized by the gods, they are entirely strangers, entirely guests.

The relationship between the three primary role players, cult head, supplicant, and shaman, changes abruptly when possession takes place. What until then had all the features of a friendly gathering of intimates, is transformed into the rigid rituals of formal Chinese greeting behavior. Eye contact is no longer sought, and quickly dropped when it accidentally occurs. The spatial relations between a number of loosely interacting sets of two or threes is swiftly formalized by the movement of the shaman to a position in which he occupies the "inferior host" position vis-à-vis the god (who is imagined as sitting at the head of the table facing out the door). Henceforth, dialogue takes the form of shaman-cum-deity talking and all others speaking only when spoken to. As soon as the shaman begins to speak, Mr. Lim loses control of his domestic economy. The decisions about when, where, and how to perform the ministrations to the gods are taken out of his hands and delegated freely by the shaman/god, who may peremptorily order him to un-do or re-do some aspect of caring for the altar, the amount or timing of offerings, etc. Others present may be instructed to take certain activities out of his hands. The whole range of Mr. Lim's rights over the cult and his household are partly or wholly abridged by the shaman/god, and the usual small deferences shown by the unpossessed shaman as a guest in his house are completely forgotten.

As an example of the kinds of problems for which the villagers seek out the intervention of the gods, I want to present a short description of a séance which occurred in the winter of 1972. The case involved a native of the village who had moved away about twenty years before to take up a job with the railroad in a small town. He had married and had two sons. Both of them were now grown, and the eldest had been married for two years, but no children had been born as the wife could not get pregnant. In searching for the reasons for her barrenness, which included examinations by doctors trained in Western medicine, the railroad man returned to his natal household in the village. There he made the arrangements for a séance to determine if any of his ancestral spirits were angry at him and thus had caused his daughter-in-law to be barren. The railroad man recruited a cousin who was a shaman to help in arranging the séance. This cousin in turn went to see Mr. Lim and asked his help in mobilizing several other shamans to attend. On the appointed evening, Mr. Lim and several others, about a dozen men in all, appeared at the main hall of the railroad man's natal household. A divining chair supplied by Mr. Lim was possessed and it developed that the spirit of an uncle was indeed responsible for the troubles that the railroad man was experiencing. The uncle had died before having any children of his own, and his portion of the estate, along with his wife, had been inherited by the railroad man's father. The dead uncle was now demanding that one of the railroad man's sons be adopted out to him as his descendant. Only by reestablishing the uncle's line of descent and restoring the proper ancestral sacrificies to him, could the daughter-in-law's barrenness be cured.

On thing in particular was angering the uncle's ghost: this was the fact that his grave had never been dug up and his bones given a "new house," where they would be protected from further decay and dissolution. The uncle's spirit demanded not only that the railroad man adopt out a son to him, but that he also provide the uncle's bones with a new grave, so that the son could perform the proper rites for the uncle, especially at *Ch'ing Ming*[2]. The railroad man agreed to do this, taking on a considerable financial burden in order to come to terms with the spirit of his dead uncle, who felt as though he had been disinherited and turned into a hungry ghost. The specific events connected with this case can be seen in my film *Blood, Bones and Spirits* (Seaman 1974a). What is important to note is the fact that reproductive failures are related to the actions of ancestral spirits. When the specific ancestors who are intervening in human affairs are identified, and their complaints specified, the solution is achieved through making an agreement so that the proper forms of the relationship are restored. In this case it required the actual removal of a person from one line of descent and his transfer to another, plus a considerable expenditure on a new grave, in order to restore the proper features of an ancestral cult to the dead uncle. The gods, through possessing their shamans and other mediums, acted as the means of communicating with the dead uncle's spirit. The gods also acted in the role of guarantors of the agreements which were reached, and they even insisted that the railroad man correct the inscription on the gravestone made for the uncle's grave. The inscription had originally been phrased so that it was not clear that the railroad man's son was in fact adopted out to the uncle. The gods, by insisting upon the uncle's rights, gave both sides confidence that the terms of the agreement would be observed: on the one hand that the uncle would cease to interfere with the fertility of the railroad man's daughter-in-law, and on the other hand that the railroad man's son would in fact observe the ritual duties becoming a son of the dead uncle.

For the duration of the medium's possession, the supplicant can attain to direct communication with the source of centralized authority. He does not have to deal with intermediaries, go-betweens, yamen servants or running dogs. He can question the god about every conceivable source of and solution to his problems, discuss and even argue with the god about them. When the séance comes to an end, the shaman's status reverts to that of an essentially disinterested observer. Mr. Lim again takes control of the normal administration of cult affairs, and it is left up to the supplicant whether or not to let his behavior conform to that enjoined upon him by the authority of the god. The institution of spirit medium thus serves to relieve both the shaman (in his unpossessed state) and Mr. Lim from serving at once as mediator and as administrator. Since the god, when he is present, accepts the responsibility for serving in both these roles, much of the burden is removed from the shaman and Mr. Lim. The god has "high responsibility" since he lays out correct behavior, but he also has a great deal of "policy authority", since he occupies a very high status position.

Of course, the institution of shaman as means of relieving the cult leadership from being personally responsible for administering policy decisions only works when the cult ideology of spirit possession is accepted. That is, that the normal personality of the shaman is completely displaced by a "guest spirit", the spirit of a god. One aspect of this displacement has already been discussed, that of spirit adoption. It is extremely interesting that in other cultures where spirit possession is a prominent feature of the cultural landscape, the shaman is the medium for a spirit that "Often represents what the possessed is not – men are possessed by women, women by men" (Crapanzano 1977:19). In China, the possessed shaman represents what most peasants are not: the rich, the learned, the powerful, and, one might add, the fortunate.

In possessing a shaman, the gods are related to their peasant hosts by means of familiar idioms of expression: as a father to the shaman and as a guest to the cult head. The idiom of a father-son relationship between the shaman and his possessing deity is a pivotal one, since it accounts for the transformation of the shaman's personality. It obviously strains credulity for a peasant farmer to act like a military mandarin, and only the strongest ideological underpinnings will make such a change in role acceptable. It is the borrowing of the idiom of descent, which grants the father complete control over his son, that allows the shaman to act in ways appropriate to the powerful personages of the court and bureaucracy. Likewise, for the cult head, the employment of an idiom of host/ guest relationship with the gods allows a readily understandable way of express-ing a connection with powerful figures. The cult head builds a relationship as a client of the god by providing the services which are necessary to existence: food, shelter, money, incense, etc. In making these things readily and regularly available to the gods, the cult head extends the idiom of ancestor cult, with which all villagers are familiar, to encompass figures far more powerful than the ancestors. Thus the shaman and cult head are both utilizing structural features of household and kinship organization to express their relationships with powerful gods in terms that are familiar to all villagers. It is the familiarity of this idiom that supports the credibility of spirit possession.

The "credibility factor" of the shaman's possession brings us to one final con-sideration. Is the shaman's behavior classifiable as "socially deviant" or "abnormal"? At the beginning of this paper I referred to the social structural approach as avoiding the labeling of the shaman as "abnormal". For China, at least, possession must be an abnormal state if the shaman is not to be suspected of self-interested manipulation. Indeed, the abnormality of the possession state is frequently commented upon by the cult participants, and the episodes of self-mortification which accompany possession are taken as direct proof that a com-plete transformation of personality has, in fact, taken place. In reading Yap's (1960) descriptions of possessed patients in Hong Kong, which he characterizes as abnormal, it seems to me that the only feature which distinguishes his patients from the behavior of shamans of my acquaintance, is the presence of an on-going, structured relationship with other cult members during possession. The expressed identification with rich and powerful figures of legend and history is the same in both cases. But such behavior, hysterical, abnormal and inappropriate though it may be at many times and places and for certain individuals, is accommodated within the context of a shamanistic séance. It is accommodated because the shaman has a function to fulfill as a mediator and guarantor in necessary adjustments of relationships with the spirits of other, parallel worlds. The "role reversals" which occur during séances invite behavior on the part of shamans which is only appropriate to very high status individuals and which would be condemned in them if they were not in an abnormal state. However the *content* of the role which the shaman plays when possessed is *not* deviant, but rather only appropriate to an authority figure. Self-evidently, the *psychic state* of the shaman is abnormal, but his *social role* is not.

The conclusion of this paper is a simple one. It seems to me that the shamanistic cult functions in a way that allows the average villager to approach figures of distant, autocratic authority in an idiom which makes sense in terms of their own social reality. The Chinese peasant household is an entity which does not easily admit outsiders to participate in its affairs, and which jealously guards its estate. The conceptualization of gods in the form of honored guests and mediums in the form of adopted sons who have left their ancestral line of descent is an effective way for the ordinary villager, whose personal network can never extend very far up the social hierarchy, to relate himself to forces outside his direct control.

Morton Fried has a theory of the tribe which makes it, in essence, a creation of the imperialistic state. Tribes, are, in his view, "the product of processes stimulated by the appearance of relatively highly organized societies amidst other societies which are organized much more simply" (Fried 1967:170). I would suggest that the institution of shamanism has a similar relationship to the state. Just as tribes are a preliminary response to the existence of stratified societies, and are a way in which fringe groups on the *outside* of the state adapt themselves to their altered environment, so shamanism (in China, at least) is a similar adaptation *within* the state. It is, however, an adaptation which recognizes the legitimacy of the claims of the political center to power and authority, in contradistinction to the institutions of tribal societies, which are often evolved in order to avoid making that concession. The functioning of the shamanistic cult in China allows personal, direct access to authority, and thus to the really virtuous ruler, the god who has the combined powers of administrative responsibility and policy making authority. Since the god is not to be suspected of the materialistic self-interest of this worldly servants of central authority, the positive aspects of the ideology of the virtuous official can be realized. Everyday encounters with the venality of officials and their running dogs are thus made more endurable, when such despicable minions can be circumvented through attendance at a shamanistic séance. And, too, the cult leadership is relieved of some of the tension generated by the combining of high responsibility for results and the relative lack of policy authority.

The close link between the cult of the ancestors, which serves as the base of parental authority, and the cult of powerful gods and their shamanistic mediums, is clearly to be seen in the way that both cults are expressed in idioms of kinship and householding. The integration into these cults of concepts of the continued existence and identity of the individual soul over numerous rein-carnations is also a very important aspect of the utility of shamanistic séances in dealing with all sorts of psychic and social problems. Since the living are linked with the dead by ties of kinship and descent, by the interwoven strands of fate over the generations, indeed over millenia, the resolution of many of the afflic-tions of the living are to be sought in the restitution of balance in relationships with the souls of the dead. It is in this context that the shaman can serve as the medium for figures of prestige and power. The gods, in turn, can serve as guarantors of the accords which they also negotiate. As in the example given above, the supplicant can determine the details of some grudge or enmity of the ancestors, then negotiate a settlement of the conflict directly with the aggrieved party. These agreements across different planes of existence are reached by employing shamans who, in their possessed state, act out the roles of high-status personages concerned with high ideals and moral standards. The behavior of these shamans does not conform to the limits of their roles as kinsmen or neighbors when they are not possessed. As a result, a shaman, when he is possessed by a god, can give direct and peremptory commands in a fashion completely beyond his ability to exercise authority while in a normal, unpossessed state. At the same time, however, the shaman is protected from negative sentiments by the idiom of kinship in which his relationship with the gods is expressed.

NOTES

1. *Tâng-ki* (Hokkien, divining youth) is the common term for shaman in Taiwan – the Editors.
2. *Ch'ing-Ming* (Mandarin, clear and bright) is the annual festival of the tombs – the Editors.

REFERENCES

Adams, R. N.
  1975 Energy and Structure. Austin: University of Texas Press.
Baity, P. C.
  1975 Religion in a Chinese Town. Taipei: Orient Culture Services.
Chang, Chung-li
  1967 The Chinese Gentry. Seattle: University of Washington Press.
Crapanzano, V. (ed.)
  1977 Case Studies in Spirit Possession. New York: Wiley.
Dimond, E. Grey
  1975 More Than Herbs and Acupuncture. New York: Norton.
Fei, Hsiao-tung
  1968 China's Gentry. Chicago: University of Chicago Press.
Freedman, M.
  1958 Lineage Organization in Southeastern China. London: Athlone.
  1966 Chinese Lineage and Society. London: Athlone.
Fried, Morton
  1967 The Evolution of Political Society. New York: Random House.
Kilson, M.
  1972 Ambivalence and power: Mediums in Ga traditional religion. Journal of Religion in Africa 4:171–177.
Lewis, I. M.
  1971 Ecstatic Religion. London: Pelican.
Seaman, Gary
  1974 Blood, Bones and Spirits (Super 8 film). Cedar Park, Texas: Far Eastern Audio Visuals.
  1977a The Divine Palanquin (16mm film). Cedar Park, Texas: Far Eastern Audio Visuals.
  1977b A Child of the Gods (16mm film). Cedar Park, Texas: Far Eastern Audio Visuals.
  1978 Temple Organization in a Chinese Village. Taipei: Orient Culture Services.
  n.d.   Spirit Money: An Imaginary Currency of China (ms.).
Silverman, J.
  1967 Shamans and acute schizophrenia. Amer. Anthropologist 69:21–31.
Stover, L. E.
  1974 The Cultural Ecology of Chinese Civilization. New York: Pica Press.

Yap, P. M.
  1954 The mental illness of Hung Hsiu-ch'uan, leader of the Taiping rebellion. Journal of
        Asian Studies 13:287–304.
  1960 The possession syndrome: a comparison of Hong Kong and French findings.
        British Journal of Psychiatry 106:114–137.

MARTHA LI CHIU

5. INSANITY IN IMPERIAL CHINA:
A LEGAL CASE STUDY

I. INTRODUCTION

Written records spanning over two thousand years of China's past attest to
eruptions of a form of insane behavior which threatened both society and the
individual. As described in the *Huang-ti nei-ching*, a classical source for Chinese
medical theory,[1] initially the person became emotionally labile, "despondent,
happily forgetful, bitterly angry, easily frightened." As the illness developed,
sleeplessness, loss of appetite, delusions of grandeur, and incessant scolding
appeared (*Ling-shu* 1910 4:3). When the illness was extreme, euphoric hyperactivity was the overriding feature.

> ... then he will discard his clothes and run about, mount heights and sing, or get to the
> point of not eating for several days. He will leap walls and ascend rooftops. In short, all the
> places he mounts are beyond his ordinary abilities ... he will talk and curse wildly, not
> sparing relatives or strangers. Not wishing to eat, he will run about wildly. (*Su-wen* 1910
> 3:36)

Despite wide variation in theories of etiology, the clinical picture of what
came to be labeled *k'uang* 狂 continued basically unchanged in the long tradition of subsequent medical texts.* The only notable addition is found in the
Chou-hou pei-chi fang (3:8), which dates in part to the fourth century. It
portrayed the most extreme variant of all, with unkempt hair, loud yelling, and
murderous and self-destructive tendencies.

The medical viewpoint offers the most detailed descriptions of *k'uang*
symptomatology. However, it cannot begin to do justice to the great diversity
characterizing the response of the Chinese throughout their past to this particular kind of human crisis. A thorough treatment of this subject awaits a close
investigation of such varied sources as the philosophic classics, poetry, folklore,
and novels, but in this paper I propose to explore *k'uang* through the eyes of
official representatives of the law. I have chosen to look only briefly at the pre-
Ch'ing documents and to concentrate primarily on the Ch'ing Code, its commentaries, and the Ch'ing legal casebook, the *Hsing-an hui-lan* (HAHL).[2] The
relationship between the law and the insane not only is a significant example of
an interaction between normal and abnormal members of any society, but in
the case of China and many other cultures it is also one of the few which can be
examined out in the open.

While professional interest enabled officials to talk freely about their dealings
with the insane, it also influenced the nature of the information they provided.
First of all, like the physicians, they had an obligation to actively suppress

75

A. Kleinman and T.-Y. Lin (eds.), Normal and Abnormal Behavior in Chinese Culture, 75–94.
Copyright © 1980 by D. Reidel Publishing Company.

outbursts of insanity. The former resorted to an assortment of therapies to heal the afflicted; the latter tried to restore general order through coercive punishments and confinement. In both cases, the preoccupation with controlling deviancy left little room for admiring fascination possible in other roles.[3]

A second consequence of their vocation was that, even more so than many medical text authors, the officials who wrote the legal codes and casebooks were self-consciously Confucian elite. Hence, as the late Ch'ing legal scholar Hsüeh Yün-sheng[4] (1820–1901) frankly admitted, they deliberately omitted references to the spirit possession explanation of insanity (Hsüeh 1970:861).

Another constraint of the legal outlook is that it tended to filter out individual dimensions of the experience of insanity in China and to focus on its social and legal aspects. This was especially true by the time reports on cases reached up through the bureaucracy to the Board of Punishments. Nevertheless, the little detail which the legal texts did provide accords in general with the medical description of k'uang. This leads me to believe that despite a shift in legal terminology from the classical term k'uang or tien-k'uang 癲狂 to feng ping 瘋病 by the Ch'ing, the legal and medical spokesmen across the centuries were discussing more or less the same phenomenon of insanity.

The translation of Chinese labels into English inevitably raises the issue of cross-cultural implications. I use vaguer words like "insanity" and "madness" in order to avoid the more culturally specific refinements of contemporary psychiatric concepts. At the same time I believe that there is a range of outward-acting, occasionally violent conduct which violates the norms of all cultures. How the Chinese articulated and managed this slice of universally shared reality is my present focus. Their attitudes toward quieter, less obvious forms of abnormal behavior is the subject of future investigation.

A central issue that insane criminals presented to officials in imperial China was how much leniency their special condition deserved. According to Karl Bünger, the stance through the dynasties was total exemption from punishment due to unchanging compassion. Other scholars have disputed this generalization. In this chapter I will argue that the response of Chinese lawmakers to the insane was complex, ambivalent, and variable.

II. PRE-CH'ING LEGAL ATTITUDES

A. The Debate

The controversy began in 1948 with M. H. Van der Valk's sharply critical book review of Bünger's first effort in legal history, *Quellen zur Rechtsgeschichte der T'ang-Zeit*. Bünger's 1950 article on 'The Punishment of Lunatics and Negligents According to Classical Chinese Law' essentially set out to refute two specific points that Van der Valk raised. Here I am mainly concerned with the first.

Was it a general principle in Chinese law to assign responsibility to every offender, even if afterwards his penalty was reduced? Van der Valk's affirmative answer grew out of the belief that in the Chinese legal world view crimes upset the harmony of the cosmos. It could only be restored by seeking redress from the one at fault. Bünger disagreed, using leniency toward insane offenders as prime evidence. Thus, he concluded, "We may safely say that the exemption of lunatics from punishment is a fundamental notion of ancient China and a principle of the Chinese law from the Chou dynasty until nowadays" (Bünger 1950:8–9). This assertion glossed over subtleties of which even Bünger himself at times seemed aware and invited A. F. P. Hulsewé's continued attack in *Remnants of Han Law* (1955).

Instead of supporting one or another large generalization, there is a basic need to distinguish between legal attitudes toward individuals suffering from *k'uang* who committed serious crimes like murder and those guilty of lesser offenses. Let us turn now to evidence supporting this view, drawn from Chinese sources up through the Ming.

B. *Inconclusive Evidence (Up Through the Former Han)*

Bünger extended his claim for the exemption of lunatics from punishments back to the Chou because of the *Chou li* passage concerning the Three Amnesties (*san she* 三赦) (*Chou li* 1929 36:2). Besides the very young or old, the third category deserving special consideration before the law was what Edouard Biot translated as "idiots and imbeciles" (*ch'ung yü* 惷愚) (Biot 1939 2:356). Influenced by the T'ang Code's interpretation, Bünger took this *Chou li* reference to the mentally deficient as applicable to the emotionally ill, without stopping to consider the differences between the two kinds of handicaps. In addition, although he admitted that the exact meaning of *she* was ambiguous, he was prepared to argue, "But if it does not mean complete exemption from criminal prosecution, it certainly means a lessened criminal liability" (Bünger 1950:6). Given the meagerness of the data, others are not so willing to make such assumptions about the Chou legal stance toward the insane.

Hulsewé interpreted two Former Han sources as proof that the classical attitude toward insanity was far from compassionate. In my opinion, they too remain inconclusive on the issue of whether or not all lunatics, both serious and light offenders, were exempted from penalties. They do, however, pertain specifically to *k'uang*. Consequently, from this point onward, at least we can be sure we are dealing with attitudes toward a form of insane behavior.

Hulsewé directs our attention, therefore, first to the *Han Shu* record (1962: 1475) of an incident which occurred in 7 or 8 B.C. A former conscript suffering from "*k'uang* transformation" (*k'uang yi* 狂易) was caught within palace walls. Although he claimed that "the Heavenly Emperor" made him dwell there, he was sent to prison, where he died. Hulsewé contended that the reference to this case of "wildly insane and transformed" dying in prison actually implied that he was executed (Hulsewé 1955:301). I prefer to leave this matter open to debate.

The next piece of evidence concerning legal reactions to *k'uang* seems more substantial. Based on the *T'ai-p'ing yü-lan*'s version (1960 646:6b) of the Han text *Decisions of the Commandant of Justice*, we learn of a commoner named Chang T'ai, who during an attack of *k'uang* illness killed his mother and younger brother. When the offense came before the Commandant of Justice, no heed was given to the occurrence of an imperial amnesty. Instead the legal official insisted that the penalty of decapitation and having one's head displayed be carried out as usual. Hulsewé accepted this as strong proof that in early Han there was no special treatment accorded to any insane criminal (Hulsewé 1955:301). However, I wish to stress that this is an instance of one of the gravest transgressions possible in imperial China, namely the murder of a parent. As a result, while it reveals that leniency toward *k'uang* seemingly did not extend to the commission of serious crimes in the early Han, I feel the record remains silent concerning lesser offenses.

C. Firmer Ground (Late Han Onward)

Firmer ground on which to take a stand in the debate concerning the legal treatment of insanity in imperial China is first found in the biography of Ch'en Chung 陳忠 in the *Hou-Han shu* (1965:1556). Among the legal reforms which this high official recommended to the emperor around 100 A.D. was the following: "When a wildly insane and transformed person kills people he should be enabled to be sentenced to the decreased extreme penalty" (Hulsewé 1955:301). His proposal was approved and thus became the first law explicitly directed toward cases of *k'uang*, notably those guilty of the serious crime of murder. In line with Hulsewé and Van der Valk's orientation, this reference indicates that *k'uang* killers were held responsible enough for their actions to merit a penalty being set; but out of compassion for those who acted when they were not really themselves, the sentence was reduced.

Apparently not everyone agreed with the idea of lenient punishment for *k'uang* murderers. In commenting on this passage, Fan Yeh (398–445), the compiler of the *Hou-Han shu*, criticized it as "a great mistake". Hsüeh Yün-sheng suggested that perhaps opposition of this strong sort was the reason why no other laws specifically dealing with the subject appeared until the early Ch'ing (Hsüeh 1970:863).

Although the policy concerning penalties for homicide due to insanity was to remain unsettled for dynasties to come, in the T'ang a set of general legal provisions for the special consideration of *tien k'uang* became established. In the T'ang statutes (Inoue 1976:227) *tien k'uang* was explicitly listed along with leprosy, total blindness, and two broken limbs, as a form of the most serious category of invalids, the "incapacitated" (*tu chi* 篤疾). Scattered in the T'ang laws are many references to the specific privileges extended this group. For example, *tu chi* individuals were exempted from taxes (Inoue 1976:226). In addition, they could not be forced to give testimony in a trial (*T'ang lü shu-yi* (TLSY) 1965 4:75).

In the Terms and General Principles section of the T'ang Code (TLSY 1965 2:3–4) are found the most complete guidelines pertaining to the actual penalties meted for crimes committed by the *tien k'uang* and others. It reads:

Among those who are eighty years old and above, ten years old and below, or incapacitated, if they commit rebellion, sedition, or murder, and deserve the death penalty, they may send up a petition. As for those who have robbed or wounded people, their penalty can be commuted by monetary redemption. All other cases are not liable for punishment.

Notice that the imperial Chinese legal attitude of leniency was a finely graded one. Earlier attempts to stress either absolute mercy or severity toward the *tien k'uang* fall short of describing the complicated truth.

My own interpretation of this passage is that first of all, for those guilty of the most serious offenses, such as rebellion or murder, the penalty was left vague and up to imperial discretion. Whether this ambiguity arose from a lack of consensus surrounding this issue, as Hsüeh Yün-sheng suggested, is not certain but indeed plausible. Secondly, the interlineary commentary makes clear that monetary redemption for thefts and wounding by *tu chi* was definitely seen as an extension of leniency without full exemption of responsibility. "Since such offenses encroach on and injure others, of course we cannot permit a total exemption (from penalties)." This point seems to accord with Hulsewé and Van der Valk's positions. However, Bünger's view is also substantiated in part by the third line which excused from punishment all other lighter crimes committed by the *tu chi*.

No doubt subtle shifts in the legal response to insanity took place in the thousand years intervening between the T'ang Code (653 A.D.) and the Ch'ing. Because an in-depth investigation of this topic is not my concern here, a glance at a late edition of the Ming Code must suffice. An impression of stability is conveyed by the fact that even on the eve of the Manchu invasion the aforementioned T'ang principles for setting penalties for *tu chi* were still generally intact (*Ming lü chi-chieh fu li* (MLCCFL) 1969:286–287).

As a sign of change, included among the 382 new Ming substatutes was one promulgated in 1595 designed to prevent taking advantage of the special provisions for *tu chi* (MLCCFL 1969:291–293). In order to avoid the death penalty and gain their release, criminals apparently were intentionally blinding themselves, breaking their limbs, as well as pretending to be *tien k'uang*. As a result, the emperor decreed, "Henceforth, when serious criminals are labeled *tu chi*, (officials) must thoroughly investigate and verify its actuality. Only then can one memorialize for their release." This mood of heightened vigilance regarding the *tien-k'uang* and others in the *tu chi* category brings us into the Ch'ing.

III. CH'ING LEGAL ATTITUDES

Addressing the topic of Ch'ing legal attitudes on homicide due to insanity. Hsüeh Yün-sheng wrote, "In the past sentencing was very lenient but confinement was especially severe. Recently, sentencing has become severe but confinement very lenient" (Hsüeh 1970:861).[5] The specific meaning of this analysis will become clearer as we go along. The main point which it conveys is that the Ch'ing legal answers to the problem of insanity not only shifted over the years but also could be at one time both lenient in one respect and severe in another! As we shall see, the type of crime committed by the insane was not the only factor influencing how much leniency they received from the imperial Chinese judicial system. Concern for the danger they posed to others, as well as wider legal and socio-political trends, helped to shape their fates.

A. The First Phase: "In the past sentencing was very lenient . . . "

When the Manchu rulers first took over China, the pace of legal change was for the most part cautiously slow. The 1646 edition of the Ch'ing Code was largely a copy of the Ming Code and sub-statutes, with some subtle differences in the commentary (Bodde and Morris 1965:65,70). Yet, one should not conclude that even in this early period there were no modifications in specific areas of law. Indeed, it is precisely in this opening phase of the Ch'ing that a major step was taken in legislation relating to *feng ping*.

In 1669, seven years after the K'ang-hsi emperor ascended the throne, a new "currently operative sub-statute" was approved which stated, "In cases of homicide due to insanity seek a monetary redemption of 12.42 ounces of silver from the offender to give to the victim's relatives for funeral expenses" (Philastre 1967 2:226; *Ta Ch'ing lü-li* (TCLL) 1870 26:45). It was raised to the level of a supplementary statute in 1727 (Wu 1886 26:72). The significance of this development is that the procedure for sentencing an insane murderer was now made explicit instead of left up to imperial discretion. None of the sources consulted throw light on the particular causes precipitating this action. The general explanation given again and again was an awareness of a previous lack of clear patterns in the law to deal with homicide due to insanity (Hsüeh 1970:860; HAHL 1968:2114).

One possible reason so little interest was placed in the details lying behind the emergence of the new sub-statute could be that to the Ch'ing legal mind it was not a radical innovation. On the one hand, the new ruling amounted to extending to the specific category of homicide due to insanity the privilege of monetary redemption permitted since the T'ang to the broader group of *tu chi* guilty of the less serious crimes of theft and wounding. On the other hand, it involved recognizing a similarity between serious crimes committed unintentionally during an attack of insanity and "by accident". As a result, it was possible to apply the specific amount of 12.42 ounces of silver for monetary redemption already worked out in the Ming Code for the latter to the former case. This new sub-statute and the multiplying numbers which followed on homicide due to insanity, were all placed in the "homicide by accident" category of the Ch'ing Code.

B. "... but confinement was especially severe"

In *Law in Imperial China*, Derk Bodde stated, "What is prized above all in this kind of society is social and political stability" (Bodde and Morris 1967:184). In my opinion, this concern for preserving and regularizing order was probably the most important motivation for the proliferation of legislation concerning insanity during the first half of the Ch'ing. This impulse is clearly reflected in the move toward stricter confinement to accompany the light sentence of monetary redemption.

In the absence of public institutions for the care of the insane[6] this task had probably all along been mainly shouldered by the Chinese family. Still, there was nothing to force them to do so beyond their own consciences and informal local pressure. As long as their duties remained vague and unlegislated, the possibility of families which either were unable or unwilling to restrain those with insanity remained great. A particularly shocking case involving the murder of four persons in one family heightened the fear of the homicidal potential in all with this illness and helped convince the Ch'ing legislators that this situation of unregulated responsibility was intolerable (Hsüeh 1970:859).

To guard against future atrocities of this sort, in 1689 (Wu 1886 26:73) a sub-statute was enacted, spelling out clearly the obligations of relatives, community, and officials. Relatives were given the initial duty to report the existence of an insane family member and keep him in strict confinement. If the family failed to report to the authorities or the insane had no family, then neighbors, clan heads, and local leaders were explicitly instructed to take charge. The district magistrate was expected to exert verbal pressure by ordering the family and the like to keep the insane under strict surveillance. To top it all off, any one who neglected to do his part, resulting in the insane killing himself or others, was subject to specified penalties (*Ta Ch'ing lü-li an-yü* 1847 57:22; TCLL 1870:45a-b).

This sub-statute was never a popular one. Its history of repeated revisions already underway in 1723 signifies that a wide gap existed between the new law and deeply embedded social and legal attitudes. First of all, to insist that families report insane members to the local officials defied the pervasive wariness of entanglements with the law. Secondly, according to Hsüeh Yün-sheng, it forced families to make public a fact which they would rather keep secret. He added that it would be even harder to obey this ruling if it required younger people to violate sentiments of filial piety in order to report insane elders (Hsüeh, 1970: 859); As for legal objections, these included the fact that this sub-statute contradicted the right to concealment of the crimes of relatives recognized by the law as far back as the Han (Ch'ü 1961:70).

Hsüeh Yün-sheng at one point voiced another concern. If the unpredictable occurrence of other categories of murder did not implicate relatives, neighbors, and officials, why then should homicide due to insanity? (Hsüeh 1970:859). He answered this question more fully elsewhere and in a way which corroborates the view that in Chinese law responsibility had to be assigned for every serious crime. As Hsüeh explained, since in the first phase monetary redemption for cases of homicide due to insanity seemed too light, others were called on to bear part of the blame. However, during the second phase when there was a move toward harsh penalties for the insane themselves, even this justification for punishing relatives and others disappeared (Hsüeh 1970:863).

Another incident involving the murder of four people in one family by an insane member led to the significant decision in 1753 that henceforth all insane persons guilty of homicide would be first put in prison instead of kept confined at home. Only in the event of a recovery from the illness, after waiting one more year to make sure it didn't recur, were the officials permitted to instruct the relatives to bring the former deviant home under surveillance. This sub-statute was entered into the Code in 1756 (Wu 1886 26:77a-b).

Still a lot of dissatisfactions and questions concerning the handling of the insane remained unsettled. The package of legislation which was taking shape in 1762 and finally entered into the law books by 1768 represented a major effort to put these issues to rest. In the process the 1669 ruling requiring merely a monetary compensation was weakened, parts of the 1689 law were eliminated, and the sub-statute of 1753 was set aside as no longer operative. These changes will become clearer in the following analysis of the specific provisions included in this new group of laws (Wu 1886 26:74a–75b; TCLL 1870 26:46–47; Philastre 1967 2:226–227).

Who was responsible for actually confining the insane person so as to keep him out of trouble? As in the controversial 1689 law, the family was again given priority but only on the conditions that they had enough room to lock up the insane family member securely and also that he had not killed anyone. Whereas previously in the absence of relatives, the neighbors were forced to undertake this task, they were spared in this new ruling. Instead it was the magistrate who now shouldered a much heavier burden for imprisoning the insane in the district jail if they were murderous, had no family, or their relatives lacked the means to keep them at home. In addition, if an insane person created a disturbance while he was in prison, from the gaoler on up to higher officials in charge, all would be penalized.

This collection of articles elaborated further on how the district magistrate was to proceed after receiving a report on an insane individual from the family or neighbors. In order to insure that the family strictly confined this potential menace to society, the official was now expected to go beyond verbal orders to the much more active role of personally issuing the chains and fetters with which to restrain him. In the event of cases of homicide due to insanity and feigned insanity arising, guidelines for how to investigate and try them were provided.

The 1753 ruling had made the first effort to address the problem of what to do if the insane returned to normalcy. Now, over a decade later the Ch'ing lawmakers arrived at new, much more detailed answers, which marked the official start of a strict isolation policy. First of all, if the insane were not guilty of homicide and were enchained at home, only after the district magistrate had conducted a careful investigation verifying their cure, could they be freed. The arm of the law plainly was meant to extend quite deeply into the private life of the insane person, for there was an explicit warning that if the family released him on their own initiative, they would be punished. Secondly, if a non-murderous individual who was insane was in prison and recovered, after several more years elapsed an inquiry was to be conducted and only then could he be released under surveillance.

The most noteworthy decision of all stated, "In case of an insane person guilty of homicide, besides seeking a monetary redemption, he is to be imprisoned for life. Even if cured, he is never to be freed." Note that the old "by accident" pattern of monetary redemption, though minimized, was still mentioned, at the same time as the idea of lifelong imprisonment was first advanced. In this provision, therefore, we find the culmination of the first phase which Hsüeh Yün-sheng observed. "The sentencing was very lenient but confinement was especially severe." Already the unsettling tension between pity for and fear of the insane was fueling dissatisfaction with this particular compromise and moving the lawmakers into the second phase.

That attitudes were even then shifting toward greater severity is reflected in an 1806 Board of Punishments memorandum explaining the reasoning behind the decision to imprison for life cases of homicide due to insanity. It was apparently made with a clear awareness that it amounted to great suffering for those who acted in a temporary fit of insanity and later recovered. Yet, feelings of compassion were overriden by the stronger fear that the illness would recur even after an apparent cure and result in further disorders and deaths. The refrain "exclude future calamities and avoid additional murders" (HAHL 1968:2115, 2117) was to become a familiar one in the years shead.

C. Second Phase: "Recently, sentencing has become severe . . . "

Efforts were soon underway to circumscribe the leniency in sentencing introduced by the old "by accident" analogy for homicides due to insanity. The general strategy was to apply distinctions warranting severe penalties in legislation for ordinary individuals step by step to those for insane.

(1) Multiple Homicide

"The killing of three or more persons in one family", listed as one of the Ten Abominations in the Ch'ing Code, had long been considered a circumstance meriting especially heavy punishment in laws for normal people (Bodde and Morris 1967:93). Nevertheless, in the first half of the eighteenth century, cases of multiple homicide owing to insanity were routinely permitted monetary redemption of the deserved death penalty according to the "by accident" analogy (Hsüeh 1970:862). Apparently, the prevailing attitude in the early

Ch'ing was that no matter how many murders were committed during an attack of insanity, since all were unintentional, there was no reason to increase the penalty.

As time passed, this argument was no longer persuasive. In 1766, while the 1762 package of legislation was barely in the books, a Szechwanese judicial commissioner requested that cases of multiple homicide due to insanity be judged in accordance with the ordinary sub-statutes covering multiple killings (Hsüeh 1970:862–3). The Board reversed its decision at that point, but by 1776 the tendency toward increasing strictness and the desire to refine the laws for insanity according to "normal" distinctions won out.

In that year, in reply to the memorial of a Censorate official a ruling was handed down, stating, "Those who due to insanity successively murder two or more ordinary people are to be sentenced to strangulation after the assizes." (Wu 1886 26:77; Philastre 1967 2:227) In the light of the complexity of legislation in the Ch'ing Code relating to "multiple homicide" by "the sane" (see Philastre 1967 2:195–199), this one-line ruling left vague many critical issues.

The *Hsing-an hui-lan* casebook testifies to the results of this ambiguity. As late as 1809 (HAHL 1968:2125) and 1812 (HAHL 1968:2122), the 1776 sub-statute had not only failed to penetrate effectively to the provincial level but also the Board itself remained undecided as to when to apply it. In an 1824 memorandum, after a detailed investigation of the past record of judgments in cases of multiple homicide due to insanity, the Board confessed, "There is no clear pattern for setting penalties" (HAHL 1968:2125–2126).

Analysis of the guidelines set forth at that juncture (TCLL 1870 26:49b) reveals that at last distinctions in the "normal" laws for multiple homicide regarding the number and family ties of the victims were made explicit. In doing so, the old monetary redemption procedure was not only left far behind but there was even an extension in severity over the 1776 blanket penalty of strangulation after the assizes. In the most extreme case of an insane person killing three or more members in one family, he ran the risk of actual decapitation. Yet, the impulse toward compassion was not entirely lost. Instead of suffering immediate execution as was the norm, those judged insane were at least permitted another hearing at the autumn assizes.[7]

(2) A New Distinction

The established pattern of monetary redemption and lifelong imprisonment for cases of homicide due to insanity was further undermined by increasing numbers of "crafty and cunning rogues" (HAHL 1968:2117) who hoped to escape their death penalties through the loophole of feigned insanity. Around the turn of the nineteenth century the problem had reportedly reached such proportions as to cause genuine alarm (HAHL 1968:2114). In reaction, in 1802 the Board of Punishments decided to "act with severity" to deter such imposters, even at the expense of harsher treatment for borderline cases of insanity.

Instead of regarding alike all insane murderers and routinely sentencing them to life confinement, two kinds were distinguished. First there were those who were ill long enough prior to the homicide to enable their relatives to report them to the authorities beforehand and who remained confused in speech from the beginning to the end of the legal process. Under such circumstances the monetary redemption and life imprisonment judgment was still in effect.

There also was provision for a new type of insane murderers. They were those who were affected by an abrupt onset of insanity, which was so sudden that there was no time to inform the authorities before they murdered someone. At some later point, they recovered, if not by the time of the first trial, then at least by the retrial, where they confessed in a sane state of mind. These were no longer allowed monetary redemption but instead were to be punished according to whatever statute was normally applicable. The rationale was that besides genuine cases of acute onset of insanity, imposters would tend to fall into this latter category. Thus, they would no longer gain from their subterfuge.

At the time the intention was merely to change the lightness of monetary redemption, leaving the strict isolation policy intact. A decision in the following year makes this point abundantly clear. A Szechwan case came before the Board involving a man who in a fit of madness killed his younger brother with a sharp instrument and regained his sanity by the retrial (HAHL 1968:2114). If the 1802 decision was followed to the letter, he would have been released from prison to be sent into life exile in accordance with the usual light penalty for elder brothers who committed such a crime. However, once more the deep-set fear of recurring insanity leading to further violence, even in the far-off border areas, intervened. As a result, the Board made a new ruling which was again circulated to all the provinces. If murders committed during an attack of insanity did not merit the death penalty according to "normal" statutes, even if the offender later confessed in a sane state of mind, one should keep him in lifelong confinement. Furthermore, those sentenced to death penalties but spared the actual execution were to be imprisoned for life. They were not eligible for reconsideration on the occasion of an imperial amnesty (HAHL 1968:2117).

When the polished version of the 1801 and 1802 rulings was entered in the volume of sub-statutes in 1806 (Shen 1909 12:93a–b; TCLL 1870 26:50a–b), there was only a slight hint that the conflicting tendency toward leniency still remained beneath the surface. As Hsüeh Yün-sheng pointed out (Hsüeh 1970: 862), a measure of special consideration was shown by treating all verified cases of "confessing in a sane state at the trial" as "murder during an affray", requiring strangulation after the assizes. Only those lacking the proper evidence and thus suspected to be imposters felt the full force of the severer penalty of decapitation after the assizes meted to the category of "premeditated murder".

(3) Homicide Within the Family

Bodde and Morris have stressed that the legal codes recognized intra-family distinctions based upon sex, generation, degree of kinship, and age that were even more complex than their model in society at large, i.e., the five-degree mourning system (Bodde and Morris 1967:37). In keeping with the general trend toward severe penalties for cases of homicide due to insanity, in the late 1700's the endeavor to apply some of these familial considerations in rulings pertaining to the insane was begun. However, given the complications of normal Chinese family law, as well as relatively defined ideas concerning how insane criminals should be handled, the Ch'ing lawmakers never got very far in their effort to accommodate one to the other. Confusion, controversy, and inconsistency bogged them down from beginning to end.

(a) Juniors killing senior relatives The Board of Punishments initially relied on the painful accumulation of specific precedents to signal a change in policy from light to severe sentences for insane family members who murdered senior relatives. When such a case arose in 1786, and again in 1792, the provincial authorities first followed the usual monetary redemption and life imprisonment pattern established for general circumstances of homicide due to insanity (HAHL 1968:2120). Insisting on taking even distant blood ties into account, the Board unexpectedly overturned the lower courts' decisions and condemned the insane to decapitation after the assizes, in accordance with the normal family laws.

By 1799 the Board's message had apparently finally gotten through to the provincial level; for there is no indication of any hesitation in sentencing to immediate decapitation a Shantung man who due to insanity chopped to death his aunt and a kitchen servant. The proposal that the emperor reduce the penalty to decapitation after the assizes was apparently the only concession to special consideration for his illness (HAHL 1968:2122). Again, in 1808 and 1812 two more cases of juniors who killed their senior relatives were routinely assigned decapitation after the assizes (HAHL 1968:2124).

All this while the Board had not set forth any general principles for the sentencing of insane individuals guilty of killing their senior relatives. Monetary redemption had not been explicitly ruled out, and tough·penalties according to normal family laws were not yet institutionalized in a sub-statute. Therefore, as late as 1828, in the case of an insane person who stabbed to death his distant uncle, a confused Szechwan governor-general made the mistake of seeking a monetary redemption, as well as setting a death penalty (HAHL 1968:2127).

It was not until 1845 that a ruling was entered into the Code, clearly defining the procedures which had become gradually accepted through individual cases (Hsüeh 1970:863). It was slightly revised in the 1870 edition of the Ch'ing Code (TCLL 1870 26:50f–51).

(b) Wives killing husbands An 1806 imperial edict recorded in the *Hsing-an hui-lan* provides us with a glimpse of the controversy involved in formulating the official Ch'ing policy toward wives who killed their husbands during psychotic

excitement (HAHL 1968:2123). The problem was essentially deciding at what point, if any, the circumstance of insanity merited some form of special consideration. Earlier judges had chosen to forego any measures of leniency and to treat such offenders exactly as their "normal" counterparts; for by the time the case of Mrs. Tuan née Li arose, the established procedure was to sentence degenerate wives of this sort to immediate decapitation. The insertion of proposal slips for reduction of this penalty was not even permitted. Mindful that the mourning relationship of wife to husband was among the closest possible, the Board of Punishments and lower courts had recommended the same fate for Mrs. Tuan.

As had occurred occasionally in the past, the issue was raised concerning whether to allow her execution to be postponed in some way. The Chia-ch'ing emperor rejected the Grand Secretariat's initial suggestion that the customary penalty of immediate decapitation for wives killing their husbands be changed to decapitation after the assizes, in accordance with the "younger brothers beating to death their older brothers" sub-statute. In so doing, he implied that there was no need to twist the usual ordering of society merely to accommodate insanity. Eventually, because he felt that the condition of insanity did offer "some slight excuse", the emperor set down new guidelines which made the insertion of proposal slips a formal requirement. This imperial edict was incorporated almost in its entirety into a sub-statute first added into the Code in 1852 (Hsüeh 1970:860–861).

(c) Other categories The obstacles encountered in reconciling normal family law with insane criminals were even greater in situations where light penalties were ordinarily warranted, such as seniors killing their junior relatives or husbands murdering their wives. Consequently, it is not surprising that no explicit laws were promulgated in this period for such categories of homicide due to insanity.

The 1796 case of Liu Tsu-ch'ih (HAHL 1968:2119) provides some insight into the problems entailed. Although the ordinary family laws had been rigorously applied to sentence the insane who killed their senior relatives, to do so when insane seniors murdered their juniors would have meant releasing them without any penal consequences at all! This was precisely what the lower courts had recommended in Liu's case. The Board of Punishments, however, feared above all the potential for future disorder represented by the freely roaming insane. It reversed the earlier decision and returned to the general sub-statute for homicide due to insanity requiring lifelong confinement. In short, in order to keep a *k'uang* murderer safely isolated from society, the Board was even willing to contradict its supposed concern for the normal mourning rules.

(4) Less Serious Crimes

Though overshadowed by murders, less serious crimes were committed by the insane in Ch'ing China. Such cases are found scattered throughout the *Hsing-an hui-lan*. Judging from the handful included alongside homicides due to insanity, as well as the few appropriate sub-statutes, it appears that the fate of all insane offenders was affected by developments in legal attitudes toward those guilty of homicide.

During the initial phase, while the Ch'ing lawmakers were primarily occupied with establishing light sentences and strict confinement for homicide due to insanity, procedures for handling less serious crimes followed suit on the side. It was assumed from the start that the 1669 statute allowing monetary redemption for homicide due to insanity naturally also applied to cases of injury (Hsüeh 1970:860, 893). Moreover, along with the decision to imprison insane killers for life, the 1762 package of laws also decreed that even those insane who had not yet committed any crime were to be fettered until officials verified their cure.

How did the insane guilty of less serious offenses fare in the move in the late 1700's toward both severe penalties and imprisonment for murder? The *Hsing-an hui-lan* records that on the one hand, at least up until 1826, as long as life imprisonment was being upheld in cases of homicide due to insanity, strict confinement still remained effective for insane persons who committed misdemeanors (HAHL 1968:2113, 2127–2128).

On the other hand, as the monetary redemption pattern fell into disfavor for cases of homicide due to insanity, for a time it continued to be used for judging wounding due to insanity. Indeed, a separate sub-statute was added into the "Affrays and Blows" section of the Ch'ing Code to institutionalize this apparently popular procedure (Hsüeh 1970:890). Yet, the pull to follow the homicide due to insanity precedents in setting severe penalties according to "normal" law at last proved too great. As reflected in an 1827 Board of Punishments memorandum, the eventual decision to sentence by normal family law those who injured their relatives due to insanity took into account how similar cases of murder were handled (HAHL 1968:2120–2122).

D. "... but confinement became very lenient"

The final phase which the late Ch'ing legal authority Hsüeh Yün-sheng observed in legislation regarding homicide due to insanity seems to have developed in the latter half of the nineteenth century. Since the *Hsing-an hui-lan* casebook breaks off in the 1830's, deep understanding of the complex motivations behind the shift back to lenient confinement lies beyond the scope of this study. At best, we are left with a few hints that more than a mere "outflow of compassion" (Bünger 1950:6) was responsible.

(1) Imperial Amnesties

There is no denying that a few individuals here and there may have been primarily inspired by humanitarian impulses. This was perhaps true in the case of one Shantung governor (HAHL 1968:2114–2115). In 1796 on the occasion of an imperial amnesty he raised the issue of whether it could apply to special cases of homicide due to insanity imprisoned for life. In his memorial he confessed that he felt "extreme pity" for those who had been in jail for over ten to twenty years, were over seventy years old, and recovered long ago. In keeping with Morris' idea of "structured" clemency (Bodde and Morris 1967:534), by the time his proposal had gone up the bureaucratic hierarchy and been approved by the Board and the emperor, it had taken on a much more restrained and regulated form.

Close study of Board of Punishments memoranda reveals that ordinarily those responsible for regularizing clemency were moved by two major concerns. Foremost in their minds was the preservation of social order. In the 1796 case, the Board first responded to the Shantung governor by reiterating the old fear that seemingly cured insanity could recur. It ended up making twenty years the minimum and requiring careful investigation before formerly insane murderers could be released. Secondly, because the officials were motivated to avoid inappropriate sentences and take distinctions of normal law into account, at that point they acted out of special concern for old age. In 1808 even this slim hope of eventual freedom was retracted for those who killed senior relatives or their husbands (Hsüeh 1970:861; TCLL 1870 26:50c).

(2) Remaining at home to continue the ancestral line

The practice of permitting only sons, no matter what their crime, to return home to care for aged parents or to continue the ancestral line upheld the Confucian values of filial piety and ancestor worship. It dates back as far as the Northern Wei dynasty and was first incorporated into the T'ang Code (Ch'ü 1961:76). In 1801 it was explicitly extended for the first time to include those who once murdered due to insanity, were sentenced to life imprisonment, and later recovered (Hsüeh 1970:861; TCLL 1870 26:49a–b). No minimum number of years in jail was necessary.

Demonstrating in this way a willingness to comply with established norms, the Board still made every effort to minimize the danger to society. It encouraged district magistrates and relatives to fulfill their duties conscientiously by setting penalties for them in the event of the insanity recurring and causing further disturbances. It further stated that under such circumstances the insane offender would be returned to prison for life. After adding a deterrent to imposters and excluding cases of multiple or family homicides, an 1811 sub-statute extended this ruling to include insane murderers who later confessed in a sane state of mind (Hsüeh 1970:863; TCLL 1870 26:50c–d).

The *Hsing-an hui-lan* tells a story of cautious reluctance to broaden too far the applicability of this privilege. Time and again when lower officials raised cases which they felt merited such leniency, their superiors on the Board of Punishments disagreed on the grounds that the actual specifics did not fit the legal ideal (HAHL 1968 32:2116–2119). Only one instance is reported in which this measure of mercy was actually approved. It involved a Shantung man who killed his wife during an attack of insanity, later recovered, and testified that his only son had died while he was in prison (HAHL 1968:2119). The Board ruled in 1819 that if further inquiry substantiated his claim he was to be freed to go home and continue the ancestral line.

(3) Practical Necessity

The ground for the swing back to lightened imprisonment for insane offenders may have been laid in the early 1830's. Thus, in 1831, due to a general New Year's amnesty the Board released to the care of her family a woman who during an attack of insanity had killed her daughter-in-law and later recovered (HAHL 1968:2124). Indicating that this was not necessarily just an isolated incident, the following year the Kwangtung supervisory department allowed yet another imprisoned insane, a high provincial official in this case, to be returned to his home (HAHL 1968:2126–2127). Of course, the especially low status of the daughter-in-law and the particularly high position of the official probably affected the outcome of these two instances. However, they may also reflect a general loosening of the strict isolation policy toward the insane that Hsüeh Yün-sheng noted.

In petitioning for the release of the insane Kwangtung official, the governor-general argued, "Since Kwangtung presently lacks quarters in which to restrain him, hand him over to his mother . . . " (HAHL 1968:2126). When one recalls that South China in the 1830's was caught in the midst of deepening internal and external pressures, this comment takes on added meaning and leads to the hypothesis that the move toward greater leniency in confinement in the subsequent decades of the Ch'ing was motivated more by practical necessity than by "simple compassion".

The message of disinterest in further elaboration of the laws pertaining to insanity is unmistakeably clear in one last Board memorandum. In 1833, a Kiangsi censor petitioned for clarification of laws regarding the responsibility of relatives who kept the insane at home, penalties for allowing the insane to cause disturbances in prison, and the "remaining at home" provision (HAHL, 1968:2128). The fact that he felt there was a need to do so at that time may be significant. Perhaps more of the insane were being entrusted to the care of their relatives. Those who remained behind in crowded prison conditions may have become more agitated. Whatever the reasoning behind this proposal, after 150 years of multiplying laws concerning insanity, the Board betrayed a sense of weariness and indifference in its reply. It agreed that the sub-statutes in question were vague but argued that increasing details only complicated affairs further. As a result, "there was no need for further discussion."

Probably due to the deliberate design of its compilers, it is on this note of curt finality that the major section on insanity in the *Hsing-an hui-lan* ends. The case on insanity appeared to be closed for the time being in Ch'ing China.

IV. CONCLUSION

The historical study of the Chinese response to insanity not only should illuminate a facet of the past not normally seen but also should deepen our understanding of the behavior of contemporary Chinese. Both of these objectives underlie the preceding legal case study.

For those interested in a fuller picture of imperial China, the fluctuation in official policy toward the insane has proven to be a unique gauge of shifting governmental priorities. As we have learned, from at least the Latter Han on, representatives of the law tried to control psychotic outbursts. However, it was only in the first half of the Ch'ing that a sustained effort was made to eliminate such disruptions of the social order by legislating the responsibilities of family, community, and officials. This interlude of determined intervention coincided with an especially vigorous phase of an established state with the resources to attend to this problem. The waning of legal interest in individuals suffering from insanity suggests in an indirect way the impact of more pressing threats to stability in the nineteenth century.

As for implications of use to mental health professionals dealing directly with Chinese in the present, this paper has shown that for the most part, Chinese families shouldered the major responsibility for the care of insane members. Even at the risk of defying Ch'ing law, many persisted in their deeply ingrained habits of hiding such sick relatives at home and resisting the intrusion of "outsiders". As for the community, it seemed reluctant to involve itself and greatly relieved when the law shifted its responsibility onto the shoulders of the district magistrate. Tsung-yi and Mei-chen Lin described a strikingly similar pattern of social relations in their recent article on help-seeking behavior of Chinese living in Vancouver, Canada (Lin and Lin 1978; and Chapter 20 in this volume). Separated by time and space from their forebears in imperial China, the response of the Vancouver Chinese to the insane in their midst still falls recognizably within the broad parameters of a longstanding cultural tradition.

ABBREVIATIONS

HAHL	*Hsing-an hui-lan*	TCLL	*Ta Ch'ing lü-li*
MLCCFL	*Ming lü chi-chieh fu-li*	TLSY	*T'ang lü shu-yi*

NOTES

*Editors' Note: The term *k'uang* refers to a condition consistent with acute psychotic excitement which can be caused by mania, schizophrenia or organic psychosis. In certain translated texts the word "mania" was often used but in the view of the editors this term, *k'uang*, is not limited to the manic condition.

1. Scholars agree that the *Huang-ti nei-ching* is the cumulative product of many authors. Some place the period of formation in the late Chou, but on the basis of recent archaeological findings Yamada Keiji argues that it was compiled between 100 B.C. and 100 A.D. (Yamada 1979:67–89).

2. The *Hsing-an hui-lan* is a collection of over 5,650 penal cases dating from 1736 to 1834 taken from the archives of the Board of Punishments. It was compiled by two officials who served many years in the Board and were convinced of the need to provide jurists with a body of precedents in readily accessible form. For more information, see Bodde and Morris (1967:144–159).

3. For example, Lu Hsün's 'Diary of a Madman', which depicts *k'uang* as the ultimate form of social protest, seems based on a long intellectual tradition that imparts a sense of nobility to this particular kind of nonconformity. Similarly, the popular belief in a Boddhisattva in the guise of a "mad monk" named Chi Tien 濟顛 attaches reverence to insanity. I am indebted to Dr. Loh Wai-fong for having pointed out these interesting avenues for further research. I also wish to warmly thank Prof. Yang Lien-sheng for having first directed me into the legal record out of which this chapter stems.

4. Hsüeh Yün-sheng (1820–1901) was an eminent scholar-official whose forty years of service in the Ch'ing judiciary system included the post as Chinese president of the Board of Punishments. Among the number of works he edited was the *Tu-li ts'un-yi*, in which he set out to produce a comprehensive evaluation of the Ch'ing sub-statutes as a guide for overall revision (Hsüeh 1970:1).

5. Since the sixth century the Chinese legal definition of punishment was, strictly speaking, limited to five standard categories, ranging from beating with a light stick up to some manner of death. Neither monetary redemption nor imprisonment was formally recognized as a separate penalty. Instead, the former was seen as a substitute for one of the accepted forms of punishment; and the latter was usually a corollary of the lengthy judicial process. (Bodde and Morris 1967:77–79). This is the context behind Hsüeh's contrast between "sentencing" (or "applying the penalties" *chih tsui* 治罪) and "confinement" (or "restraining in chains" *suo chin* 鎖禁).

6. According to Joseph Needham in *Clerks and Craftsmen in China and the West* (1970:277) some hospitals did exist before the Ming and Ch'ing but declined thereafter. At any rate, the first insane asylum by western standards was established in 1897 by an American medical missionary, Dr. John Kerr.

7. Beginning in the Ming dynasty, the autumn assizes was an annual assembly which reconsidered all capital cases in which there was any doubt about carrying out the execution. See Bodde and Morris (1967:134–142) for details on its elaborate procedures.

REFERENCES

1. Western Sources

Biot, Edouard
    1939 Le Tcheou-li. Peking reprint of Paris, 1851 ed., Imprimerie nationale.
Bodde, Derk and Morris, Clarence
    1967 Law in Imperial China. Cambridge, Massachusetts: Harvard University Press.
Bünger, Karl
    1950 The punishment of lunatics and negligents according to classical Chinese law.
          Studia Serica 9:1–16.
Ch'ü, T'ung-tsu
    1961 Law and Society in Traditional China. Paris and the Hague: Mouton and Co.
Hulsewé, A.F.P.
    1955 Remnants of Han Law. Vol. 1. Leiden: E.J. Brill.
Lin, Tsung-yi and Lin, Mei-chen
    1978 Service delivery issues in Asian-North American communities. American Journal
          of Psychiatry 135:4:454–456.

Needham, Joseph
  1970 Clerks and Craftsmen in China and the West. Cambridge: Cambridge University Press.
Philastre, P. L. F., trans.
  1967 Le Code Annamite. Taipei: Ch'eng-wen Publishing Co.
Van der Valk, M. H.
  1948 Review of Bunger's Quellen zur Rechtsgeschichte der T'ang-Zeit. *T'oung Pao* 38:339–343.
Yamada Keiji
  1979 The formation of the *Huang-ti Nei-ching*. Acta Asiatica 36:67–89.

2. Chinese and Japanese Sources

Chou-hou pei-chi fang 肘後備急方 (Prescriptions for emergencies), attributed to Ko Hung 葛洪, 8 chüan in the *P'ing-hua shu-wu ts'ung-shu* 瓶華書屋叢書 1848 ed., ts'e 28, 3:6–9.
Chou li 周禮 (Institutes of the Chou)
  1929 42 chüan. Shanghai: Chung-hua Shui-chü 中華書局.
Han shu 漢書 (Standard History of the Former Han)
  1962 Pan Ku 班固. Peking: Chung-hua Shu-chü 中華書局, in 8 volumes with continuous pagination.
Hou-Han shu 後漢書 (Standard History of the Latter Han)
  1965 Fan Yeh 范曄, comp. Peking: Chung-hua Shu-chü 中華書局, in 18 volumes with continuous pagination.
Hsing-an hui-lan 刑案滙覽 (Conspectus of penal cases)
  1968 Chu Ch'ing-ch'i 祝慶祺 and Pao Shu-yün 鮑書芸. Reprint of Shanghai, 1886 ed., Taipei: Ch'eng-wen Publishing Co., in 11 vols. with continuous pagination.
Hsüeh Yün-sheng 薛允升
  1970 *Tu-li ts'un-yi* 讀例存疑 (Concentration on doubtful matters while perusing the substatutes). Reprint of Peking, 1905 ed., Taipei: Ch'eng-wen Publishing Co., in 5 vols. with continuous pagination.
Inoue, Mitsusada 井上光貞, et al., eds.
  1976 Ritsuryo 律令 (T'ang Code and Statutes). Tokyo: Iwanami shoten 岩波書店.
Ling-shu 靈樞 (Divine Pivot) in *Huang-ti nei-ching Su-wen Ling-shu ho-p'ien* 黃帝內經素問靈樞合編
  1910 Shanghai: Yi Hsueh Kung Hui 醫學公會.
Ming lü chi-chieh fu-li 明律集解附例 (Ming Code with collected commentaries and appended sub-statutes)
  1969 Reprint of 1908 ed., Taipei: Ch'eng-wen Publishing Co., in 5 vols. with continuous pagination.
Shen Chia-pen 沈家本, et al., comp
  1909 *Ta Ch'ing hsien-hsing hsing-lü an-yu* 大清現行刑律案語 (Commentary on the currently operative penal code of the great Ch'ing), 37 ts'e. Peking: Fa lü kuan 法律館.
Su-wen 素問 (Candid Questions in the Inner Classic of the Yellow Emperor) in *Huang-ti nei-ching Su-wen Ling-shu ho-p'ien* 黃帝內經素問靈樞合編
  1910 Shanghai: Yi Hsueh Kung Hui 醫學公會.
Ta Ch'ing lü-li 大清律例 (Statutes and sub-statutes of the great Ch'ing)
  1870 revised edition. 47 chüan. Ta Ch'ing lü-li kuan 大清律例館.
Ta Ch'ing lü-li an-yü 大清律例按語 (Commentary on the statutes and sub-statutes of the great Ch'ing)
  1847 104 chüan. Hai-shan hsien kuan 海山仙館.

T'ai-p'ing yü-lan 太平御覽 (Imperially reviewed encyclopedia of the T'aiping era)

    1960 Li Fang 李昉. Peking: Chung-hua Shu-chü 中華書局, in 4 volumes with continuous
         pagination.

T'ang lü shu-yi 唐律疏義 (T'ang Code with commentary).

    1965 Taipei: Shang-wu yin-shu kuan 商務印書館, 4 volumes in one with continuous
         pagination.

Wu T'an 吳壇 , comp.

    (preface dated 1886).

        40 chüan. *Ta-ch'ing lü-li tung-k'ao* 大清律例通考 (General Annotations on the
        statutes and sub-statutes of the great Ch'ing).

6. TRADITIONAL CHINESE MEDICAL BELIEFS AND THEIR RELEVANCE FOR MENTAL ILLNESS AND PSYCHIATRY

After more than one hundred years of contact with the West and importation of Western medicine into China, traditional Chinese health beliefs and practices continue to exert important effects on the symptom manifestations and health-related behaviors of Chinese patients (Kleinman et al. 1975, 1978; Topley 1976; Chan and Chang 1976). This is particularly true when the problems they experience are psychiatric or psychosocial in nature (Kleinman 1979). In this paper, I will review some key traditional Chinese health concepts, especially as they relate to mental illness, and discuss their implications for contemporary psychiatric practice among Chinese populations.

As will be seen in the sections that follow, Chinese medical concepts generally reflect the central theme of Chinese culture, which can best be characterized by a dialectic interaction between the idea of *Tao* and a strong pragmatic material orientation. The concept of *Tao* connotes a continuous search for the proper way of conducting one's social and personal life. Compared to Western civilization, Chinese culture has been less concerned with ontological issues such as the existence of God or the ultimate fate of the human race. Its two dominant philosophical traditions, Confucianism and Taoism, both focused their efforts in delineating *Tao* in different spheres: Confucianists have been mostly concerned with the proper way of conducting a person's social life; while Taoists have persistently devoted attention to searching for the optimal way for an individual to live a harmonious personal life in relation to cosmological and natural spheres (Hsu 1934). This concentrated interest in the well-being of the individual as an integrated organism within the context of his cosmological, natural and social environments has shaped and permeated Chinese thoughts all through the centuries. The pragmatic aspect of the concept of *Tao* leads Chinese to be less concerned about the absolute, supposedly "objective truth" of events than their Western counterparts, and also more willing to try apparently contradictory approaches as long as they work. The coexistence of scholarly traditional Chinese medicine ("the great tradition") and various folk healing practices ("the little tradition") demonstrates well their pragmatic and pluralistic tendency (Li mimeographed report). Both of them were largely fostered by the Taoist tradition, yet developed along divergent lines. In this chapter I will review the two traditions separately.

TRADITIONAL CHINESE MEDICINE

Although not formally scientific in the modern sense, the Chinese medical system, as revealed in its classics (*Huang-ti nei-ching Su-wen, Ling-shu; Shang-han*

A. Kleinman and T.-Y. Lin (eds.), Normal and Abnormal Behavior in Chinese Culture, 95–111.
Copyright © 1980 *by D. Reidel Publishing Company.*

lun; Chin-kuei yao-lüeh), presents a rational, empirical and systematically synthesized healing tradition largely devoid of supernatural components. Scholars have shown that it went through a critical, ongoing developmental process involving observation and speculation as well as conceptual elaboration, and was often surprisingly objective and therapeutically effective (Agren 1975; Porkert 1974; Tseng 1973), although in later years it suffered from an overgrowth of theory and too literal and rigid interpretation of the originally dynamic, allegorical principles formulated in earlier phases (Wong and Wu 1936; Chen 1937).

Microcosm-macrocosm correspondences (*tien-jen-hsiang-ying*) and dynamic balancing or harmony (*t'iao-ho*) appear to be the two most central concepts of Chinese medicine (Nan-Tung City Chinese Medical School 1959; Agren 1977; Bennett 1978). As noted above, the early Taoists were devoted naturalists. They saw human "beings" (the terms "body" and "psyche" should be avoided, as they represent a Western dichotomy)[1] as part of the natural world, and believed that what was observed in the macrocosm should have its counterparts in the microcosm. Thus, whatever happened in the larger natural and social environments should also have its effect on the smaller human sphere of the individual.

An elaborate system was developed to describe the correspondences between astronomical systems, seasons, weather, and time on the one hand, and the internal organs, functions, sensations, and emotions on the other hand. From this framework three main themes of fundamental importance evolved: the *yin-yang* system, the Five Evolutive Phases, and the *ching-lo* (meridian) system.

The concept of balance and harmony is the fundamental principle governing both macrocosm and microcosm. Since changes are regarded as not only unavoidable but a basic rule of the universe, balance (harmony) is not static but constantly dynamic. However, as there is always a certain degree of regularity involving both macrocosm and microcosm, "cyclicity" and "circulation" are prominent considerations in maintaining this balance (harmony).

The etiology of diseases is classified into two categories: those operating internally and those originating externally. Internal etiology includes 7 kinds of excesses of emotions. External etiology is further classified into 6 categories: "wind" (*feng*), "coldness" (*han*), "hotness" (*shu*), "dampness" (*shih*), "dryness" (*tsao*), and "fire" (*huo*). While the middle four are closely related to the weather and are reminiscent of Galen's humoral system, the concepts of "wind" and "fire" are more abstract and generic, and consequently have even wider applications. Besides its literal meaning, "wind" also refers to any pathogenic force acting swiftly and therefore potentially more damaging. Symbolically, "wind" is thus implied in many diseases with acute onset or with an unpredictable nature. In combination with cold/hot/damp/dry conditions, "wind" provides the qualities of their being "actively invading" and rapid, and hence makes them even more dangerous. "Fire" as used here, is apparently different from the "fire" in the Five Evolutive Phases which will be described later, and denotes a more passive, complementary factor aggravating any conditions caused by the first five factors.

Since these "meteorologic" factors are always present in a person's surroundings, the important thing is not to avoid them, but to avoid sudden exposure and change of the environment, and to adjust the individual's physiological and psychological condition in advance or in response to these changes, so as to avoid adverse effects from them.

YIN AND YANG

These are a pair of polar terms used to describe qualitatively contrasting aspects inherent in the universe. They are relativistic, functional and dynamic. The use of these two terms invariably infers a comparison. They are at the same time contradictory, but also complementary and interdependent with each other (i.e., the idea of darkness is necessary for the concept of brightness). The interaction of *yin* and *yang* serves as the basis of all change in the universe, both macrocosmic and microcosmic. Owing to their interaction and the changes that result, temporary imbalance is unavoidable. But ultimately if balance cannot finally be achieved, the result will be a situation of dysfunction.

Briefly described, *yang* signifies not only the apparent, active, excited, external, upward, forward, aggressive, volatile, hard, bright, hot, but also the abstract and functional. In direct contrast, *yin* signifies not only the passive, inhibited, unclear, inward, downward, retrogressive, cold, dark, soft, unaggressive, but also the material and concrete.

The theory of *yin-yang* has broad application in Chinese medicine. It is used to describe anatomico-physiological relations and pathological conditions. But it also details the nature and phase of disease, as well as the categorization of medication, dietary considerations and other therapeutic measures. The primary concern of diagnosis in Chinese medicine is to delineate imbalance between *yin-yang* and treatment is primarily aimed at the restoration of this balance. A particularly important outgrowth of *yin-yang* balance theory is that through its relationship with "hot" and "cold" and other polar oppositions, diet and herbs have been dichotomized accordingly, and patients and even healthy people often exercise extreme caution in eating proper diets based on balancing these polar constituents of individuals, their sicknesses, and their foods. The use of tonic, diet and other "balancing" interventions, such as special foods, also plays an important role in health maintenance.

FIVE EVOLUTIVE PHASES (WU-HSING)

The dynamic and functional nature of Chinese medical theory is apparent in the choice of the term, *hsing,* which, rather than the often mistranslated term "element," actually means a condition of constant change and progression. Since the concept originated from astronomical observation (from the five planets which can be seen by the naked eye) and from the composition of the inorganic world (metal, wood, water, fire and earth), its macrocosm-microcosm correspondence is evident when it is applied to human beings and to medicine.

The simple rules of sequential facilitation and inhibition, as applied in the Five Evolutive Phases, results in an intricate system of interdependence and mutual regulation (Figure 1).

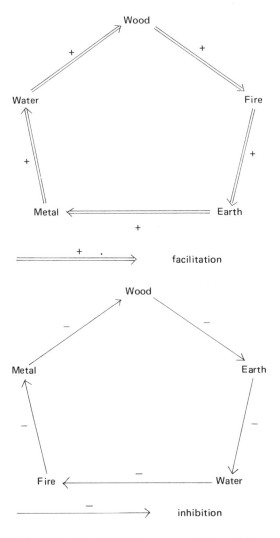

Fig. 1. The facilitative and inhibitory routes of the *wu-hsing* system.

Besides its apparent facilitative and inhibitory functions, implied in this system is another rule called *chih-hua* (rule of regulation of change) which is comparable to a negative feedback system in the modern sense. Figure 2 shows the complete *wu-hsing* system, including both its facilitative and inhibitory routes. The five *chih-hua* subsystems are inherent although somewhat concealed in this figure. Figure 3 depicts a subset of Figure 2 and thereby illustrates one of the five *chih-hua* subsystems.

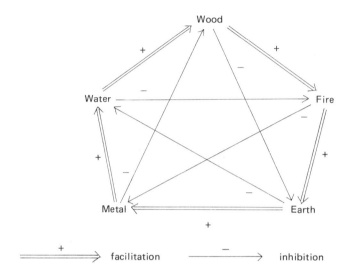

Fig. 2. The complete *wu-hsing* system.

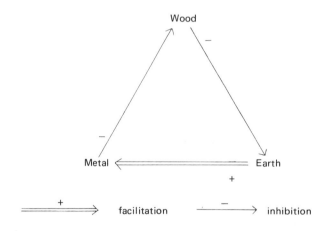

Fig. 3. A subset of the *wu-hsing* system showing a *chih-hua* circle.

Chinese applied this system extensively to both macrocosm (astronomical movement, seasons, geographic orientation, weather, colors, geomantic configurations) and microcosm (internal organs, sensory organs, secretions, tastes, psychological functions). Table 1 presents some of the more important correspondences:

TABLE 1

Five Evolutive Phases	Internal Organs	"Orifices"	Tastes	Colors	Psychological Functions
Wood	liver, gall bladder	eye	sour	blue	anger
Fire	heart, small intestine	tongue	bitter	red	happiness
Earth	spleen, stomach	mouth	sweet	yellow	desire
Metal	lung, large intestine	nose	spicy	white	worry
Water	kidney, urinary bladder	ear	salty	black	fear

It is not exactly clear how these correlations were established. Often they appear to have been based on superficial similarities. For example, lung, like metal, can produce sounds, thus the two were coupled together. On the other hand, some correlations appear to be based on functional considerations. For example: water is excreted through the kidney, so the two belong to the same system. In any event, the important point to note is that the Five Evolutive Phases theory has deeply affected Chinese medical thought and practice. Many practical insights and misconceptions in anatomico-physiology, diagnosis and therapeutics are incorporated into this intricate and closed system. Although too rigid an interpretation of such a complicated symbolic system could conceivably lead to ridiculous conclusions at variance with experience, this early focus of Chinese medicine on the integration of different "bodily" systems and the awareness that treatment should not be aimed only at target organs probably made Chinese medicine a more sophisticated and dynamic system of traditional medical beliefs than its prescientific Western counterpart. For example, both affect and mental illness would be viewed in this perspective in ecological terms and related to potentially important environmental infleunces.

CH'I AND THE CHING-LO (MERIDIAN) SYSTEM

Another important outgrowth of the system of macrocosm-microcosm correspondences is the *ching-lo* (meridian) system and the circulation of *ch'i* (vital energy) and its myriad variants (*hsüeh, ying, wei, chin, i, ching-chi, shen-ch'i, yüan-ch'i, yang-ch'i, yin-ch'i* and many others).

Ch'i is the vital energy for all parts of the body. It has its main origin from the stomach which grinds foodstuff into minute particles and transforms them into "energy." When this energy is combined with the air ("energy" from the surrounding air) from the lungs, *ch'i* (vital energy) is formed. *Ch'i* is circulated sequentially via all the meridian tracts to provide nourishment and vitality for all parts of the body. Blood (*hsüeh*) and the cardiovascular circulatory system in the modern sense are regarded as the more substantive parts of the *ch'i* circulation system. Blood is viewed as mainly containing "constructive" energy (*ying*) while *ch'i* is viewed as containing more "defensive" energy (*wei*).

Since *ch'i* is so important in the maintenance of all vital functions, and also is virtually irreplaceable, any loss of *ch'i*, or obstruction of its circulation, is considered to have grave consequence. The manifested symptoms of dysfunctions of *ch'i* are organized and recognized according to the meridian system.

It is asserted that there are 12 regular meridians, 8 "unusual" tracts, and numerous emissaries, connecting various parts of the body surface and/or sensory organs. This system is not only of preeminent importance for acupuncture, but also is highly relevant to diagnosis, herbal therapy, other treatment methods, and *ch'i-kung* (phase energetics − a special kind of exercise and method of "meditation" to strengthen *ch'i*).

FUNCTIONAL APPROACH

All the above mentioned principles indicate that Chinese medicine is basically holistic and focuses predominantly on function rather than structure. This is not only true in the area of normal physiology (including psychology − the two are not differentiated), but also in concepts concerning pathology, diagnosis, disease classification and therapy. Chinese medicine is much less concerned with specific pathological changes and more preoccupied with the restoration of balance according to the theories of *yin-yang*, Five Evolutive Phases, *ching-lo*, and the circulation of *ch'i*. The apparent remoteness of the acupuncture sites from their target symptoms is an evident example (Porkert 1976).

PSYCHIATRIC IMPLICATIONS OF TRADITIONAL CHINESE MEDICAL CONCEPTS

The most psychiatrically relevant aspect of traditional Chinese medicine is its unwillingness to differentiate between psychological and physiological functions. Contrary to popular impression, Chinese do not appear to lack psychological awareness. Rather, they show ample evidence of awareness of psychological factors in all aspects of health and illness. Their tendency toward extreme somatization (Tseng 1975; Kleinman 1979) may be qualitatively different from that of other cultures. I will discuss three aspects of this problem.

1. Although psychological factors are clearly indicated in all the major classics of Chinese medicine as one of the two major categories causing imbalance and disease, they are dealt with differently. Excess and incongruence of seven kinds of emotions (happiness, anger, worry, desire, sadness, fear, and fright) are regarded as pathogenic. However, contrary to the Greek and European tradition which stresses the therapeutic value of emotional catharsis, Chinese directed their efforts to avoid excesses of emotions and fit their emotional states to their natural and social milieu. Since excesses, rather than emotions per se, are regarded as pathogenic, high value is placed on moderation and inhibition of affective expression. Also, to prevent psychosomatic-somatopsychic imbalance, the Taoist and Chinese medical traditions developed ways that were supposed to be effective in training Chinese not to respond to

hazardous stimuli with excessive emotions (*lien-ch'i*: mental exercise, meditation) (Yan and Xu mimeographed report). Since Confucianism also teaches that
maintaining harmony in familial and other social relationships requires inhibition
and avoidance of emotional expression (Yeh 1971), these Chinese philosophical
traditions worked together to reinforce the quality of equanimity among
Chinese and to legitimate suppression as a psychoculturally adaptive coping
mechanism. This tends to give the superficial impression that Chinese are not
psychologically-minded (Tseng 1975).

Disappointing perhaps for Western-style psychotherapists is the reverse
emphasis of the Chinese psychosomatic model on somatopsychic effects. Once
physiological functions are disturbed, the logical methods of treatment become
physiological or pharmacological interventions, even if excess of emotions is
held as the initial reason for the disturbance. Training body-mind together is
basic as a traditional Chinese method of psychological intervention, but its value
was held to be greater for prevention than therapy. It is also of interest that the
principle of moderation is not only applied to the six negative emotions, but to
the positive one – happiness – too. It is evident that psychological health was
believed to be maintained through this culturally approved system of somatopsychic training of moderation.

2. Internal organs (again these should refer to the 12 functional organ
systems rather than anatomical structures)[2] are viewed as centers for combined
physiological and psychological functions. Of special importance are the heart,
kidney, lung, liver and gallbladder. These organs are still often used for colloquial expression of feeling states (e.g., *k'ai-hsin*: "opening heart" – happiness;
tan-ch'ieh: "cowardly gallbladder" – fearfulness). Of these organs, the heart,
kidney, and lung appear to be of special importance in regulating the psychological functions. "Heart" is regarded as the organ harboring *shen* ("spirit" or
"mind") which is the governing body or integrative center of all the psychological functions. "Kidney" is the reservoir of *ching* ("essence" – purified,
concentrated *ch'i*). *Ching-shen* as a term is used to denote the mental function
of an individual. Thus, if taken literally, *ching-shen ko* (Chinese term for
psychiatry) would mean the study of the function of "heart" and "kidney." As
described previously, *ch'i* (vital energy) is regarded as the product of the concerted efforts of stomach and lung. Thus dysfunction of either of them tends to
diminish *ch'i* and slow down general vital processes. Probably this is why lung is
described as susceptible to "worries" and "sadness," and stomach and spleen to
"thinking too much." Liver and gallbladder are believed to be especially predisposed to "anger."

These ideas have greatly affected Chinese concepts of psychological problems
which have persisted up to the contemporary era. When a patient suffers from
psychological difficulties, and is aware of his predominant emotional state, his
attention is thereby easily channeled to preoccupation with the alleged physiological function of the "related" bodily organ (e.g., a patient suffering from anger
may be worried about his liver and insist on having liver function tests done).

The importance of the kidney in psychological functioning was probably further enhanced when Chinese began to understand the psychological relevance of the spinal cord and the brain. A theory was developed to connect the kidney, sexual function (regarded as belonging to the kidney), and the central nervous system. It was asserted that sperm (which is also called *ching*, the essence of *ch'i*), optimally conserved, is sifted into the spinal cord to nourish both the cord and the brain. A condition called *shen-k'uei* ("kidney insufficiency") is regarded as resulting from excessive loss of sperm (*ching*), and thus, also the essence of *ch'i*, which produces psychological, psychosomatic and sexual symptoms such as difficulty in concentration, forgetfulness, weakness, backpain, tiredness, dizziness, nocturnal ejaculation and impotence (see Chapter 18).

3. Another consequence of its psychosomatic integration is that Chinese medicine relies equally on behavioral as well as physiological observations for diagnosis and therapeutic action. Examples are abundant; the following offers just one illustration. The syndrome of hand-minor *yin*-pericardium meridian includes symptom manifestations of hot palms, flexed arms, lumps in the axilla, a feeling of fullness in the chest, palpitations, flushing of the face, yellowish sclera, and *constant laughing, elevated mood, troubled mind.*

Since one of the axioms of diagnosis is that the patient does not need to manifest all the symptoms to be classified into a particular syndrome, there is a great degree of laxity which allows either the primarily organic or the primarily psychological condition to be included in a certain diagnosis. In the same fashion, treatment can also be directed at either one or both of these aspects.

These characteristics of Chinese medicine, working together, must have exerted a retarding influence on the development of psychiatry and psychology in Chinese culture. No separate attention was paid to mental illnesses, especially to minor ones; instead they were fully integrated with other physiological problems, and treated in the same way. Emotions were regarded as important etiological factors for both types of illness.

This is also true for depression. Although its psychological precipitants may be well recognized, it is not regarded as a psychological condition. The lack of energy and fatigability often associated with it are neatly explained as disturbances of *ch'i* which could be produced by: (1) excessive sadness or worry hurting the "lung," or (2) too much deliberation damaging the stomach and spleen. The latter would also explain the loss of appetite, a cardinal symptom of depression.

However, the major psychiatric problems producing dramatic or erratic effects posed difficulties for this highly developed and usually self-sufficient explanatory system. Although attempts were still made to interpret them according to the system, they were sometimes treated separately. Thus, a separate chapter of the classic *Huang-ti nei-ching Ling-shu* was devoted to the problems of *tien-k'uang* (craziness) which originally included both psychosis and seizure disorder. The clinical description of psychosis (*k'uang*) is compatible with either schizophrenia or the manic phase of manic-depressive psychosis. Descriptions of psychotic symptoms or delirium associated with fever were scattered in many other chapters of the two volumes of *Nei-Ching* (*Su-wen* and *Ling-shu*).

Observations continued to accumulate that helped later authors to divide the *tien-k'uang* (functional psychoses) into three categories: *tien, hsien,* and *k'uang*. *Hsien* is used for epilepsy/seizure, and is excluded from the other two. *Tien* is used for psychotics who are more passive and apathetic, while *k'uang* is used for those who are more excited and agitated. *Feng*, a colloquial term commonly signifying "craziness," is written with a character that is composed of "sickness" and "wind" radicals, perhaps reflecting the rapidity of onset of some psychoses and the unpredictiveness of the behavior of affected patients. The term is apparently related to two terms: *feng-tien* and *feng-k'uang*, first used by Fang Chau-yen in the T'ang dynasty. Another commonly used term, "flower insanity," or "peach flower insanity," was described in young unmarried women. Manifestations include hypomanic or catatonic excitement and hypersexual behavior. Frustrated sexual desire was viewed as the cause.

Illnesses with clinical pictures suggestive of hysterical attacks were described quite early. Chang Chung-ching in the Han dynasty described the "hurrying-pig sickness" and the sickness of the "hasty-organ." The former starts with a sensation of air arising from the lower abdomen, progressing quickly to the chest and then the larynx. The patient may appear seriously ill, but recovers in a short period of time. The latter has a predilection for women, who manifest unstable emotions, are easily saddened, cry freely, and yawn frequently. The organ involved was thought to be the uterus or the heart. Both terms denote a temporary crisis situation breaking the rhythm and peace of life. In the Ming dynasty, hysterical attacks were described as "deceiving sickness," a psychological etiology was implicated, and the problem treated accordingly.

FOLK HEALING BELIEFS AND PRACTICES

Similar to the classical Chinese medical tradition, folk healing theories and practices have been heavily influenced by Taoist ideas, with a strong emphasis on macrocosm-microcosm correspondence and dynamic balance. This was particularly true for the earlier Taoist movement which tended to focus on natural rather than supernatural interpretations of the human environment. Later Taoism (from the late Han dynasty) showed a gradual reunion with the animistic indigenous tradition involving shamans and other ritual experts and also adopted ideas from Buddhism. The naturalistic Taoist tradition was responsible for the development of fortune-telling, astrology, physiognomy and geomancy. Native shamanism has survived under the umbrella of a syncretic integration of Taoism and Buddhism up to the contemporary era. This combined influence is responsible for the supernatural tradition of Chinese folk beliefs and practices, including divination, sorcery, spirit loss, and spirit possession (by ghosts and by fox-fairies).

Similar to Chinese medicine, Taoist ideas of *yin-yang*, Five Evolutive Phases and *ch'i* are fundamental in the practices of fortune-telling, astrology, physiognomy, and geomancy. Additionally, the system of celestial stems (*t'ien-kan*) and terrestrial branches (*ti-chih*) provides a reference system for time-space coordination. Health, and in a broader sense, fortune or fate of all kinds, are regarded as determined by these principles. The determinants of fortune or health status, however, vary for the different folk healing disciplines. For the Chinese version of fortune-telling, it is the exact timing of a person's birth that determines his or her fate. For astrology, the correspondence between the movements of celestial bodies and the individual's fortune or health status is crucial. In physiognomy, bony configurations and the location of moles on the body serve as determinants. In geomancy, the same principles are applied to the study of geographic configurations to select a site for a house or a tomb that will maximally capture the *ch'i* flowing through the earth, in order to bring fortune, wealth and health to the owner of the house or the descendents of the deceased. All these practices have persisted over the centuries and are often still utilized by Chinese when facing health or other life problems.

Ch'ien drawing closely resembles fortune-telling except that the help of a god is implied. When a person is troubled by emotional, health, or other life problems, he may go to a temple to pray to a god, then randomly draw one of the numerous bamboo sticks from a container. With the number on the stick, he then finds a poem which is believed to provide an answer to his problem (Hsu 1975).

In the supernatural realm in Taiwan, the most popular folk healing practice is shamanism, which has its historical root in the animistic belief of early Chinese, and can be traced back to the term *wu* which was invariably mentioned with *i* in early Chinese classics to mean a physician who conducted ritual healing (*wu-i* literally means a "witch doctor") (Lu and Needham 1976). In contemporary Taiwan, a shaman, who is called a *tâng-ki* (Kleinman 1975), enters into trance states in which he is possessed by a supernatural power. The client can then consult with the supernatural agency (god, ghost, ancestor) through the shaman for instructions in dealing with life problems (Tseng 1972; Kleinman 1979).

Belief in spirit possession by "hungry" ghosts and fox-fairies has haunted Chinese for centuries. Such ghosts are usually the spirits of those who died earlier than assigned by the king of the hell, those who were wronged in their lives (e.g., murdered), or those who were denied ancestor worship owing to inattentive families or the absence of heirs. Sometimes no explanation is given, and the haunting ghost is regarded as just a wandering evil spirit. Folk concepts of demonic possession as the cause of mental illness apparently gradually infiltrated the originally naturalistic medical theories and started to appear in major medical textbooks of later times, such as Koh Hung's *Chou-hou pei-chi-fang* and Chau Yuan-fang's *Chu-ping yuan-hou lun* (Tseng 1973; Li mimeographed report).

In contrast to ghosts, belief in the ability of foxes to transform themselves into human form and to harm people through possession and sexual activities is unique to East Asians (Veith 1975). Both kinds of possession are often used to explain the occurrence of emotional and/or physical illnesses. Rituals of exorcism are performed by Taoist priests and shamans to expel or destroy these evil forces.

Divination through spirit mediums is a method of communicating with special supernatural agencies that is used in many cultures to deal with illnesses and misfortunes generally. A special kind of divination, derived from Buddhistic belief in the existence of hell, is called ch'ien-wan. The divination specialist, usually a middle-aged woman, travels to hell for her client(s) to meet with his (her) deceased relative. Then supposedly possessed by the spirit of this relative (usually a parent), she gives her client(s) his advice. The content of the conversation usually involves admonitions and suggestions to modify current familial relationships, and may have inherent psychotherapeutic effects.

Sorcery is also sometimes encountered in traditional Chinese settings. It involves sympathetic magic (e.g., drawing a picture of a person and putting arrows through the heart of the picture in order to hurt the person) and is conducted either by a Taoist priest or by a shaman.

Amulets are often obtained from Buddhist or Taoist temples for protection of the wearer's spirit and body against attack by evil spirits.

STIGMA

The extent of stigma of mental illness in Chinese culture is still a controversial issue. While contemporary attitudinal surveys and clinical observations seem to indicate that stigma is exceedingly strong, surveys of historical records tend to give conflicting opinions. It is apparent that Chinese, with their characteristic focus on pragmatism, did not show the same degree of fascination and psychological fear of "craziness" as occurred in Western cultures. This, coupled with the strong Chinese family institution, prevented the development of large psychiatric asylums in China. The ultimate rejections of lunatics in medieval Europe, as evidenced by the epidemics of ships of fools and the assimilation of the insane into the highly stigmatized lepers' role (Foucault 1965), did not appear to happen in traditional China. However, ample evidence exists to indicate that pity and compassion towards the mentally ill were often overshadowed by the need to safeguard society from the unpredictive behavior and occasional violence of the psychotic population. On this pragmatic level, fear has long been operative and has often led to harsh, inhuman confinement, either initiated by the family, or mandated by local governments (see Chapters 5 and 20 in this volume). We also do not know if in the family context the insane were poorly cared for and allowed to succumb to diseases of starvation and neglect, especially in times of famine and social disorganization.

It is likely that in traditional China, the burden of the stigma of mental illness tended to fall more on the family than the individual. Contrary to the assertion of Veith (1975), the hereditary basis of the functional psychoses seems to have been well recognized by the Chinese, and the family with a psychotic member was often excluded from the marital pool in traditional society. Also, Chinese cultural norms held the family as responsible for the individual's behavior and welfare. The erratic and asocial behavior of the psychotic patient brought extreme shame and guilt to the family. The shame for the individual's behavior even extended to the ancestors. When a person suffered from psychosis, neighbors might have shown sympathy toward the sick individual, but they also would have indicated that either his ancestors had done something immoral or his family was responsible for his problem in some other way. Families with mentally ill members feared being ridiculed and "losing face," and therefore attempted to deny the existence of mental illness or disguise the problem under a more socially acceptable label, such as eccentricity or physical illness. This family oriented stigma undoubtedly has presented one of the biggest obstacles to providing optimal mental health care to Chinese communities all over the world right up to the present.

CONCLUSION

This brief review illustrates the cultural specificity of traditional health beliefs. It indicates that most, if not all, of traditional Chinese health beliefs regarding mental illness are deeply rooted in the Chinese core culture and have evolved along with the historical development of that culture. Their content cannot be comprehended without adequate understanding of this cultural background. Yet, despite this emphasis on cultural specificity, it should also be pointed out that when comparing traditional health beliefs about mental illness in different societies the similarities are often striking. For example, psychotic conditions are categorized similarly in societies with drastically different cultural roots. Although they employ different terminology, the description of hysterical symptoms in traditional Chinese medical texts is very similar to that of Hippocrates. Chinese humoral theory is comparable to that of the Indians as well as Galen's version (Temkin 1973). These particular similarities may well be the result of cultural diffusion. Supernatural phenomena are also implicated in different cultures in explaining and categorizing mental illnesses, and similar supernatural treatment methods (e.g. shamanism, divination) are found in societies with greatly different cultural heritages and no history of contact or diffusion. Similarly, the lack of psychological orientation, although possibly more prominent in Chinese culture, is also a common feature in most traditional societies.

Both Tseng (1973) and Westermeyer (in press) have devoted their attention to this kind of comparison and conclude that the similarities in "folk psychiatry" among different peoples in different historical times and cultural places suggest that mental illness is a universal human experience, that there is a common need for understanding, categorizing and explaining mental conditions, and that there are a limited number of ways of responding to them.

For the practice of modern psychiatry in Chinese cultures an adequate understanding of the relevant Chinese medical and folk religious beliefs and treatment approaches is of utmost importance. This is not only because indigenous health beliefs often produce cultural barriers to the practice of Western-style psychiatry in Chinese setting, but more importantly, through these concepts and categorizations, Chinese culture continues to influence the way symptoms are perceived, expressed, and reacted to. Adequate understanding of these beliefs is the key to the indigenization of Western psychiatry in Chinese settings, and the successful planning and provision of culturally appropriate mental health services for Chinese patients. The present paper reviews only historically documented beliefs and concepts. Since beliefs evolve not only out of people's cultural heritages but are also affected constantly by concurrent social conditions, and since modernization has been a far reaching and still ongoing process in most Chinese societies, it is likely that in the present day popular culture of Chinese societies, beliefs about mental illness represent a mixture of traditional Chinese and modern Western ideas. Research on these contemporary beliefs is of both theoretical and clinical significance. Such research should seek to understand their practical effects on illness behavior, help seeking, clinical communication, compliance and other clinically salient issues.

NOTES

1. Chinese medicine did not differentiate psychological from physiological function. In this paper, "human" or "human being" is often used to denote this holistic notion of the total existence of a person as an integrated biopsychosocial system. However, in several places, this usage seemed awkward, and I have employed the term "body," albeit reluctantly. The reader should be cautioned that this term does not refer purely to anatomical part or physiological function.
2. The term "functional" is used because in Chinese medicine these "organs" are not thought of in a strictly anatomical sense. Instead, they are meant to be interpreted as individual anatomico-physiological-psychological systems that constitute the total human being. For the sake of simplicity, the significance of these "organs" in Chinese medicine is not discussed in detail. Interested readers should refer to Porkert (1974) or the standard Chinese medicine texts.
3. From: Chang, C. P.: *Ching-Yue chueng-shuh* (*Ching-Yue's* Collected Work) (In Chinese).

REFERENCES

Agren, H.
    1975   A new approach to Chinese traditional medicine. American J. of Chinese Medicine
           3: 207–212.
Agren, H.
    1977   Empiricism and speculation in traditional East Asian medicine. Journal of
           Japanese Medical History 23: 300–318.
Bennett, S. J.
    1978   Chinese medicine: Theory and practice. Philosophy East and West 28: 439–453.
Chan, C. W. and Chang, J. K.
    1976   The role of Chinese medicine in New York City's Chinatown. American J. of
           Chinese Medicine 4: 31–45, 129–146.

Chen, P. S.
1937 The History of Chinese Medicine. Shanghai: Commercial Press (In Chinese).
Foucault, M.
1965 Madness and Civilization; A History of Insanity in the Age of Reason. Translated by Richard Howard. New York: Vintage.
Huang-ti nei-ching Su-wen
1949 (The Yellow Emperor's Classic of Internal Medicine; Elementary Questions). Translated by I. Veith. Baltimore: Williams & Wilkins.
Hsu, T. S.
1934 The History of Taoism. Shanghai: Commercial Press (In Chinese).
Hsu, J.
1975 Counseling in the Chinese temple: Psychological study of divination by *ch'ien* drawing. *In* Culture-Bound Syndromes, Ethnopsychiatry, and Alternative Therapy. Vol. IV of Mental Health Research in Asia and the Pacific. W. P. Lebra, ed. Honolulu: University Press of Hawaii.
Kleinman, A. M.
1975 The Symbolic context of Chinese medicine. A comparative approach to the study of traditional medical and psychiatric forms of care in Chinese culture. American J. of Chinese Medicine 3:103–124.
Kleinman, A.
1979 Patients and Healers in the Context of Culture. Berkeley: University of California Press.
Kleinman, A. et al., eds.
1975 Medicine in Chinese Culture. Washington, D.C.: U.S. Government Printing Office for Fogarty International Center, N.I.H.
Kleinman, A. et al., eds.
1978 Culture and Healing in Asian Societies: Anthropological, Psychiatric and Public Health Studies. Cambridge, Massachusetts: Schenkman.
Li, M. E.
mimeographed report Mental Illness in China: A Window for Cultural Change.
Lu, G. D., and Needham, J.
1976 Records of disease in ancient China. American J. of Chinese Medicine 4: 3–16.
Nan-Tung City Chinese Medical College
1959 Introductory Lectures of Chinese Medicine. Nanking: People's Publishing Company (In Chinese).
Porkert, Manfred
1974 The Theoretical Foundations of Chinese Medicine: Systems of Correspondence. Cambridge, Massachusetts: The MIT Press.
Porkert, Manfred
1976 The intellectual and social impulses behind the evolution of traditional Chinese medicine. *In* Asian Medical Systems, Leslie, C., ed. Berkeley: University of California Press; pp. 63–76.
Temkin, O.
1973 Galenism, Rise and Decline of a Medical Philosophy. Ithaca: Cornell U. Press.
Topley, M.
1976 Chinese traditional etiology and methods of cure in Hong Kong. *In* Asian Medical Systems, Leslie, C., ed. Berkeley: University of California Press; pp. 243–265.
Tseng, W. S.
1972 Psychiatric study of shamanism in Taiwan. Arch. Gen. Psychiatry 26: 561–865.
Tseng, W. S.
1973 The development of psychiatric concepts in traditional Chinese medicine. Arch. Gen. Psychiatry 29: 569–575.

Tseng, W. S.
    1975 The nature of somatic complaints among psychiatric patients: The Chinese case.
          Comprehensive Psychiatry 16: 237–245.
Veith, I.
    1975 The Far East, reflections on the psychological foundations. *In* World History of
          Psychiatry, Howell, J. G., ed. New York: Brunner/Mazel; pp. 662–703.
Westermeyer, J.
    (in press) Folk concept of mental disorder among the Lao: Continuities with similar con-
          cepts in other cultures and in psychiatry. Culture, Medicine and Psychiatry.
Wong, K. C., and Wu, L. T.
    1936 History of Chinese Medicine: Being a Chronicle of Medical Happenings in China
          from Ancient Times to the Present Period. Shanghai: National Quarantine Service.
Yan, H. and Xu, S.
    mimeographed report Traditional Chinese Medicine and Psychiatry. Shanghai Psychiatric
          Hospital.
Yeh, E. K.
    1972 The Chinese mind and human freedom. The International Journal of Social
          Psychiatry 18: 132–136.

GLOSSARY OF SELECTED TERMS

Romanization	Definition	Character
Huang-ti nei-ching	Yellow Emperor's Classic of Internal Medicine	黃帝內經
Su-wen	Elementary Questions	素問
Ling-shu	Divine Pivot	靈樞
Shang-han lun	Treatise on Ailments Caused by Cold	傷寒論
Chin-kuei yao-lüeh	Golden Box Summary	金櫃要略
t'ien-jen hsiang-ying	microcosm-macrocosm correspondence	天人相應
t'iao-ho	balance, harmony	調和
yin-yang	male and female forces	陰陽
ching-lo	meridian system	經絡
feng	wind	風
han	coldness	寒
shu	hotness	暑
shih	dampness	濕
tsao	dryness	燥
huo	fire	火
wu-hsing	Five Evolutive Phases, Five Elements	五行
chih-hua	rule regulating change	制化
ch'i	vital energy	氣
hsüeh	blood	血
ying	constructive energy	營
wei	defensive energy	衛
chin	bodily fluid	津
i	secretion	液
ching	essense of energy	精
shen	spirit or mind	神
yüan-ch'i	fundamental energy	元氣
ch'i-kung	phase energetics; exercise of the *ch'i*	氣功
lien-ch'i	mental exercise; exercise of the *ch'i*	練氣
k'ai-hsin	happiness; "opening heart"	開心

Romanization	Definition	Character
tan-ch'ieh	fearfulness; "cowardly gallbladder"	胆怯
shen-k'uei	kidney insufficiency or weakness	腎虧
tien-k'uang	craziness	顛狂
hsien	seizure	癇
feng	craziness, madness	瘋
feng-tien	craziness	瘋顛
feng-k'uang	craziness	瘋狂
t'ien-kan	celestial stems	天干
ti-chih	terrestrial branches	地支
tâng-ki (Taiwanese)	shaman	童乩
ch'ien-wang	"directing the dead" (spirit mediumship)	牽亡
ch'ien	a lot for divination	籤
wu-i	"witch doctor," or shaman	巫醫
i	doctor (or to heal or cure)	醫
ching-shen ko	psychiatry	精神科
ching-shen	mental functions	精神
i-ping	"deceiving sickness"; hysteria	癔病

SECTION II

CHILD DEVELOPMENT AND
CHILDHOOD PSYCHOPATHOLOGY

INTRODUCTION TO SECTION II

In this section the perennial question of how culture affects child development and child psychopathology is examined by three contributors. Wilson looks at the socialization of children to become Chinese in terms of their moral development. First, he reviews the two major approaches to the study of moral development, and then he sets out his own theoretical model of this core socialization process. This provides a framework for Wilson to analyze moral development among Chinese and compare it with moral development in other culture groups. The upshot is a refreshing examination of well-known psycho-cultural dimensions of Chinese society (e.g., the importance of learning moral rules that emphasize conformity to and unity with both large-scale culture-wide and small-scale social network-wide groups; and undergoing affective manipulation and role training that reaffirm these norms and monitor behavioral response to them). Wilson's highly original approach to old themes is nowhere better seen than in his persuasive discussion of why social deviance is so threatening for Chinese and in his well-documented argument that there is a higher degree of internalization of behavioral norms among Chinese than among Americans, a notion which is calculated to upset long-held views on the consequences of modernization for psychological development. Readers also are given an opportunity to review some of the empirical findings from Wilson's field research that support his analytic framework. The editors believe that this article advances our understanding of how Chinese cultural categories and norms affect children, the socialization process, and reactions to social deviance including mental illness, and that it infuses new blood into a subject that has languished under the long-term influence of outmoded personality theories and sinological obscurantism.

Ho's article is an attempt to accurately present the conflict between relativist and universalist perspectives in clinical psychology and psychiatry when applied to the understanding of childhood psychopathology among Chinese. Some readers may share the editors' experience of recognizing aspects of their own work in both protagonists, Dr. Relativist and Dr. Universalist. In the course of playing out this archetypal dialogue, Ho reviews the limited evidence about what are universal and culture-specific features of child psychopathology, along with conflicting interpretations concerning its nature and determinants among Chinese. Just as the author does not attempt to resolve the conflict, if it is resolvable, so too readers are likely to come away with a better appreciation of the strengths and weaknesses on each side and, more importantly, of the potential for bridging certain features of both perspectives, testing discrepant

A. Kleinman and T.-Y. Lin (eds.), Normal and Abnormal Behavior in Chinese Culture, 115–116.
Copyright © 1980 *by D. Reidel Publishing Company.*

hypotheses, and moving ahead to a more discriminating and informed discourse for assessing this subject.

In the last contribution to this section, Soong and Soong review sex differences in school adjustment in Taiwan. Their findings reveal that, though boys are clearly privileged in Taiwan, they have more problems in school adjustment than girls. The authors review the major difficulties boys experience in Taiwan's educational system and relate these to both traditional and contemporary stresses to which Chinese culture subjects them to a greater degree than girls. In addition to discussing educational and family pressures on students, the authors also briefly review the development of child mental health services in Taiwan, cite some of the clinical and research studies that have emerged from these services, and make a few recommendations for improving mental health aspects of Taiwan's educational system. Their article covers only one component of a much broader subject. We need many more empirical studies of the socialization of learning in Chinese families, social networks, and schools if we are to understand how Chinese acquire cultural attitudes and values about educational and job performance, household work, and learning generally. We also require further studies that examine, as in the Soongs' chapter, maladaptive effects of traditional and contemporary forms of social control applied to learning, such as corporal punishment and shaming techniques. To what extent do current educational practices represent a carryover from times when education was limited to formal tutoring in the classics? What are the positive and negative consequences of these practices on the individual child's cognitive, emotional and personality development? What are the psychological consequences of poor school performance or failure? What is the status of learning disorders among Chinese? These and many more issues that are important for understanding child development have yet to be examined to any significant degree for Chinese.

Whereas there is a literature on childhood in Chinese society, albeit scientifically limited and usually consisting of personal accounts, very little has been written about abnormality and deviance. It is our belief that these articles review the basic questions and point to the many areas where better theories, more data, and more powerful methods are required to adequately research this subject. Notwithstanding this early stage of development, these three articles already represent an advance in the way investigators are conceptualizing the critical issues and operationalizing their researchable components. This should rapidly become apparent to readers whose interest leads them to review the literature reviewed by these contributors. The editors regard this subject as absolutely crucial to the development of our knowledge about normal and abnormal behavior in Chinese culture, and believe that it is essential that systematic research investigation rigorously address the important questions raised in these articles.

RICHARD W. WILSON

7. CONFORMITY AND DEVIANCE REGARDING MORAL RULES IN CHINESE SOCIETY: A SOCIALIZATION PERSPECTIVE

Why some people come to hold socially approved values and why others, consciously or unconsciously, choose in some degree to violate these values are questions addressed by scholars of both moral development and deviance. These queries are often posed in a framework that includes analysis of the learning process, that is, how the individual or group came to acquire the particular dispositions that are the subject of examination. As such, analyses of this type are one part of the general study of socialization, broadly defined.

It is the purpose of this paper to examine aspects of the Chinese learning process and attempt to uncover dynamics that may help explain patterns of conformity or deviance with regard to moral rules. In order to do this I shall initially and briefly set forth current alternate theories in the field of moral development and suggest the attributes of an integrative moral development model. In subsequent sections I will then examine the relationship between Chinese socialization practices and moral development, and, finally, the relationship between Chinese socialization practices and deviance. This exposition, while necessarily somewhat abstract, will hopefully be logically compelling.

CURRENT THEORIES IN THE FIELD OF MORAL DEVELOPMENT

Mature moral judgment requires cognitive maturation and is characterized by the internalization of certain value orientations, especially those that relate to interpersonal relations. There is a corollary assumption that the values underlying mature moral judgment are usually learned during childhood socialization and derive from specific norms and more ultimate values of the social system. In seeking to understand moral development, therefore, what we examine are both the social rules themselves, their form and content as guides and as ends for behavior, and the socialization process whereby these rules are transmitted to new generations. We also analyze socialization as an experience whereby values are internalized, and ask to what degree and in what sequence this occurs. Such analysis entails inquiry concerning the nature of the relationship between this type of socialization and other characteristics of learning including, as one aspect, awareness of the child's cognitive capability at any given age to understand the meanings within value statements, especially their abstract qualities, and to understand toward whom these values apply.

Although moral development studies are clearly only one small part of the now voluminous literature that exists in the general area of socialization, they have one special characteristic that distinguishes them. While the studies differ from one another in terms of which learning features are of most importance,

117

A. Kleinman and T.-Y. Lin (eds.), Normal and Abnormal Behavior in Chinese Culture, 117–136.
Copyright © 1980 by D. Reidel Publishing Company.

the major and central emphasis in all such works is on the ways children, over time, slowly acquire internalized structures of control over behavior.

Although it is possible to construct a relatively detailed definition of moral judgment and behavior, the most appropriate one for the purpose of this paper defines mature moral judgments as more complex cognitively and more internalized than immature judgments and mature moral behavior as that which is guided by a mature moral judgment capability (Weinreich 1975). This definition is especially useful as it is at a high enough level of abstraction to be applicable for moral development approaches that place primary emphasis on either cognitive restructuring or the influence of social variables.

Moral development studies can be loosely divided between those which adhere to a social learning paradigm and those which utilize a cognitive development model. Cognitive development theorists (best exemplified by the works of Lawrence Kohlberg) discuss how children's internal judgmental capability develops with cognitive maturation in a universal pattern from an initially self-centered and strictly rule-abiding stage (egocentricism) to later stages characterized by internalized responses to events and by reciprocity among individuals (autonomy) (Bloom 1974; Gibbs 1977; Kohlberg 1964, 1969a, 1971a, 1971b, 1976; Piaget 1962; Turiel 1966, 1969). For social learning theorists, on the other hand, the norms of particular societies and the structure of the socialization environment, broadly defined, are major concerns (Aronfreed 1968; Bandura and Walters 1963; Berkowitz 1964; Bronfenbrenner 1962; Hoffman 1970a, 1970b; Maccoby 1968; Sears, Rau and Alpert 1965; Skinner 1971; Whiting and Child 1953; Wilson 1974, 1976). Social learning theorists seek to understand how culturally idiosyncratic normative structures and patterns of rewards and punishments are related to the development of particular types of moral reasoning and behavior.

Social learning theorists and cognitive development theorists differ in the degree of importance granted to external events as antecedents for the learning of moral rules. Cognitive development theorists are not unmindful of punishments and rewards and, indeed, are particularly concerned with role playing as it may help to develop mature moral judgment. Beyond such social influences, however, they feel that the brain undergoes a critical and preeminently important progressive capacity in the maturation process to integrate and logically order information. Since acquiring moral judgment involves the progressive learning of complex value abstractions, cognitive development theorists have posited culturally invariant stage development models where the learning of moral rules by children takes place consonant with the restructuring of cognitive capability.

Social learning theorists, on the other hand, while not unmindful of the importance of cognitive restructuring, feel that the learning of moral rules is not a process that is culturally invariant but is, rather, critically related to particular learning environments and to the distinctive normative code of the society in question. For them the major influences on moral development are what B. F.

Skinner calls "contingencies of reinforcement" and they look to these contingencies as culturally variable factors that explain why different peoples acquire different types of moral orientations (1971).

At the present time, there is no resolution in the field of moral development between the cognitive development and social learning approaches. While Lawrence Kohlberg and his associates in the cognitive development school are perhaps more widely known, their views are nevertheless vigorously challenged and debated and evidence favoring one approach over another is not clearcut for either side. Empirical studies, some based on Kohlberg's stage development model, indicate that different social systems do indeed have different moral orientations; still, Kohlberg and his associates have produced evidence from a number of societies indicating that the sequence in which moral learning takes place is invariant in nature (1964, 1969a and 1969b).

In the dispute between the two moral development schools implications for definitions of deviance are also revealed. For social learning theorists moral behavior results from acting in accordance with internalized normative standards. To the extent that this behavior is in accordance with relevant values from the society's normative structure or ideology, behavior is then not deviant. For cognitive development theorists, on the other hand, behavior in terms of society's rules is at a lower moral stage than behavior which is independent of these rules in the sense that at higher moral stages behavior is in terms of autonomously derived principles rather than any specific body of norms. As a consequence, although one may not be deviant from society's standpoint one may be deviant in terms of some presumably higher order set of principles.

Regardless of the school of moral development, little effort has been made by theorists in this area to discuss deviance. Questions regarding how deviance is defined in a particular social context, how and why some individuals or subgroups are labeled as deviant, how deviance is dealt with by agents of social control, what the relationship of deviance and its labeling is to the central belief sytem of the society in which it occurs are queries that are often addressed at a sociological level of analysis rather than at the more restricted psychological level of analysis of most moral development studies (Wilson, Greenblatt and Wilson 1977). As a consequence, although moral development and deviance studies would seem from a common sense standpoint to be inextricably linked, there is at present a hiatus between them. I believe that this hiatus can best be bridged through a re-definition of moral development and by subsequent examination of both moral development and deviance in terms of the general socialization process.

AN INTEGRATIVE MORAL DEVELOPMENT MODEL

In a recent study that attempted to bridge the gap between the social learning and cognitive development schools, a model of moral development was set forth that sought to integrate certain features from both schools (see Figure 1)

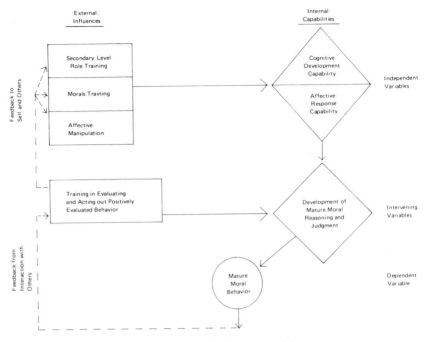

Fig. 1. Moral development model.

(Wilson 1978). In this model cognitive development is assumed to be a necessary condition for the development of mature morality; it is not, however, considered to be a sufficient condition. In terms of personality characteristics it is assumed that along with the individual's capacity for cognitive development there must also be a capability for affective response and that this affective response capability is a crucial factor in that it explains the motivation for behaving in terms of certain valued ends. To the extent that highly valued social ends become learned and become invested with a quality of good or bad, they also become aspects of a person's self-esteem. When behaving in terms of values the individual's self-esteem is also activated and in the attempt to maintain or enhance self-esteem, powerful feelings are generated. The assumption is that cognitive development alone will not provide the motivation to stimulate certain types of moral judgments and responses. Only cognition and affect together can provide both a directive and dynamic quality to behavior. Although analytically separable, therefore, cognitive development and affective response are inseparably involved in moral judgment and behavior. These two types of capabilities are not randomly stimulated, however. They are activated with regard to particular values and particular means to realize these values as the result of a culturally idiosyncratic learning process which is composed of three analytically distinct but in practice interrelated learning influences.

The first of these learning influences is affective manipulation. For instance, children (or other learners) will receive some type of positive reinforcement for judgments and actions that conform with desired moral ends. Positive reinforcements can take a number of forms but the most common are praise, nurturant tactile contact, and the giving of certain kinds of material rewards such as food or prizes. In addition to positive reinforcements, children are also subjected to various types of punishment. These may vary from aversive physical expressions, such as slapping, spanking, or pinching (which are usually more effective in suppressing undesirable behavior than in developing desired behavior), to punishment methods that fall into a large category known as love-oriented techniques of discipline. In this latter form of punishment the aversive content is not physical in nature but emotional. The child is subjected to loss of approval by important authority figures, such as the mother or the father, or to shaming or ridicule by group members. A third form of punishment, sometimes but not always thought of as a sub-category of love-oriented techniques of discipline, is induction training where the child is "induced" to experience the unhappy feelings which his socially inappropriate actions may cause in others. By this technique of training it is thought that children slowly acquire an understanding of the ramifications of their actions for others and thereby gradually internalize rules that will guide future conduct.

The second influence is morals training. Standards for moral behavior may be acquired in two analytically distinct ways (Dawson and Prewitt 1969). In the first place there may be structured learning, particularly in formal education, in which learners are brought together and are introduced systematically to socially appropriate goals and to sanctioned types of behavior. The obvious form of such learning in American society is Sunday school training, but other examples, applicable for many other societies, include civics instruction, some kinds of television programs and the content of books. Of perhaps equal importance is training that is more random in nature. In this latter learning context children are introduced to normative requirements in a more haphazard way; introduction to moral injunctions is but an intermittent aspect of interaction with others during the growth process. For instance, in peer interaction or in interaction with parents or with other authority figures injunctions may be very informally transmitted to children concerning what goals they ought to prefer and what means they should use to achieve these goals. Although most modern societies require that children receive some type of formal morals training, it is undoubtedly true that many important aspects of moral learning also take place in unstructured daily activities.

The third influence, and one which is essential for learning that moral responses may apply to unknown others, is secondary level role training. In this type of training the child is taught that moral behavior is applicable towards persons of whom the child has no knowledge, i.e., to people at the secondary social level. Only by experiencing this particular learning influence, which cannot occur without a developed capability for abstract reasoning, does the child come to realize that moral rules apply beyond specifically known others and beyond defined contexts. The specific effect of this influence is to foster the internalization of moral rules through stress in learning that these rules are relevant for unknown others and cannot be situationally activated as the result of interaction with known others in familiar contexts.

Lastly, of course, the child must also be encouraged to act out moral judgments that are considered appropriate and to have the opportunity to evaluate this behavior in terms of the moral rules that have previously been acquired. As an example, an important aspect of learning involves copying the actions of others. It would appear that children spontaneously engage in modeling behavior and to the extent that this behavior can be characterized as a pattern of set procedures relevant toward certain ends we call it role playing. For instance, the small child playing at being a mailman or at being a nurse is engaged in specific kinds of role playing. Playing certain kinds of roles may introduce children to moral rules. Playing at being a mother or father, for instance, or at being a policeman may involve play-acting within situations where relationships between individuals are governed by explicit normative require- ments. In role playing, therefore, the child may be exposed to a training process involving acting out the ways in which moral rules apply in given social contexts. Such training gives the child the opportunity to evaluate actual behavior against moral judgments and to assess through practice the relevance of particular actions for obtaining moral ends.

CHINESE SOCIALIZATION PRACTICES AND MORAL DEVELOPMENT

If the integrative model developed above is used as a framework for examining Chinese socialization practices, it is then possible to highlight certain significant aspects of moral development in that society. Turning first to affective manip- ulation, it would appear that the most powerful source of emotion within Chinese socialization emanates from the overpowering influence of the mother as both a source of dependency feelings and as the agent of socialization who has the largest impact on the child in shaming (or punishment) situations. Much attention has been focused in studies of Chinese socialization on the relationship of the child with the father (Pye 1968; Solomon 1971). This, I believe, is essentially an error, not because the influence of the father is unimportant, which is not the case, but because his influence as a primary agent of socializa- tion is essentially secondary to that of the mother. In Chinese families the mother is preeminently involved with the giving of affect, while fathers are generally thought of as rule enforcers. This, of course, is a gross oversimplifica- tion of overlapping roles, but it seems quite plausible that the emotionally heightened attention that is focused on proper conduct in the Chinese learning process has its origin in a highly affectively-charged relationship with a very powerful, and at the same time nurturant, maternal figure. The father does not fill this nurturant role to anywhere near the same degree. Indeed, it is primarily the mother who in caring for the bodily needs of her children and also in establishing a generalized goal of pleasing her, creates a personality predisposition such that subsequent interaction by the child with others is linked to the early acquired desire to obtain the mother's approval and approbation. Although physical forms of punishment are obviously not unknown, the most powerful techniques used by mothers are generally love-oriented ones. Frequently the use of these techniques is quite unknown to the mothers themselves. They, for instance, are usually not familiar with the fact that in seeking behavioral conformity by their children they will use such emotionally-laden terms as "if you do that, I will not love you." Phrases such as this, I believe, develop anxieties in Chinese children with regard to interpersonal relations in which fear of loss of affection or of approval from significant others is highly accentuated. One way to reduce the tension that derives from these anxieties is to structure behavior in accordance with explicit precepts. In this regard, fathers as models are extraordinarily important, for they ideally act as guides for that type of proper behavior that will secure approval from important others and help avoid anxiety about potential shaming.

When a child enters school these patterns of affective manipulation are continued and, if anything, intensified. While teachers to some extent take over the roles of the mother and, to a lesser extent, the father, the major source of anxiety during the school years is transferred from household authority figures to the school group itself. The greatest source of anxiety during this period is not loss of approval by the principal or teacher (although these are important) but loss of approval by one's peer group, and this threat of generalized social opprobrium is consciously manipulated by teachers. For instance, children who make errors may be required to stand at their seats for a period of time. Bad marks on quizzes may be publicly noted by posting a different color to differentiate children in this category from those with passing grades. Activities are structured in group terms such that the child begins to develop a notion of the group as the ultimate source of approval or rejection for behavior (Wilson 1970).

Regardless of whether we look at schools in the People's Republic of China, in Taiwan, or in Hong Kong, morals training of a type not seen in American schools for fifty years is a noticeable aspect of the learning environment. This morals training is at times highly specific with stories in reading texts consciously constructed to elucidate moral rules. For instance, in an elementary level text book used on Taiwan there is a story of a small goose who flies away from the rest of the flock (*Kuo-li Pien I Kuan* 1964). Twice the small goose does this and twice other members of the flock fly after him to attempt to persuade the small goose to return. The third time that the small goose departs, however, a hawk spies and seizes him. The admonitions given by other members of the flock to the small goose during this story contain injunctions such as, "such wild flying is not permitted," "you must follow the rules of the group," "being with the group is most important," and, of course, the tragic ending is designed to provide confirmation that departing from group rules and norms is highly undesirable and dangerous. However, stories such as this one are not simply childhood parables. When the official in charge of compiling these textbook tales was queried concerning the story of the small goose, he replied that this parable had been deliberately chosen since the formation that geese fly in is roughly the same as the Chinese character for people. In class, therefore, the teacher could use this character as a simple device to bring the story of the small goose into a human context and thus impress upon the children the importance of proper group behavior.

In visits to schools in the People's Republic of China in 1978, skits prepared by children for the visitors also exhibited emphasis on the desirability of group solidarity, conformity and loyalty. For instance, in a kindergarden in Canton, a puppet show was put on by the children in which an industrious bee working hard for the group was counterpoised to a beautiful fly whose true identity, however, was early signaled by the rasping manner of his "speech." As the show unfolded it was revealed that, although the fly might be lovely to look at, in fact his attitude toward work for the group was bad. As a result, the fly was ultimately labeled as a "bad element" that must be reformed. In a primary school in Shanghai, a performance put on by first to third graders concerned a small lamb (played by a girl) looking for friends. One after the other the lamb rejected the rabbit, rooster, horse, etc., as not fit for her friendship. When the rooster invited her to do physical labor, she haughtily declined. The other "animals" all appeared worried about her. Finally, the little lamb was approached by a wolf who enticed her by placing a wreath of flowers around her neck. Eventually, however, the wolf was exposed; the other animals united to fight the wolf who was beaten to death. At the end of the play, the lamb returned to the fold of the good animals. In this play group solidarity was heavily stressed, individual haughtiness was condemned, cooperation was praised, and stress was placed on being ever alert to determine genuine from fake behavior, on clearly differentiating enemies from friends. Again, at a kindergarden in Shanghai, a skit performed by children aged five and six concerned the tending of ducks by two small girls. While the two girls were telling each other stories, one duck ran away and, when the children went to find the missing duck, yet another then left the group. The ending, however, was predictably happy. Both missing ducks were found and returned and, in the finale, the group was shown as intact and all the ducks were happily being tended by the two little girls. The moral lessons intended to be imparted to the children were set forth by the adults who were present. First was the emphasis on group solidarity; second, the stress on helping others (elders in the production team) by tending the ducks; and third, the importance of being responsible and brave and fearing no difficulties.

In coming to school, the child has already taken one large step in terms of learning about behavior in various group contexts. From experiences that are largely within a nuclear family the child abruptly becomes a member of a school, and, in particular, a member of a class. In the early school years morals training sets forth precepts that initially describe behavior that is optimal within a small group context. As the years pass, however, stories with moral content take a more impartial stance with regard to the targets for moral behavior. For instance, stories which in first or second grade have their focus within a family or small classroom context begin, by fifth or sixth grade, to stress citizenship behavior which is applicable at the secondary level for society as a whole. The moral precepts that are stressed, of course, may, in fact, be very much the same. Take, as an example, loyalty. Loyalty is stressed in the early years of schooling as a fundamental virtue in group behavior. The child learns that in his classroom, as in his family, loyalty is an essential attribute. By the time the child has reached fifth or sixth grade, however, he learns that this loyalty should also be manifested as a citizen for society as a whole. In other words, there is a very conscious effort in current Chinese socialization practices for highly stressed moral values to be raised from an initial focus that is largely directed toward other primary group members to a focus toward other secondary group members who are mainly unknown. To date, however, the largest secondary level group which is normally stressed is that of the society or nation, of Chinese taken as a whole, and does not extend to an international context. It should also be noted that while most other members at the secondary level may be unknown the name of the group itself is very explicitly known. Children are encouraged to develop a self perspective with regard to a particular group (such as a school, for instance) rather than with friendship groupings or other amorphous bodies which do not have a formal structure.

Chinese children are expected to carry out in practice the precepts that they learn. Thus, for instance, a child in Taiwan may be appointed to oversee smaller children on their way home from school. In carrying out this responsibility the older child is expected to behave in such a manner that moral precepts concerning proper leadership are punctiliously followed. Should they not be, it is further expected that the older child will report back to his or her group and will proclaim a greater effort in the future to carry out such assignments in the appropriate manner.

Several years ago, a comparative study was made of the socialization of Chinese children in Taiwan, Hong Kong, Chinatown (New York City) and of Caucasian and Negro children in New Jersey. This study of third, fifth and seventh graders, divided equally between both sexes, involved long hours of observation in each locale, the use of a variety of written questionnaires with many hundreds of children, and selected interviews with a smaller sample from each area (Wilson 1974). Part of the tests included showing the children six large posters divided into three sets of two posters each. In the first set, one poster depicted a situation where a child is being punished by a father alone and the other a situation where the child is being punished by the teacher in front of his classmates. The children were asked to judge both situations and determine which they thought would be the worst way to be punished. In the second set, the first poster shows a speaker on a platform being questioned by individuals from a large audience; in the second poster the speaker is shown being questioned by two people alone in an empty auditorium. For this set the children were

asked which of the two situations would be most agreeable for them in expressing disagreement to a speaker. In the last set, the children were shown two
posters each depicting a group of young people. In the first poster, the young
people are all dressed similarly and in the second poster the young people are
shown dressed in varied types of clothing. In this case, the children were asked
which group they would prefer to join. Significant statistical differences (.05
level or better) were indicated for the first and third sets using an analysis of
variance technique. The results of these tests are summarized in Figure 2 (Wilson
1974: 151–155, 172–174, 191–196).

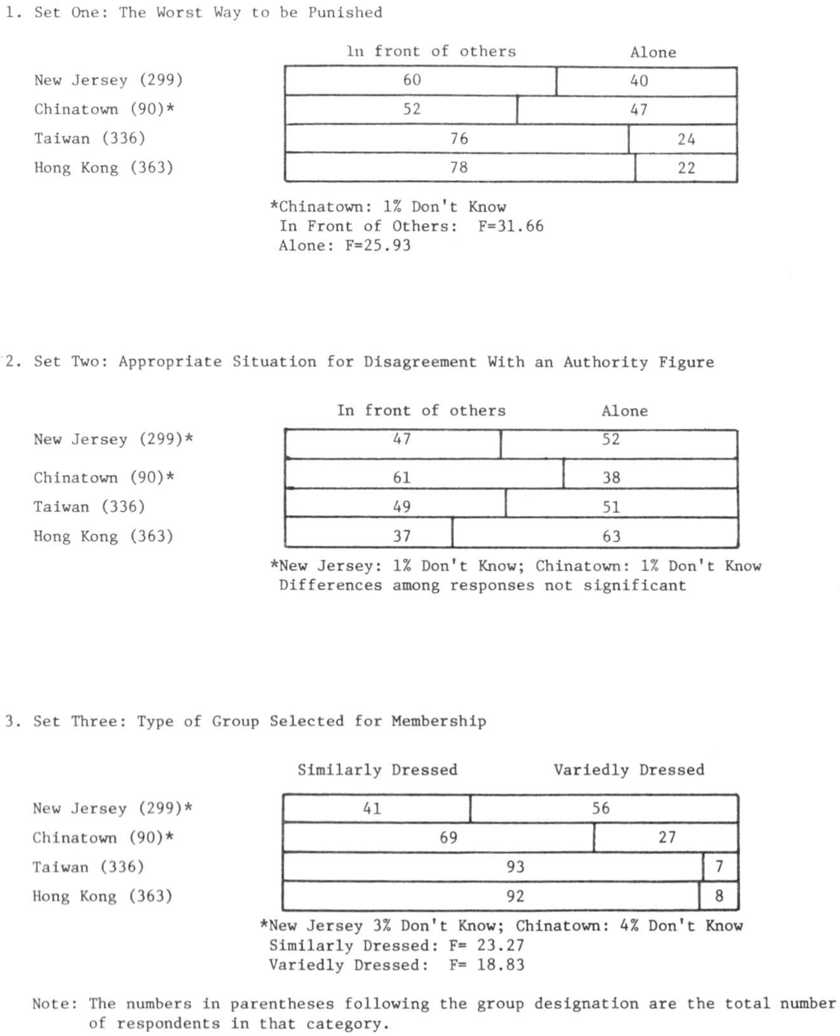

1. Set One: The Worst Way to be Punished

	In front of others	Alone
New Jersey (299)	60	40
Chinatown (90)*	52	47
Taiwan (336)	76	24
Hong Kong (363)	78	22

*Chinatown: 1% Don't Know
In Front of Others: F=31.66
Alone: F=25.93

2. Set Two: Appropriate Situation for Disagreement With an Authority Figure

	In front of others	Alone
New Jersey (299)*	47	52
Chinatown (90)*	61	38
Taiwan (336)	49	51
Hong Kong (363)	37	63

*New Jersey: 1% Don't Know; Chinatown: 1% Don't Know
Differences among responses not significant

3. Set Three: Type of Group Selected for Membership

	Similarly Dressed	Variedly Dressed
New Jersey (299)*	41	56
Chinatown (90)*	69	27
Taiwan (336)	93	7
Hong Kong (363)	92	8

*New Jersey 3% Don't Know; Chinatown: 4% Don't Know
Similarly Dressed: F= 23.27
Variedly Dressed: F= 18.83

Note: The numbers in parentheses following the group designation are the total number
    of respondents in that category.

Fig. 2. Responses to poster situations: percent.

Although no significant differences among the groups were found on the poster questionnaire for set two (concerning whether questioning an authority figure before a group or alone is most appropriate), interview data using this set suggests that questioning authority figures (and the group as a whole) is much more difficult for Chinese than for American children. Figure 3 summarizes

	New Jersey (18)	Chinatown (6)	Taiwan (18)	Hong Kong (18)
1. Regarding the Permissibility of Making an Authority Figure Lose Face				
Should not lose face	33	67	100	50
Can lose face	67	0	0	17
No indication	0	33	0	33
2. Regarding Whether One Can Disagree with an Authority Figure				
Can disagree	61	100	72	61
Cannot disagree	0	0	28	33
No indication	39	0	0	6
3. Regarding Whether One Can Openly Argue with an Authority Figure				
Can Openly argue	83	33	17	22
Cannot openly argue	17	67	83	78
No indication	0	0	0	0
4. Regarding Whether One Can Go against the Group				
Can go against the group	72	50	17	33
Should not go against the group	28	50	83	67
No indication	0	0	0	0

Note:The numbers in parentheses under the group designation are the total number of interview respondents in that category.

Fig. 3. Expressions regarding opposition to authority figures and groups: percent.

interview responses to questions concerning disagreement with authority figures and groups (Wilson 1974: 171, 172, 196). Although this analysis is somewhat subjective, the great dissimilarities in response patterns appear to reveal definite cultural differences. The data appear to support a conclusion that punishment by group sanctions is early, intensely and increasingly feared by Chinese children, that conformity in group behavior is rewarded and is related to positively stressed values of unity and organization and that opposition to either the group or its authorities is viewed as threatening. For the children from New Jersey, on the other hand, while group sanctions are certainly feared, the threat seems less pervasive and both authority figures and groups are seen as challengeable.

Morever, diversity among group members is seen as positively desirable although, paradoxically, this value may be related to obtaining group approval.

Although in the context of a paper it is difficult to set forth full documentation concerning how particular socialization practices lead to certain kinds of moral outcomes, the results of a test of Chinese and American children of the degree to which values are internalized as guides for behavior is revealing (Wilson 1974). In summarizing the responses it was found that children from Taiwan and Hong Kong tended to behave in terms of internalized standards to a far greater degree than did children from Chinatown (New York City) or Caucasian and Negro children from New Jersey. The results of these findings are summarized below by location and by grade levels — three, five and seven — (see Figure 4) (Wilson 1974: 243–244).

One interesting aspect of these findings concerns the social context in which

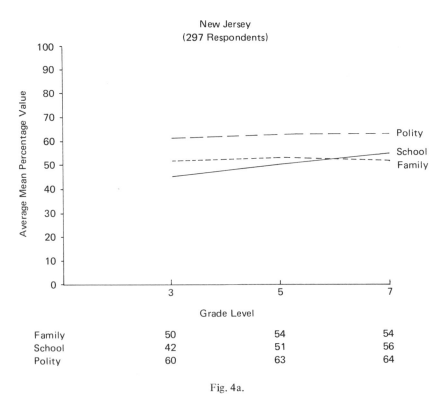

	3	5	7
Family	50	54	54
School	42	51	56
Polity	60	63	64

Fig. 4a.

Figs. 4a–d. Average Mean Percentage Values for Groups by Grade Level and Social Context for Responses Indicating Behavior in Terms of Internalized Standards. The average mean percentage values noted above were derived from a 20 item multiple choice questionnaire. Using an analysis of variance technique 11 questions showed significant differences (.05 level or better) among groups. The general pattern of responses was similar for all questions.

internalized values are most operative. For the two groups of children from America, behavior in terms of internalized standards is most apparent at the polity level, that is, for citizenship roles generally speaking. While behavior in terms of internalized standards in a family context was generally lowest for all four groups, it will be noticed for children from New Jersey that it is actually the school context which is lowest for grades three and five and this context only supersedes the family context by grade seven. In other words, I would conjecture that the kinds of learning influences which I have described for Chinese children and which apparently result in considerable internalization of values (and value uniformity among group members) are not as highly characteristic for Caucasian and Negro children in New Jersey. For children from Taiwan and Hong Kong, however, the case is markedly different and especially so for the children from Taiwan. There the school context remains highest regardless of age level. Since it is within that context that morals training is so rigorously carried out it is perhaps not strange to find that it is the same context where internalized standards are most operative with the polity context following. For children from Hong Kong the case is more mixed but even there the

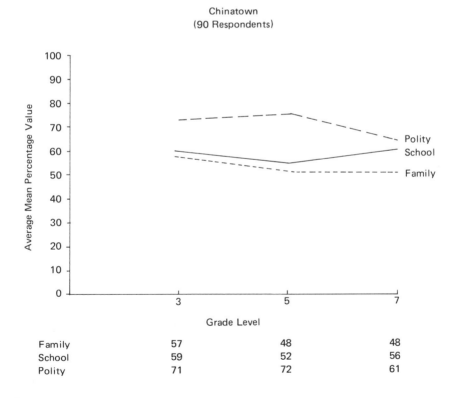

Chinatown
(90 Respondents)

	Grade Level		
	3	5	7
Family	57	48	48
School	59	52	56
Polity	71	72	61

Fig. 4b.

school becomes the primary area for behavior in terms of internalized standards by seventh grade. Unfortunately, these tests were not given to older children, nor were other types of social contexts tested for, so that the results presented here can only be preliminary and suggestive. The difference in magnitude of response among the groups as well as differences in terms of social contexts suggest, however, that powerful cultural influences are operative and that differences in degrees of internalization of normative requirements are due to different types of learning situations.

CHINESE SOCIALIZATION PRACTICES AND DEVIANCE

While clearly there is wide variety in Chinese childhood training patterns, there does appear, in general, to be a powerful manipulation of affect, a conscious effort to inculcate certain types of moral responses, and a deliberate effort to raise the level of social interaction at which these moral precepts are applicable to the secondary level. There is also considerable effort to clarify the moral criteria by which behavior will be evaluated and this clarification provides the

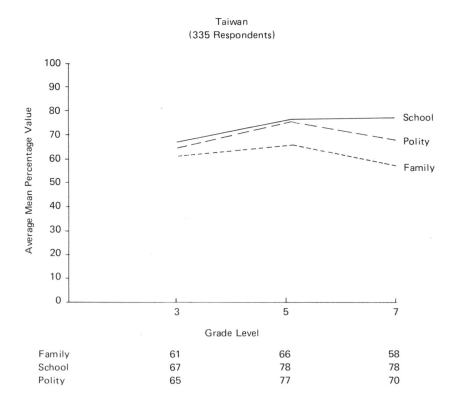

Fig. 4c.

basis for the labeling of deviance. Deviant behavior itself is seen as highly threatening since the actions of the deviant individual reflect back upon the group or groups of which he or she is a member. Since group unity is highly prized and heavily stressed, behavior which violates ideal group goals can cause shame for all other group members. As such, these deviant individuals and their errant behavior must be clearly labeled and efforts made both by the individual and other group members to transform this behavior.

Stuart Schram has stated that both Mao Tse-tung and the 19th century Chinese hero Tseng Kuo-fan both believed that "practical activity must be penetrated from beginning to end with moral values" (1963: 84) a feeling which, in my opinion, is one that is widely shared in Chinese culture as a whole. Since actions and thought are held to be closely linked, the learning of moral precepts is highly explicit and it is not conceivable that an individual will engage in objectionable actions without prior knowledge of the limits of acceptable behavior. Conformity to group patterns is a marked characteristic of Chinese social interaction, whether or not the behavior itself is actually felt by the individual to be desirable. Where efforts to restore the deviant individual to the

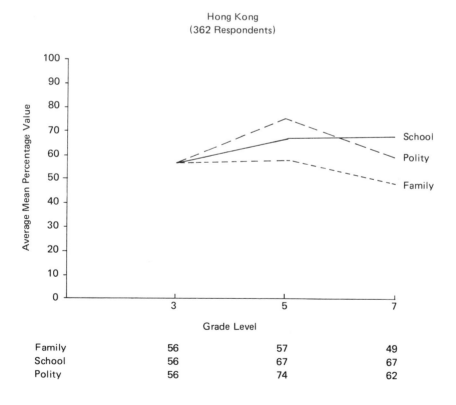

Hong Kong
(362 Respondents)

	3	5	7
Family	56	57	49
School	56	67	67
Polity	56	74	62

Fig. 4d.

group fail (by getting the individual to expunge undesirable behavior) then no recourse remains but to expel the individual from the group and subject him to several varying kinds of treatment. At best he may be simply ostracized and ignored, at worst his behavior will be labeled freakish and monsterish, of a type that does not characterize those who can call themselves humans, let alone group members. Either of these forms of treatment involve the affected individual with withdrawal of support from the group, withdrawal of affect, and abandonment. As such, the anxieties that are raised are linked with similar anxiety patterns that were developed early in the socialization process.

In a study of American and Soviet children, Bronfenbrenner found that the desire of American children for specific peer approval is sufficiently strong that, unlike Soviet children, they are more rather than less inclined to break adult norms if they know their peers are aware of their actions (1970). A finding such as this for Chinese children appears, on the face of it, inconceivable. While both Chinese and American children seek the approval of their peer group, these groups in the United States stand in a semi-autonomous relationship to the larger social setting in a manner that does not characterize Chinese social organization. If our argument concerning Chinese learning patterns is correct, proper behavior is ideally in terms of the largest social grouping of which one is a member. It is my belief that in Chinese socialization overall group unity and loyalty are values that are heavily stressed and are of greatest overall social significance when deliberately reinforced by the emotional impact of rewards and sanctions in small groups (although obviously, especially in traditional society, powerful countervailing pressures for primary loyalty to family, friends and colleagues exist). These values are almost always stated in a manner that is explicit in content, vertical in the sense that values applicable in the largest social setting should also be applicable in sub-settings, and closed in terms of alternatives. The explicit articulation of inclusive values appears to be a culturally-sanctioned technique for reducing anxiety and it is just this very stress which gives Chinese moral learning its heavily formalistic quality.

Conformity to group standards is based on adherence to internalized universalistic codes for behavior. Random expressions of hostility toward other group members or toward group leaders is muted by awareness of group sanctions, but opposition to authority is felt to be legitimate if moral standards have been violated. However, invoking these moral codes as justification for labeling another as deviant may not be sufficient if that other individual is an authority figure, for loyalty itself is considered a prime virtue, the violation of which, under normal circumstances, is justification for punishment by legitimate authority. As such, opposition to particular others, especially leaders, may appear muted or sporadic until some alternate authority figure has sanctioned this behavior. Once an individual has been authoritatively labeled as deviant, he will then have been deemed to have violated standards regarding conformism and unity and will thus achieve outgroup status. This, I suspect, is particularly the case in the People's Republic of China and in Taiwan where much effort has

been expended in the socialization of children in stressing the primacy of universalistic over particularistic moral criteria and where maintaining the form of a
relationship for the sake of the relationship itself is minimized as appropriate
social behavior.

The most severe label of deviance attaches to those individuals who are said
to have violated ideals of unity and loyalty. These values, and behavior in
accordance with them, are the *sine qua non* of inward acceptance of the group
and its leadership. To be found in violation of these values is tantamount to
being potentially lacking in virtue in all areas of behavior; moreover, if the
revelation of bad characteristics has been relatively sudden, the deviant individual may also be stigmatized as poisonous and cunning, a double-dealer as well
as a renegade. In political controversies, losers such as Liu Shao-ch'i, Lin Piao or
the Gang of Four have certainly been labeled as deviant in these terms. Indeed,
given the value orientations which lie behind such stigmatization, it is difficult to
see how such individuals could avoid being called "wolves in sheep's clothing"
and viewed as manifestations of every conceivable type of social evil.

While the general pattern of labeling deviant individuals in Chinese society
may not be unique, I do suggest that the strong pressures for group conformity
and the consequent strong pressures for behavior in terms of explicit moral
rules, make the status of deviance more anxiety provoking for the Chinese than
for members of societies where conformity and inclusive group membership are
less highly stressed. Although being labeled a deviant in the Chinese case may
clearly have no relationship whatsoever to the actual level of moral development
of the individual who is so labeled, the criteria for the label are artifacts of
socialization practices that are an aspect of moral development training.

CONCLUSION

In the material presented above a model of moral development was presented
which placed considerable stress on aspects of socialization regarding affective
manipulation, morals training, secondary level role learning, and role playing and
training. In presenting this model for the Chinese case evidence was set forth
showing how Chinese socialization practices place heavy emphasis on the learning of moral rules, on explicit affective manipulation, and on the group level
that children identify with. These learning-environment characteristics were then
hypothesized to be related to the degree to which children internalize values as
a basis for behavior. An interesting result was that data for Chinese children
indicated a higher degree of internalization than that for American children. I
infer that the reason for this is that the socialization process which Chinese
children experience places heavier emphasis on explicit moral development than
does the socialization process of American children. However, if Chinese
children develop a heightened ability to behave in terms of internalized
standards, the very process which encourages this outcome seems also to be one
that makes deviance from social rules frightening and the role of the deviant one

to be avoided if at all possible. No doubt high degrees of conformity are highly desirable in many social contexts. It would seem, however, that relative uniformity in behavioral response is bought for most Chinese at a price of considerable anxiety about deviant behavior and thus deprives society of random dissent which in other ways may have desirable social consequences.

Finally, if this essay has proved suggestive as a partial explanation for some important Chinese behavioral patterns, it may be useful to state briefly some practical applications and potential significance that stem from a focus on moral development in Chinese socialization. Whether we study Confucian or Marxist China, it is clear that the Chinese invoke moral values as guides and explanations for their behavior to a greater extent than is true for many other peoples. The question that has been too infrequently asked is why the Chinese feel the need to consciously invoke moral standards when discussing behavior and how the particular standards that are most frequently stated relate to patterns of interpersonal relationships and general social dynamics. Studies of socialization or, more narrowly, education, often appear sterile by their lack of an organizing focus around which questions and analysis may be framed. In contrast the study of moral development would appear to offer a powerful analytical framework for an understanding of the ways in which peoples acquire particular moral stances, with what intensity they are acquired, and what behaviors are sanctioned as legitimate ways to act out these value stances. As the remarks at the beginning of this paper indicate, however, work still needs to be done in the field of moral development *per se* in clarifying the potentially most powerful theoretical approaches. In this regard, data from non-Western societies and Chinese society in particular can help enrich this debate as well as provide further insights into Chinese culture itself.

REFERENCES

Aronfreed, J.
    1968 Conduct and Conscience: The Socialization of Internalized Control over Behavior.
          New York: Academic.
Bandura, A. and Walters, R. H.
    1963 Social Learning and Personality Development. New York: Holt, Rinehart and
          Winston.
Berkowitz, L.
    1964 Development of Motives and Values in a Child. New York: Basic Books.
Bloom, A.
    1974 Social Principledness and Social Humanism: A Cross Cultural Investigation into
          Dimensions of Politico-Moral Reasoning. Cambridge, Mass.: unpublished disserta-
          tion, Psychology and Social Relations Department, Harvard University.
Bronfenbrenner, U.
    1962 The role of age, sex, class and culture in studies of moral development. Religious
          Education 57 (4, Research Supplement): 3–17.
    1970 Two Worlds of Childhood: U.S. and U.S.S.R. New York: Russell Sage Foundation.
Dawson, R. E. and Prewitt, K.
    1969 Political Socialization. Boston: Little, Brown and Company.

Gibbs, J. C.
    1977 Kohlberg's stages of moral judgment: A constructive critique. Harvard Educational Review 47: 43–61.
Hoffman, M. L.
    1970a Conscience, personality, and socialization techniques. Human Development 13: 90–126.
    1970b Moral Development. P. H. Mussen, ed., Carmichael's Manual of Child Psychology (3rd ed.) Vol. 2. New York: Wiley.
Kohlberg, L.
    1964 Development of moral character and moral ideology. M. L. Hoffman and L. W. Hoffman, eds., Review of Child Development Research, vol. 1. New York: Russell Sage Foundation.
    1969a Stage and sequence: The cognitive developmental approach to socialization. D. A. Goslin, ed. Handbook of Socialization Theory and Research. Chicago: Rand McNally.
    1969b Development of children's orientations toward a moral order. R. C. Sprinthall and N. A. Sprinthall, eds. Educational Psychology. New York: Van Nostrand-Reinhold Co.
    1971a From is to ought: How to commit the naturalistic fallacy and get away with it. T. Mischel, ed. Cognitive Development and Epistemology. New York: Academic.
    1971b Stages of moral development as a basis for moral education. C. M. Beck, B. S. Crittenden and E. V. Sullivan, eds., Moral Educlation: Interdisciplinary Approaches. Toronto: University of Toronto Press.
    1976 Moral stages and moralization: The cognitive developmental approach. T. Lickona, ed., Moral Development and Behavior: Theory, Research and Social Issues. New York: Holt, Rinehart and Winston.
Kuo-li Pien I Kuan (National Compilation and Translation Office)
    1964 Kuo-yu K'e-pen (Mandarin Primer), Lower and Middle Grades, Book 5. Taiwan: Office of Education, Taiwan Provincial Government.
Maccoby, E. E.
    1968 The development of moral values and behavior in childhood. J. A. Clausen, ed. Socialization and Society. Boston: Little, Brown and Company.
Piaget, J.
    1962 The Moral Judgment of the Child. New York: Collier Books.
Pye, L. W.
    1968 The Spirit of Chinese Politics: A Psychocultural Study of the Authority Crisis in Political Development. Cambridge, Mass.: The M.I.T. Press.
Sears, R. R., Rau, L. and Alpert R.
    1965 Identification and Child Rearing. Stanford, Calif.: Stanford University Press.
Skinner, B. F.
    1971 Beyond Freedom and Dignity. New York: Knopf.
Schram, S. R.
    1963 Thought of Mao Tse-tung. New York: Praeger.
Solomon, R. H.
    1971 Mao's Revolution and the Chinese Political Culture, Berkeley, Calif.: University of California Press.
Turiel, E.
    1966 An experimental test of the sequentiality of developmental stages in the child's moral judgments. Journal of Personality and Social Psychology 3: 611–618.
    1969 Developmental processes in the child's moral thinking. O. Mussen, J. Langer and M. Covington, eds. Trends and Issues in Developmental Psychology. New York: Holt, Rinehart and Winston.

Weinreich, H.
  1975 Kohlberg and Piaget: Aspects of their relationship in the field of moral development. Journal of Moral Education 4: 201–213.
Whiting, J. W. M. and Child, I. L.
  1953 Child Training and Personality: A Cross Cultural Study. New Haven: Yale University Press.
Wilson, A. A., Greenblatt, S. L. and Wilson, R. W., eds.
  1977 Deviance and Social Control in Chinese Society. New York: Praeger.
Wilson, R. W.
  1970 Learning to be Chinese: The Political Socialization of Children in Taiwan. Cambridge, Mass.: The M.I.T. Press.
  1974 The Moral State: A Study of the Political Socialization of Chinese and American Children. New York: The Free Press.
  1976 Some comments on stage theories of moral development. Journal of Moral Education 5: 241–248.
  1978 A new direction for the study of moral behavior. Journal of Moral Education 7: 122–131.

8. CHILDHOOD PSYCHOPATHOLOGY:
A DIALOGUE WITH SPECIAL REFERENCE TO
CHINESE AND AMERICAN CULTURES

Two psychologists, Dr. Relativist (R) and Dr. Universalist (U), were having a discussion on childhood psychopathology from a cultural perspective. Dr. R's basic position was that the conceptualization, recognition, and treatment of psychopathology are ultimately rooted in the belief systems of a given culture; and to that extent, psychopathology is culture-specific. On the other hand, Dr. U believed that there are certain features instrinsic to psychopathology which are invariant across cultures and which render it recognizable within any cultural context; hence, psychopathology is a universal. They decided to focus their discussion especially on a contrast between the Chinese and the American perspectives. Their dialogue may be divided into four main sections: (a) childhood psychopathology and its relationship with how childhood and the parent-child relationship are conceptualized in different cultures, with respect to both time and space; (b) issues of culture-specificity versus culture-invariance and the conceptualization of psychopathology in general; (c) the problem of how different psychopathological conditions are differentiated and classified, together with a detailed discussion of hyperactivity and aggression in Chinese and American children; and (d) concluding remarks.

Dr. R. Let us begin our discussion by considering the following story of an eight-year-old lad who was extremely devoted to his parents. The family was so poor that they could not afford to furnish their beds with mosquito curtains. Every summer night myriads of mosquitoes attacked them without restraint, feasting upon their flesh and blood. Seeing his parents thus annoyed in their sleep, the lad felt a great grief in his heart. He took off his clothes to attract the mosquitoes. Even though he felt the pain from their attacks, he would not drive them away for fear that they might go to attack his parents instead. He would rather endure the suffering for the sake of his parents.

Dr. U. My immediate reaction is that the lad's devotion to his parents appears to be too extreme, and that the whole situation would call for its being viewed in psychopathological terms. The lad's behavior would seem to reflect a strong masochistic tendency. Equally, the parents' role would appear highly suspect. One would raise the question of whether they had been oblivious to their son's physical – and mental – suffering, in having succeeded to inculcate into his mind such a sense of filial duty at a tender age. An occasion is called for to look into their pattern of familial dynamics.

Dr. R. In actuality, the story is taken from one of the *Twenty-Four Examples of Filial Piety* from China, about the lad Wu Meng who lived during the Chin dynasty (4th to 5th century A.D.). For centuries, the *Twenty-Four Examples of Filial Piety* formed an integral part of standard educational materials in China,

A. Kleinman and T.-Y. Lin (eds.), Normal and Abnormal Behavior in Chinese Culture, 137–155.

and must have been familiar to almost every Chinese child in the past. As its
name implies, 24 stories of exemplary filial devotion are told, meant as models
to be emulated by others. (For a rendition of the 24 stories in English, the
reader to referred to Chen (1908) and Koehn (1944); see also Tseng and Hsu
(1972) for an interpretation of familial relationships as expressed in these and
other Chinese children's stories.)

Dr. U. A good many of the other stories from the *Twenty-Four* also provide
a rich source for thought in the realm of psychopathology. The filial acts were
often extreme to the point of unreasonableness, even cruelty — as in the story of
the man who divorced his wife because she failed to show reverence toward
wooden statues which he had carved in the image of his deceased parents, or the
poor man who was prepared to bury his three-year-old son so that his mother
would no longer need to share her portion of food with the child. A strong
masochistic component seems to be present in a number of the filial sons who
subjected themselves to great personal indignity, physical suffering and risk, or
self-sacrifice to satisfy what were sometimes highly unreasonable parental
demands — as in the story of the boy who, despite ill-treatment by his step-
mother, laid himself on a frozen river in order to catch fresh fish which she
desired to eat. In still other stories, the filial devotion assumed a form which
suggests an excessive, perhaps even pathological, attachment to the mother —
as in the case of the poet and calligrapher who was said to have watched his sick
mother for a whole year without leaving her bedside or taking off his clothes
(vigilance against forbidden impulses?), and who, despite his high social position,
performed the most menial tasks, like washing the stool, for her (atonement?).
Continued grief over the death of a parent was taken to be a hallmark of the
filial son: the more torturous and the more prolonged the grief, the greater the
filial devotion. In sum, filial piety took precedence at the expense of everything
else. Sensitivity to human needs, personal aspirations, and growth toward
independence were all repressed. Even dubious or wrongful acts could be con-
doned, even praised, if they were done with filial intentions — as in the story of
the six-year-old child who pocketed two of the oranges offered him by his host,
and when discovered, explained that they were intended for his mother back
home.

Dr. R. Your clinical interpretation of these stories is characteristically
American, but alien to Chinese traditional ethos. Hardly any contrast among the
ideologies concerning childhood is more explicit, and dramatic, than that
between the child-centeredness of contemporary American society and the age-
centeredness of traditional China. Filial piety was the primary guiding principle
in the socialization of Chinese children. For the family predicated on reciprocal
intergenerational dependence, it was of paramount importance that filial obligations be fulfilled.

By contrast, the contemporary American scene is the epitomy of a permissive,
growth-oriented, and child-centered culture. Benjamin Spock, psychological
testing, child guidance, Head Start . . . these are symptoms of the *Zeitgeist.* They

are distinctly the products of American society. Never before has there been such awareness of the immense potentialities for learning in the young and of the importance of early experience on subsequent development. Never before has there been such conscientiousness about parenting, the instrumental role that it plays in deciding the mental health or ill-health of the child. Childhood has been "discovered," and with it its psychopathologies. The working assumption is that the child's difficulties are reflections of disturbances in the adults around him. He is, therefore, not the culprit, but the victim of unhealthy forces in the environment, particularly in the family. In their role as the collective spokesman on behalf of the child, psychiatrists, psychologists, and social workers seem to have taken a generally antiparent stance: parents, mothers in particular, are the major cause of the child's psychological difficulties. Accusatory terms like "schizophrenogenic mother" made their appearance in the scientific literature. In traditional Chinese eyes, professionals in the field of child mental health must be most unfilial!

Dr. U. I venture to say, however, that the contemporary American scene you have described is rather unique, in both time and space. Let us not forget that the age of permissiveness has had only a short history. It was not long ago that masturbation and thumb sucking had to be stamped out with steadfast parental determination, often ruthlessly if necessary. In the heyday of early simple-minded behaviorism, mothers were advised not to cuddle their babies on the rationale that it might lead to more crying and demanding behavior; nor to feed them when they were hungry, but according to the clock. (Chinese mothers, never so advised, were free to follow their natural inclination on these matters.) The sensible way to treat children, according to John Watson (1928), was to "treat them as though they were young adults," to be always "perfectly objective . . . and at the same time kindly." Parental sentimentality had no place in parenthood: "Never hug and kiss [your children], never let them sit on your lap. If you must, kiss them once on the forehead when they say good night. Shake hands with them in the morning." (On the particular point of treating children as young adults, Watson might have met with more approval from his Chinese contemporaries than from his own countrymen today. For, in China traditionally it was the child who behaved like a miniature adult, one who was "young in years but old in style," that brought praise from adults. However, the suppression of parental sentiments, coupled with the mechanical fashion of handling children, were essentially alien to the interactional styles in the Chinese family — see Ho (1972) for a discussion of the function of affect in Chinese families.) Apparently, a fundamental change took place in the ideology of child rearing around the 1940s (see Bronfenbrenner 1958; Newson and Newson 1974; Wolfenstein 1953), away from rigid, puritanical, and authoritarian ways to the permissiveness of the present day.

Dr. R. However, a swinging back of the pendulum may be discerned. There seems to be growing sentiment that permissiveness has gone too far. Many people are putting the blame on permissiveness for the alarmingly high rates of juvenile delinquency and, more generally, social unrest. Post-Vietnam American society is undergoing a period of self-doubt and soul searching, after having experienced what might be analogous to adolescent disillusionment. It is ironical that the country which has overwhelming superiority in resources for social science research is also the one which seems to have visibly more than its share of social problems — more visible perhaps because American society is highly self-conscious and does not conceal its disgraces. Interestingly enough, Benjamin Spock himself admitted, in his 1968 edition of *Baby and Child Care,* that a principal change has occurred in his own outlook on child rearing. He now has misgivings about today's child-centered viewpoint: "the tendency of many conscientious parents to keep their eyes exclusively focused on their child, thinking about what he needs from them and from the community, instead of thinking about what the world, the neighborhood, the family will be needing from the child and then making sure that he will grow up to meet such obligations" (p. xvi). Now, this is more in tune with the Chinese than with the American ethos.

Dr. U. It is most unfair to put the blame on permissiveness. Too many irresponsible things have been done under its pretext. Permissiveness must be distinguished from indulgence or lack of concern. As to the cause of the high rates of juvenile delinquency, I believe that we must look beyond the psychology of individuals to its roots in the sociopolitical structure of American society.

An unfortunate side-effect of implicating parental responsibility in the child's psychological disturbances is that many parents have become guilt-ridden and uncertain of their roles as parents. The result is that they are unable to exercise their parental authority when the occasion requires it. Abrogating their parental roles, however, would in all likelihood lead to more destructive consequences than their continuing to function as parents, no matter how imperfectly.

Dr. R. Still, the adoption of the therapeutic orientation, rather than the punitive, represents a real advance in the work of child mental health. The problem child in America today is no longer to be regarded as the object of punishment, but treatment. This is all the more significant when we reflect on how cruelly children have been treated throughout the ages. The use of punishment has been the rule, rather than the exception. As late as the last century, for instance, in Britain children were offered mice pie as a curative for wetting the bed. It would be difficult to say whether these children endured it better than the corporal punishment they were no less likely to receive.

Recognition, however, precedes treatment. Since antiquity, various forms of childhood psychopathology have been recognized and sporadically documented. In China, for example, a classification of developmental defects, both physical and mental, can be found in *Kuo Yü (Conversations of the States)* of the Chou period. The book classifies the defects into eight categories, called the "eight diseases", and suggests different jobs suitable for each type of sufferer — probably the oldest example of occupational psychology (see Chen (1963) for details). However, on the whole, the existence of childhood psychopathology remains to be "discovered." Thus in the eighteenth century the philosopher Immanuel Kant stated categorically, in his classification of mental disorders, that there was no such thing as disturbed children. The elevation of childhood psychopathology into general social consciousness is an American achievement in the twentieth century.

Dr. U. It may seem incredible to the younger generations who have grown up in America and are accustomed to child guidance, etc., that professionally organized mental-health services for children have had only a short history. The term "child psychiatry" was introduced only in the 1930s; and prior to the 1920s, there was no body of knowledge or of clinical practice integrated enough to merit being set aside as an organized specialty (Kanner 1969: 1). The phenomenal growth in child mental-health research and services since World War II has been primarily an American and, to a lesser extent, European enterprise. In Africa and India, for instance, according to Minde (1976) child psychiatric services have been introduced only during the past seven to eight years. Minde concluded that almost all disturbed children in Africa and Southeast Asia are without any professional assistance. The consequence is that there is a near vacuum in our knowledge of childhood psychopathology outside of the European-American context. Considerable materials can be found in the literature on cross-cultural aspects of child rearing, but without focus on psychopathology, and on transcultural psychiatry, but with only passing references to children, so that the union of these sets of materials yields no systematic knowledge on childhood psychopathology from a cross-cultural perspective.

Dr. R. When it comes to contemporary investigations, the great divergence in sociopolitical backgrounds of Chinese children living in different parts of the world presents added complications to the comparative framework. However, cultural continuity with the past in many ways still enables one to speak meaningfully of *Chinese* parents and children, albeit with qualifications when necessary. Information from the People's Republic of China would be of special interest because of the profound social changes that have taken place there since 1949. Unfortunately, there is virtually no available information on the current state of child psychiatry in the Mainland. The only report I have been able to find ('Child Psychiatry in Shanghai' 1974) is quite fragmentary, telling us little beyond reiterating what has been reported on general psychiatry (see Ho 1974). As related by representatives of the Shanghai Psychiatric Institute, the treatment emphasis is placed on physical labor, ideological re-education, developing the child's own initiative and involving parents in the curative process, and the combined use of Western as well as traditional techniques (e.g., acupuncture and medicinal herbs). Among the various conditions mentioned were childhood schizophrenia (constituting 60% of child patients in the hospital), epilepsy (5%), and abnormal intellectual development (6%). It was claimed that the rate of child mental illness is continually declining because of improved maternity and postnatal care — for example, .3% of all patients in the hospital were children for the years 1970/71/72, as compared with 2% for 1963/64/65.

The majority of studies in Chinese child psychiatry have been done by research workers in Taiwan, Hong Kong, Hawaii, and North America. Hsu (1966) reported the results of a mental health survey covering 8,329 children in one of the largest elementary schools in Taipei. Several features of these results deserve attention. Firstly, in accordance with most studies (e.g., Clancy and Smitter 1953; Cummings 1944; Rogers 1942; Ullmann 1952), more boys (4.43%) were considered to be "problem children" than girls (2.48%) by their teachers. Secondly, the number of "problem children" reached its peak at the fourth grade for boys and at the fifth grade for girls, resulting primarily from a marked increase in problems associated with acting out and learning attitudes. This appears to be consistent with the results of the Mental Health Survey of Los Angeles County (1960), also based on teacher evaluations, which indicated higher proportions of emotionally disturbed children in the fourth and fifth grades than in all other grades. Further support of this finding may be derived from the report by Rosen, Bahn, and Kramer (1964), which showed that clinic termination rates reached their highest around age 9 and again at 14 for boys, and at ages 10 and 14 for girls. Thirdly, the overall prevalence rate of 3.49% is much lower than those reported in *earlier* studies in the United States (11% by Clancy and Smitter 1953; 12% by Rogers 1942; 8% by Ullmann 1952; 4 to 12% by Wall 1955; 7% by Wickman 1928) and Britain (7.7% "seriously disturbed" by Cummings 1944; 12% in the Great Britain Ministry of Education survey 1955). Hsu felt that possibly only a fraction of the children who were actually maladjusted was recognized as such by their teachers. This view is supported by the fact that a much higher prevalence rate of 12% was obtained from teachers after attending mental health seminars (as a part of the East-Gate project described by Hsu and Lin 1969). Fourthly, the acting-out type of disciplinary problems were reported with the highest frequency, about four times as frequently as asocial behavior problems (passivity, overdependency, shyness, etc.). By contrast, Bower (1963) and Clancy and Smitter (1953) reported that teachers in the United States identified the two types of problems with almost the same frequency, as did the East-Gate teachers after the mental health seminars. Fifthly, no problems related to sex, toilet habits, or obsessive-compulsive behavior were reported by the teachers, and even after the seminars these problems were identified only rarely. Hsu raised the question of whether this reflected an actually low level of psychosexual and psychophysiological urinary problems among the children, or whether it revealed an indifference or reluctance to bring such problems to the open in Chinese culture. Taken as a whole, the results of the survey give support to the contention that the Chinese orientation toward children is basically moralistic rather than psychological, that adults are highly concerned with problems of control and discipline, and that there is a high degree of insensitivity to psychological problems which do not disturb the order of things to which adults attach importance. Similar views are expressed by Singer, Ney, and Lieh-Mark (1978) when they state that, in Hong Kong, "the culture fails to recognize the sick role of children with psychological disturbance"; a good proportion of such children are regarded as having problems of discipline, or the sick role is defined in predominantly somatic terms so that psychological difficulties are usually presented as somatic and hypochondriacal complaints.

I think that we have established one point: the recognition and treatment of childhood psychopathology depend on how childhood and the parent-child relationship are conceptualized, circumscribed in both the temporal and spatial dimensions by the prevailing ethos and state of knowledge. Culture casts the frame within which the child's behavior is perceived and evaluated. To begin with, it preconditions the perceiver to be sensitized to certain aspects and sets up mental blocks against other aspects. Thus, it might be predicted that a body of knowledge concerning childhood psychopathology could not have arisen from within Chinese culture — given its moralistic, rather than psychological, orientation toward childhood. The child was conceived of as *wu chih* (without knowledge) and as a passive recipient of the teachings of adults, to be inculcated with moral precepts and molded into a personality as prescribed by the culture. In particular, it would be quite inconceivable for a pathogenetic theory which implicates parental responsibility to have been developed. Filial piety acted to create and maintain cultural blind spots against the awareness of childhood psychopathology and its connection with parent-child relationships. The cultural belief expressed in the saying that "there is no wrong (or bad) parents under the heavens" shows how deeply the Chinese conception of parenthood was rooted in filial piety (see Ho 1975).

The case of Wu Meng and others from the *Twenty-Four* have raised a central issue in any discussion of childhood psychopathology from a cultural perspective. If the same behavior can be highly valued in one culture and yet viewed as psychopathological in another, how can psychopathology be established with certainty? Is psychopathology culture-specific, definable solely according to the value system within which it occurs? Or, is psychopathology a universal, recognizable within any cultural context?

Dr. U. Plausibly, both the moralistic and the psychological interpretations of Wu Meng's behavior are valid. That is, he was beyond question a child of extreme filial devotion, yet at the same time psychologically disturbed.

Dr. R. We have no information from the story's account as to how well-adjusted or happy a child Wu Meng was. Such a question was simply not a matter of concern in any one of the *Twenty-Four*. However, one thing is certain. In terms of the criterion of social adequacy, that of meeting the primary requirements of society, Wu Meng must be judged to have been highly successful. Having learned to accept his filial obligations, he had prepared himself well for his later roles in life. The reputation he had earned as a filial son brought not only praise and respect for himself but also honor to his entire family. Thus, he had secured for himself a worthy position within his social order. As a matter of fact, in other stories of the *Twenty-Four* filial behavior was amply rewarded, in material terms or ascendancy in social status.

Nevertheless, Wu Meng's success was achieved at a considerable cost to himself, certainly physical and in all likelihood psychological as well. Does it not raise the question, then, that the requirements of social adequacy and psychological well-being are not always compatible? Certain age-honored institutionalized ways of socializing children may be in fact quite insensitive to their psychological needs. Consequently, successful adaptation to their cultural milieu can be achieved only at the price of suffering varying degrees of psychological disturbance.

Dr. U. But adaptation failures would lead to more serious problems. The necessity to meet certain vital or essential requirements of society is a universal imperative for the socially adequate adult. It is precisely the function of any culture to transform children into adults according to some prescribed image of what an adequate adult is. Culture must define, explicitly or implicitly, what constitutes this image, and make provisions for ensuring that children are raised in ways that will fit them to this image at least to an acceptable degree. It has been claimed, furthermore, that the demands of socialization are cross-cultural, i.e., "they can be measured by using folk concepts that are ubiquitous in all cultures" (Abbott 1974: 145). Using the California Psychological Inventory as the measuring instrument, data were gathered on the psychosocial functioning of two samples of families of delinquents and nondelinquents, Cantonese-speaking Chinese-Americans in San Francisco and Taiwanese-speaking Chinese in Taipei. It was found that in both instances delinquents had lower scores on the Responsibility, Socialization, and Self-Control scales.

It may be stated that failure to meet the minimum requirements of social adequacy is an intrinsic feature of psychopathology, and thus constitutes probably the most defensible culture-invariant criterion for establishing its presence. However, meeting social demands, as you have pointed out, needs not imply positive mental health; it is a necessary, but not sufficient, condition for it.

Dr. R. Yes, in fact, overcompliance to social demands may well be a neurotic trait. And what about the social innovator who refuses to conform to social demands?

Dr. U. I think that we can make a distinction between inability versus refusal to meet social demands. Inability may be the result of an inherent limitation in personality resources or a disturbance in their utilization, and may be regarded as an indication of psychopathology. On the other hand, refusal requires some degree of ego strength; when consciously made as an ethical choice, it may even represent the highest form of social behavior human beings are capable of. Still, the social innovator, as distinguished from the rebellious without a cause, is not at war with society without reason; he does not refuse to conform merely for the sake of nonformity, but discriminates between demands which he can ethically meet versus those which he feels he cannot. In time, such behavior may be even highly regarded by members of his own society.

Dr. R. Still, you have not come to grips with the question I raised. What happens when the demands of a culture are in themselves pathogenic? Let me point to some research bearing on the effects of filial piety on attitudinal and personality formation. Ho and Lee (1974) found a correlation of .5 between attitude toward filial piety and authoritarianism in school teachers in Taiwan. Although no causal relationship is necessarily implied, the finding does lend support to the contention that internalization of the precepts of filial piety is predisposing to the formation of authoritarian personalities. Boey (1976) found that father's and mother's attitudes toward filial piety were positively related to measures of rigidity and negatively related to measures of cognitive complexity. There is as yet no research linking filial piety and childhood psychopathology. Nevertheless, clinical observations can be made on typical reactions of Chinese children to absolute parental authority, justified on the basis of filial piety: distantiation between the child and his parents, especially the father; a generalized tendency to fear authority figures; the adoption of silence, negativism, or passive resistance as a behavioral style in dealing with authority demands; dissociation between affect and roles; and a tendency to displace or to turn inward aggression. Given the absolute upholding of and overriding importance attached to filial piety in traditional Chinese society, what could the child do but to conform? What room was there for the social innovator? The rebellious or nonconforming child would have an awfully hard time.

The authoritarian orientation toward children, ideologically rooted in the ethic of filial piety, has important consequences for the clinical practitioner who treats children. The dilemma is that encouraging the child to develop assertiveness and self-direction might lead him into greater conflict with adults in his immediate social circle and beyond, and consequently to become the recipient of harsher punitive measures; but helping the child to comply with parental authority demands would imply a suppression of his individual volition. If the clinician is permissive in his therapeutic relationship with the child, he must at the same time exercise great caution so that the child will not become confused about the world of adults and find himself at a loss as to what is the right thing to do. He must help the child to differentiate the permissive from other situations, and to learn what actions are appropriate or inappropriate respectively. This is because permissiveness may be a highly unfamiliar experience in the child's life. Perhaps the most one can hope for is that the child had enough resources to preserve inwardly his own sense of individuality, while meeting external demands of compliance. To be honest, there is no way out of the dilemma — unless one is prepared to attack the authoritarian orientation itself, at which point great resistance, culturally reinforced, is likely to be encountered.

More generally, the clinician will soon become aware of the societal forces which run counter to the therapeutic orientation and which work against the child in need of help. He is likely to encounter great difficulty in attempting to explain to parents that the child's difficulties might be related to faulty techniques of discipline or just plain mismanagement on their part, and that advisedly the object of treatment might not be the child alone but the entirety of his intrafamilial relationships. Here is an instance of a basic clash between incompatible cultural conceptions: the therapeutic versus the punitive, and the democratic versus the authoritarian. A culture which has a long tradition of panmoralistic orientation toward children produces psychologically illiterate parents!

Dr. U. The pathogenic demands of culture – specifically, those derived from the ethic of filial piety – to which you referred in no way negate the universality of psychopathology. Rather, it has imputed cross-cultural validity to the importance of parent-child relationships in the pathogenesis of psychiatric conditions. To be sure, culture exerts its powerful influence on defining what is regarded as abnormal; how abnormality is conceptualized, explained, and treated; the relative frequency of various types of disorders; and the manner in which these various types are manifest. But this must not blind us to the fact that mental disorders are found in all societies throughout the world (see Benedict and Jacks 1954). In every culture, there is a reservoir of potentially disturbed individuals, but the extent to which their psychopathology is manifest depends on the amount of stress exerted upon its members and the availability of means for coping with stress which the culture provides. The mentally ill person can in fact be recognized by members of his own cultural group, and by outsiders applying the norms of his culture. In short, psychopathology is one of the universals of human existence.

As regards childhood psychopathology, there is in addition to all of the above considerations a dimension of special importance, that of maturation. That human development proceeds according to an orderly sequence is one of the few universal generalizations that can be asserted with confidence. Regardless of cultural context, the child walks before it runs and learns to speak single words before it uses phrases or sentences. Behavior is expected to become increasingly differentiated along with the process of biological unfolding as the child grows older; new or higher level abilities are expected to appear at successive age levels. Thus, one of the most defensible indicators of validity for psychometric ability measures is how well the raw scores correlate with chronological age. While performance norms may vary considerably from one cultural or subcultural context to another, deviations within local norms can be detected. Marked delays or disturbances in sensorimotor, language, cognitive, and social development, when detected, would be a matter of concern in any culture.

Dr. R. We have been discussing issues involved in the conceptualization, recognition, and treatment of childhood psychopathology in general, but have not dealt with the problem of how various psychopathological conditions are differentiated and classified. That is the problem of nosology and nomenclature. Even in adult psychiatry, the difficulties involved are notorious. In child psychiatry, the question of how and to what extent childhood psychopathological conditions are distinct from adult conditions remains a central issue. Many classification systems proposed, particularly those in earlier periods, are modeled after traditional systems in adult psychiatry; childhood psychopathology is treated as downward extensions of similar conditions in the adult. From the cultural perspective, we are handicapped by the dearth of knowledge about childhood psychopathology outside of the European-American context.

Dr. U. The World Health Organization (WHO) has been wrestling for years with the problem of developing an international scheme for classifying childhood psychiatric disorders. A recent attempt by an international group of experts under its auspices (Rutter, Lebovici, Eisenberg, Sneznevskij, Sadoun, Brooke, and Lin 1969) deserves special attention. The main principle was that, in view of the variety of theoretical concepts regarding the etiology and pathogenesis of mental disorders and the paucity of evidence which might lead to a choice between theories, emphasis should be put on the use of solid clinical facts as a starting point. A triaxial classification scheme for children aged 0–12 years was proposed. The first axis concerns the clinical psychiatric syndrome; it is descriptive in nature, without regard to etiological or theoretical issues. The second axis specifies the child's current level of intellectual functioning, without regard to its nature or etiology. The third axis is concerned with any major biological, psychological, or social influence which is a contributory factor in the psychiatric disorder or which constitutes a handicap of significance in relation to it; multiple recording of factors is possible and, if present, necessary on this axis. These three axes are independent and separate. It was assumed that there is no necessary association between a child's intellectual level and the type of emotional or behavioral disorder he exhibits, or between the type of clinical psychiatric disorder and the type of etiological factor which is present. Thus, a child may be psychotic, mentally subnormal, and epileptic — each one of these three features describes a different aspect of his functioning.

The glossary of terms used in the tri-axial classification scheme, other than those for specific developmental disorders (in the first axis), are basically the same as those found in adult psychiatry. It was felt that only by using the same terms, wherever appropriate, would it be possible to bring together into a single scheme classifications developed in relation to different age periods. The underlying assumption is that there is a basic continuity in the conditions in childhood and in adult life referred to by the same terms. However, the classification scheme does provide for those conditions which are peculiar to childhood and which do not have any adult equivalent, such as infantile psychosis and the group of developmental disorders.

The WHO group expressed the hope that the tri-axial scheme will be tried out and critically assessed as a step in the development of that part of the International Classification of Diseases concerned with childhood psychiatric disorders, and it is likely that the scheme needs to be refined. Should it prove to be acceptable to practising psychiatrists throughout the world, it would mean a significant step toward having a common language in child psychiatry internationally. It would also serve as a useful research instrument, particularly in cross-national epidemiological studies.

Dr. R. Basically the tri-axial scheme is still predicated on the disease model.

Again, it has been taken for granted that psychopathology, internal to the individual, is universally present and underlies behavioral disturbances in all cultural contexts. It does not appear that special considerations have been given to the problem of cultural variations in the development of the scheme.

Dr. U. Among the various clinical psychiatric syndromes, mental subnormality would present the least difficulty. At least, the statistical criterion applies equally to any well-defined population within a culture or subculture. The broad category of specific developmental disorders would also present relatively little difficulty, since human development proceeds according to an orderly sequence which is culturally invariant, as has been pointed out above.

I think that conduct disorders would present the most difficulties. The tri-axial scheme defines conduct disorders as "abnormal behaviour which gives rise to social disapproval but which is neither part of any other psychiatric condition nor associated with personality disorder .... It is also necessary that the behavior be *abnormal* in its socio-cultural context. This may be judged by the frequency, severity and type of behavior and by its association with other symptoms (such as abnormal interpersonal relationships)" (Rutter et al. 1969).

If the term "psychopathology" were restricted to apply only to those conditions in which an underlying pathological process or defect is assumed to be present — which is closer to its original meaning — then conduct disorders, as defined in the tri-axial scheme, do not fall within its domain. In fact, a number of the WHO group members felt that conduct disorders were not within the province of the psychiatrist, but it was agreed that there must be some means of coding such cases. Two pertinent comments may be made regarding the place of conduct disorders in the tri-axial scheme. Firstly, the definition is circular. Conduct disorders are regarded as abnormal, but the criterion for their abnormality is social disapproval. It would seem that a great deal of conceptual confusion can be avoided by leaving out any reference to abnormality as far as the manifest behavior is concerned, and simply treat conduct disorders as repeated or persistent displays of socially disapproved behavior. Conceptually, then, conduct disorders are cases of behavior deviance, the criterion for which is purely social. If we were to arrange the various diagnostic categories along a continuum, ranging from the hypothetically purely medical to the purely social, conduct disorders would come closest to the latter end.

Secondly, it may be questioned as to whether there is ever a pure case of conduct disorder, one which does not at the same time implicate some degree of personality disturbance in the child. The definition is confusing as to what is meant by "association with other symptoms (such as abnormal interpersonal relationships)," in the absence of any other "psychiatric condition" or "personality disorder." Few would conceive of "abnormal interpersonal relationships" as a "symptom"; they are in themselves psychopathology. Examples of conduct disorder given in the tri-axial scheme include fighting, bullying, destructive behavior, and cruelty to animals. Persistence in such behavior, and not the mere fact that the child has committed a delinquent act, is necessary for the diagnosis. My interpretation is that the essence of conduct disorder is not marked by the acts of misconduct, but by the child's tendency to engage persistently in these acts in the face of social disapproval — a tendency which may be construed, regardless of sociocultural context, as symptomatic of some form of underlying personality disturbance. To preclude any association with personality disorder in conduct disorders is to prejudge the issue; it commits the clinician, especially if he is psychodynamically oriented, to a theoretical position which he may find difficult to accept.

Dr. R. Even if the validity of the tri-axial scheme were granted, there would still be great variations in the actual practice of diagnosis internationally. Clinicians in different countries are likely to vary considerably in their readiness to assign various diagnostic categories to the child. This variation arises from the fact that often diagnostic labeling depends not so much on the degree of seriousness of the behavior in question as it does on social expectation and the level of tolerance associated with it. Furthermore, whether or not the child is brought to the attention of the clinician in the first place is a function of the tolerance level of adults around him. The boisterous, disobedient, or delinquent child is much more likely to arouse concern in his parents and teachers than his sullen, socially withdrawn peers, not because he is necessarily more disturbed psychologically, but because his disruption to the orderly patterns of everyday life is more apparent.

Dr. U. Tolerance level is particularly relevant to the diagnosis of a condition like the hyperkinetic disorder, which, by definition, is hyperactivity beyond the normal limits of tolerance. This disorder is familiar, perhaps more than any other form of childhood psychopathology, to American parents and teachers as a source of great irritation and headaches. Masland (1965) estimated the prevalence rate to be between five to ten percent of the school population. Now, it is indeed extraordinary that there is such a sizeable number of children considered to by hyperkinetic in the United States, in view of the fact that American attitudes are generally alleged to be favorably disposed toward the outgoing, active child. By Chinese standards, the prevalence rate must be even higher!

Comparative data on prevalence rates of the hyperkinetic disorder in the non-Western world are lacking. However, let me refer to some interesting observations made by a group of American developmental psychologists who made a visit to the People's Republic of China in 1973 (Kessen 1975). What impressed these psychologists the most was the near absence of antisocial, disruptive, or aggressive behavior, and the conspicuously prosocial behavior among Chinese children:

If our observations were at all representative, the outstanding feature of childhood in China, and that which raises the most basic problem, is the high level of concentration, orderliness, and competence of the children. We were impressed by the sight of fifty children in a primary classroom quiet until addressed and chanting their lessons in enthusiastic unison when called upon, even more impressed by the apparent absence of disruptive, hyperactive, and noisy children. The same quiet orderliness, the same concentration on tasks, the same absence of disruptive behavior was to be seen in all the classrooms we visited, down to children barely able to walk. The docility did not seem to us to be the docility of surrender and apathy; the Chinese children we saw were emotionally expressive, socially gracious, and adept. (Kessen 1975: 216–217)

Obviously, these observations must be interpreted in the light of the highly constrained conditions under which they were made, as the visiting psychologists themselves have repeatedly pointed out. Nevertheless, they are observations corroborated by those made by numerous other visitors to China (e.g., Ho 1972), though subject to the same constrained conditions. The contrast between Chinese and American children in their behavior is so marked that it cannot be construed solely as an artifact of observational conditions. That hyperactivity occurs by far less frequently in Chinese than in American children is a statement which, I believe, can be safely made.

Dr. R. Differences in expectations and in the consistency of expectations may account for the dramatic contrast between American and Chinese children in hyperactive behavior. In present-day China, collectivist rather than individualist values are emphasized. The child is exposed to the collectivist style of living quite early in life, as soon as he is placed in the nursery. It is of utmost importance that he learns to exercise control over his impulses which may cause disruption in the group order. The expectation for the child to achieve self-control early is continuous with traditional attitudes toward child rearing: Chinese parents are generally more concerned with control than are their Western counterparts (Ho 1975). By contrast, American parents are inclined to be worried that their child is not socially well-adjusted unless he is outgoing, active, and, if male, assertive, perhaps even aggressive. Attention must also be drawn to the pseudopermissiveness and uncertainty over parental roles which you mentioned earlier.

Perhaps more importantly, Chinese expectations toward children are extremely stable and uniform, as if it were inconceivable that they could behave differently from what is expected of them. It is the weight of this uniformity in the expectations of adults surrounding the child – the weight of the whole culture – that bears upon him to exercise self-control. By contrast, American expectations are characterised more by heterogeneity than by homogeneity. Questions concerning how children should be treated are occasions for lively debate and controversy. As a parenthetical thought, one wonders if there is a tradeoff between self-control and individual variation. Could hyperactivity be to some extent an unfortunate by-product of the American respect for individuality? Is early self-control achieved only at the price of suppressing individual variation?

Dr. U. Let me offer an alternative explanation. To begin with, the hyperkinetic disorder entails much more than mere hyperactivity: distractibility, short attention span, impulsiveness, inability to delay gratification, need to handle and finger things, marked mood fluctuations, aggressiveness, and poor coordination are among its features. There is general agreement that subtle dysfunction of the central nervous system or what is commonly called "minimal brain injury" is responsible for the disorder in a large number of cases. Genetic contribution has also been implicated: 100 percent concordance for monozygote twins (Lopez 1965), and clustering of cases within the same family (Wender 1971). Perhaps, too, there may be racial differences in the predisposition toward hyperactivity. An interesting study by Freedman and Freedman (1969) suggests that there may be genuine racial differences in temperament. It was found that, in comparison with European-American newborns, Chinese-American newborns were less changeable, less perturbable, tended to habituate more readily, and tended to calm themselves or to be consoled more readily when upset. The investigators could find no potentially important covariables that could have accounted for these differences. Such findings should caution us against seeking an explanation too readily in the cultural realm.

Dr. R. Only further reasearch can settle the question of what accounts for the difference in frequency of hyperactivity between Chinese and American children. An interesting piece of research would be to determine the comparative rates between Chinese-American and European-American children matched on relevant variables, which should include the number of generations since immigrating to the United States and socialization practices. If no difference is found, we can then reasonably rule out genetic factors and ascribe a decisive role to the impact of culture.

Closely related to our discussion of the hyperkinetic disorder is how to account for the near absence of aggressive behavior observed in children in the People's Republic of China. I have often been pressed for an explanation by psychologists, but I really cannot offer one. Rather, I would turn the question around and ask how the high frequency of aggressive behavior in American children can be explained. This because I do not wish to be committed to the theoretical position that aggression, as distinct from the capacity for aggression, is a necessary component of man's biological nature. It may be argued that the presence, rather than the absence, of aggression is what needs to be explained. Again, the difference in cultural expectations between America and China is striking. In China, the child's aggressive behavior is regarded as antisocial, and consequently suppressed. In America, a certain amount of aggression is to be expected, particularly in the male child; an absence of aggressive behavior might even arouse concern, possibly as an indication of excessive inhibition. Chinese parents are typically upset if their children get into a fight; American parents may be worried about their son's "masculinity" if he runs away from a fight. An American visitor to China told me that he felt uneasy because he failed to see any fighting in kindergartens and schools he visited; he felt relieved when he finally observed one incidence of fighting between two boys unaware of his presence, in that his view of human nature had been reaffirmed. Many Chinese immigrants to the United States I talked with have expressed the concern that their children are in need of protecting themselves from physical fights in school; some have advocated their children to learn the art of self-defense — perhaps this explains why *kung-fu* has become particularly popular among young Chinese-Americans and why Bruce Lee was such a popular folk hero to them. The fact is that violence is very much visible in America, in the mass media as it is in real life. The violence of the frontier days has permeated and remained alive in the psyche of American society. Could the belief that aggression is inherent in human nature lead to the acceptance of violence as a way of life and hence to a greater likelihood of its occurrence?

Dr. U. We have been discussing at length issues involved in the conceptualization, recognition, and treatment of childhood psychopathology, centered around the theme of culture-specificity versus culture-invariance. Each of us can now sum up his views.

Dr. R. I have argued that our understanding of childhood psychopathology is grounded in how childhood and the parent-child relationship are conceptualized in different cultures; that certain aspects of culture may be pathogenic, with respect to both the relative frequency and manner of manifestation of various psychopathological conditions; that embodied within the sickness of each individual is a microcosm of the sickness of his culture; that the ethical dimension of value judgements and level of adult tolerance are not excluded in the recognition or diagnosis of psychopathology; and that the focus of our attention ought to be directed away from merely insisting on changing the individual child and his family to "adapt" better to existing conditions, but to changing the larger societal-cultural context in which he lives.

Throughout our discussion, I have been conscious of one thing. Given a child with manifest disturbance in behavior, the conceptualization of his condition, circumscribed by cultural belief systems concerning childhood and its psychopathologies, may have more to do with the child's future than the degree of seriousness of his disturbance itself. For, conceptualization dictates treatment. The fate of disturbed children throughout the world hinges largely on how childhood psychopathology is conceived.

Dr. U. I have no real quarrel with your arguments. An appreciation of the forces in different cultures at work protects us from provincialism and enriches our understanding of childhood psychopathology. However, I reject any exclusively culturogenic viewpoint which gives no recognition to defects or pathological processes internal to the individual child, and any extreme version of cultural relativism which denies the universality of psychopathology. The question has often been asked: Do psychopathological principles developed in the West apply in non-Western contexts? I am prepared to give personal testimony on this question. Clinical observations in both American and Chinese cultures have lead me to the conclusion that there is no sound basis for a separate set of principles or body of knowledge with respect to these two cultures. To avoid being misunderstood, I hasten to add that I do not mean a wholesale importation of Western psychology into non-Western contexts. Rather, I mean the need to base the refinement of our conceptualizations and principles on an enlarged range of observations in diverse cultures, and thus to increase our confidence in their universality. Ideally, clinical practice entails the creative union of universalistic principles and particular conditions. To seek the universals of human behavior — that is the task of the psychologist. May I conclude by formulating a set of related questions requiring empirical research which would clarify, or even eventually resolve, some of the issues in our dialogue. First, given a child psychiatric condition, is it found in all known cultures, despite variations in its manifestation? Second, are there culture-bound syndromes which are found in some cultural contexts but not in others? The debate of culture-specific versus culture-invariant conceptions has often been misdirected through pointing to the fact that behavior regarded as normal in one cultural context may be viewed as abnormal in another — which is nothing surprising, and which, in itself, answers no question. I believe that more can be gained through directing our efforts at the identification of behavioral categories which, regardless of the culture in which they occur, would be regarded as psychopathological *not only by members of that culture but also by outsiders*. A comprehensive inventory of such behavioral categories would go a long way toward achieving a universally accepted definition of the essence of psychopathology.

REFERENCES

Abbott, K.
1974 Psychosocial functioning, delinquency, and the family in San Francisco and Taipei. *In* Youth, Socialization, and Mental Health. W. P. Lebra, ed. Honolulu: The University of Hawaii Press.
Benedict, P. K. and Jacks, I.
1954 Mental illness in primitive societies. Psychiatry 17: 377–389.
Boey, K. W.
1976 Rigidity and Cognitive Complexity: An Empirical Investigation in the Interpersonal, Physical, and Numerical Domains under Task-Oriented and Ego-Involved Conditions. Unpublished doctoral dissertation. University of Hong Kong.
Bower, E. M.
1963 Primary prevention of mental and emotional disorders: A conceptual framework and action possibilities. American Journal of Orthopsychiatry 33: 832–848.
Bronfenbrenner, U.
1958 Socialization and social class through time and space. *In* Readings in Social Psychology. E. E. Maccoby, T. M. Newcomb, and E. L. Hartley, eds. New York: Holt.
Chen, C. K.
1963 Some psychopathological thoughts in the Book of Tso Chuen. Acta Psychologica Sinica 2: 156–164. (In Chinese, with an English abstract.)
Chen, I.
1908 The Book of Filial Duty. Translated. London: John Murray.
Child Psychiatry in Shanghai.
1974 International Child Welfare Review 22–23: 16–20.
Clancy, N. and Smitter, F.
1953 A study of emotionally disturbed children in Santa Barbara County Schools, California. Journal of Educational Research 4: 269–278.

Cummings, J. D.
  1944 The incidence of emotional symptoms in school children. British Journal of
       Educational Psychology 14: 151–161.
Freedman, D. G. and Freedman, N. C.
  1969 Behavioural differences between Chinese-American and European-American
       newborns. Nature 224: 1227.
Great Britain Ministry of Education.
  1955 Report of the Committee on Maladjusted Children. London: Her Majesty's
       Stationery Office.
Ho, D. Y. F.
  1972 The affectional function in contemporary Chinese families. In Mental Health and
       urbanization. Hong Kong: Mental Health Association of Hong Kong.
Ho, D. Y. F.
  1974 Early socialization in contemporary China. In Science Council of Japan, Proceed-
       ings of the Twentieth International Congress of Psychology, August 13–19,
       Tokyo, Japan. Tokyo: University of Tokyo Press.
Ho, D. Y. F.
  1974 Prevention and treatment of mental illness in the People's Republic of China.
       American Journal of Orthopsychiatry 44: 620–636.
Ho, D. Y. F.
  1975 Traditional Chinese approaches to socialization. In Applied Cross Cultural Psycho-
       logy. J. W. Berry and W. J. Lonner, eds. Amsterdam: Swets and Zeitlinger.
Ho, D. Y. F. and Lee, L. Y.
  1974 Authoritarianism and attitude toward filial piety in Chinese teachers. Journal of
       Social Psychology 92: 305–306.
Hsu, C. C.
  1966 A study on "problem children" reported by teachers. Japanese Journal of Child
       Psychiatry 7: 91–108.
Hsu, C. C. and Lin, T. Y.
  1969 A mental health program at the elementary school level in Taiwan: A six-year
       review of the East-Gate project. In Mental Health Research in Asia and the
       Pacific. W. Caudill and T. Y. Lin, eds. Honolulu: East-West Center Press.
Kanner, L.
  1969 Trends in child psychiatry. In Modern Perspectives in International Child
       Psychiatry. J. G. Howells, ed. Edinburgh: Oliver and Boyd.
Kessen, W., ed.
  1975 Childhood in China. New Haven: Yale University Press.
Koehn, A.
  1944 Filial Devotion in China. Peking: Lotus Court.
Lopez, R. E.
  1965 Hyperactivity in twins. Canadian Psychiatric Association Journal 10: 421–
       426.
Masland, R.
  1965 Testimony before a Subcommittee of the Committee on Appropriations, House
       of Representatives, 89th Congress, First Session, Part 3. Washington, D.C.: U.S.
       Government Printing Office.
Mental Health Survey of Los Angeles County, 1960.
  1970 Cited in The behavior disorders of childhood. E. J. Anthony. In Manual of Child
       Psychology, 3rd ed., Vol. 2. P. H. Mussen, ed. New York: Wiley.
Minde, K.
  1976 Child psychiatry in developing countries. Journal of Child Psychology and Psy-
       chiatry 17: 79–83.

Newson, J. and Newson, E.
1974 Cultural aspects of childrearing in the English-speaking world. *In* The Integration of a Child into a Social World. M. P. M. Richards, ed. Cambridge: Cambridge University Press.

Rogers, C. A.
1942 Mental health findings in three elementary schools. Education Research Bulletin 21: 3. Ohio State University.

Rosen, B. M., Bahn, A. K., and Kramer, M.
1964 Demographic and diagnostic characteristics of psychiatric clinic outpatients in the U.S.A., 1961. American Journal of Orthopsychiatry 34: 445–468.

Rutter, M., Lebovici, S., Eisenberg, L., Sneznevskij, A. V., Sadoun, R., Brooke, E., and Lin T. Y.
1969 Journal of Child Psychology and Psychiatry 10: 41–61.

Singer, K., Ney, P. G., and Lieh-Mak, F.
1978 A cultural perspective on child psychiatric disorders. Comprehensive Psychiatry 19: 533–540.

Spock, B.
1968 Baby and Child Care. New York: Pocket Books.

Tseng, W. S. and Hsu, J.
1972 The Chinese attitude towards parental authority as expressed in children's stories. Archives of General Psychiatry 26: 28–34.

Ullmann, C. A.
1952 Identification of Maladjusted School Children (Monograph No. 7, U.S. Public Health Service.) Washington, D.C.: U.S. Government Printing Office.

Wall, W.
1955 Education and Mental Health. New York: Columbia University Press.

Watson, J. B.
1928 Psychological Care of Infant and Child. New York: Norton.

Wender, P. H.
1971 Minimal Brain Dysfunction in Children. New York: Wiley Interscience.

Wickman, E. K.
1928 Children's Behavior and Teachers' Attitudes. New York: Commonwealth Fund.

Wolfenstein, M.
1953 Trends in infant care. American Journal of Orthopsychiatry 23: 120–130.

9. SEX DIFFERENCE IN SCHOOL ADJUSTMENT
IN TAIWAN

INTRODUCTION

In the patrilineal culture of the Chinese, boys are definitely the preferred sex. They receive preferential treatment at home, enjoy many privileges denied to girls and are often given a central position in the familial interaction. They should, in theory, have security and self-respect, which should enable them to develop ego strengths to withstand stresses in their lives.

In contemporary Taiwan, schools have become increasingly a source of serious stress for children. Owing to incredibly keen competition and over-crowded classes, adjustment, personality development and behavior of school children are serious concerns for educators and mental health professionals. The Taipei Children's Mental Health Center (CMHC) of National Taiwan University Hospital recently conducted a study on school absenteeism and also a prevalence study of school maladjustment (Soong et al. 1978; Shen et al. 1978). In both studies significant sex differences were found. This chapter discusses these sex differences in their sociocultural context in current Taiwan.

Since the above two studies were carried out as part of the school mental health program in Taiwan initiated in 1954, the authors would like first to present a summary review of the program.

Back in the 1950's, the Taipei Children's Mental Health Center was the only professional agency concerned with mental health of children in Taiwan. The establishment of the Chinese National Association for Mental Health in 1954 marked the beginning of an organized effort to interest school teachers in mental health. In 1959, CMHC organized a weekly mental health mobile clinic, in collaboration with the Provincial Public Health Nursing Training Center. This mobile clinic, originally designed for public health doctors and nurses, attracted the attention of many elementary school teachers. In response to popular request, subsequently a separate program was set up for teachers on mental health for school children.

The above experiences helped CMHC in planning for its later programs. From 1960 to 1966 a six-year pilot project was conducted at the East-Gate Elementary School in Taipei. It was conceived in two major parts. The first part aimed at imparting basic knowledge and skills in mental health to all teachers of the School by means of a 9-month mental health seminar for a group of 15 teachers each year. The second part consisted of training teacher-counselors and the establishment of a counselors' office in the School. The first counselors' office at elementary school level in Taiwan was established in 1963 (Hsu and Lin 1969). This office was also used to train teacher-counselors for other schools in the city.

157

A. Kleinman and T.-Y. Lin (eds.), Normal and Abnormal Behavior in Chinese Culture, 157–165.
Copyright © 1980 *by D. Reidel Publishing Company.*

This East-Gate Elementary School mental health program still continues to lead the school mental health program in Taipei.

The model school mental health program developed at the East-Gate Elementary School was thereafter adopted and further developed at other elementary schools in Taipei, notably at the West-Gate Elementary School. The emphasis in the West-Gate Elementary School and other elementary schools lies in making every teacher of the school responsible for mental health of children under his/her care, rather than relying on the assistance of teacher-counselors or specialists, except for the seriously disturbed. The development of standardized tools, e.g., Raven's Colored and Standard Progressive Matrices (CPM/SPM) (Hsu et al. 1976) and Bower's Screening Tools for the Emotionally Disturbed Children (Hsu 1970), have greatly facilitated these teachers' ability to identify and help problem children. The junior high schools in the city also followed suit in 1972 and now every junior high school in Taipei has a counselors' office responsible for its mental health program.

In addition, CMHC was also instrumental in the establishment of special classes for the mentally retarded. The Special Education Program included training teachers in teaching and handling special classes, developing curriculum and teaching tools, and designing concrete methodologies for screening and recruiting children (Hsu et al. 1968).

To sum up, CMHC has played a key role in the past 25 years' history of school mental health in Taiwan. It initiated, organized and helped carry out important programs, and after schools and government agencies assumed administrative and financial responsibilities for them, CMHC transferred its leadership role to research. Among the researches that have been carried out are Hsu's study on child development (1978), Soong's on physiological maturation (1977), Hsu et al. on cognitive tasks (1976) and Chen (1979) on group psychotherapy with maladjusted school children.

THE ABSENTEEISM STUDY

In order to understand the epidemiology of absenteeism and to develop some guidelines for the work of school mental health, Soong et al. conducted a study on 5,605 students (2,863 boys and 2,742 girls) from the first to the sixth grades of the East-Gate Elementary School. The five-week study consisted of three stages. In the first week attendance records were gathered. Classes with matching absentee rates for each grade were assigned randomly into either the "experimental" or control group. Thus experimental and control groups had a comparable mean absentee rate. In the second stage (two weeks), trained senior medical students made immediate home visits to the absentees of the experimental group, assessed students and enquired about the circumstances of their absenteeism from parents, using standard questionnaires. In addition, information about learning potential, school achievement, and school adjustment of these students was obtained from school teachers. The visiting medical students also discussed with parents the ways to get the children back to school as soon as possible. In the third stage (two weeks), attendance records were monitored to assess the influence of home visits to the experimental group compared to the control group. The following are some of the findings related to sex difference:

1. *Daily absence rate:* Among the 2,863 boys, 81 did not attend school and contributed a total of 161 days of absence. While among the 2,742 girls, 55 missed school and contributed a total of 85 days of absence. Hence the average daily absence rates are 0.937% for the boys and 0.516% for the girls. The difference is highly significant (X^2 = 20.472, df = 1, p<0.001, Table 1).

TABLE 1

Daily absence rate

	Boys (N=2,863)	Girls (N=2,742)
Total attendance (person-day)	2863 x 6	2742 x 6
Total absence (person-day)	161	85
Daily absence rate*	0.937%	0.516%

X = 20.472, df = 1, p<0.001
* Daily absence rate = total absence (person-day/week) ÷ total attendance (person-day/week)

2. *Teachers' rating of maladjustment:* 56 boys and 50 girls from the experimental group were absent from school for one day or more. Of these, 20 boys (35.71%) and 9 girls (18.00%) were rated by their teachers as maladjusted using a 4-point rating scale. The sex difference is significant (X^2 = 4.170, df = 1, p<0.05, Table 2).

TABLE 2

Teacher's rating of maladjustment among absentees

Maladjustment	Boys	Girls	Total
No	36 (64.28%)	41 (82.00%)	77 (72.64%)
Yes	20 (35.71%)	9 (18.00%)	29 (27.35%)
Total	56 (100.0%)	50 (100.0%)	106 (100.0%)

X^2 = 4.170, df = 1, p<0.05

3. *The result of clinical examination:* During the home visit, clinical examination was performed on those students whose absence was attributed to physical illness by their parents. Thirty-nine boys and fourteen girls were found to show no objective physical signs to account for being absent from school. The difference is statistically significant (X^2 = 7.918, df = 1, p<0.005, Table 3).

TABLE 3

Result of clinical examination

Objective signs	Boys (N=58)	Girls (N=37)
Yes	19 (32.75%)	23 (62.16%)
No	39 (67.25%)	14 (37.84%)

X^2 = 7.918, df = 1, p<0.005

4. *Reported management of absentees by parents:* Upon inquiry only 23 of 58 boys (39.65%), whose absences had been attributed to physical illness, were reported to have seen physicians. Twenty-four out of 37 girls (64.86%) were reported to have done so. This is in inverse relationship to the use of over-the-counter drugs, 22 boys (37.93%) versus 9 girls (24.32%). Thirteen boys and four girls received no treatment. Again the sex difference is significant (X^2 = 5.883, df = 2, p = 0.05, Table 4).

The third and fourth findings above can be interpreted as follows: among those children on sick leave, more boys had either very mild physical illness or no objective signs, and thus received little treatment at home. In other words, more boys' sick leave seemed unjustified medically.

TABLE 4

Management of claimed illness

Management	Boys (N=58)	Girls (N=37)
seeing doctor	23 (39.65%)	24 (64.86%)
buying over-the-counter drug	22 (37.93%)	9 (24.32%)
no management	13 (22.41%)	4 (10.81%)

X^2 = 5.883, df = 2, p=0.05

5. *Reasons for absence:* Based on all the information gathered from school teachers, parents, and the clinical examination of the child, the investigators made an overall assessment, without knowledge of the sex of the child, of the most probable reasons for absence. The results showed again more boy absentees (52, 55.31%) than girls (21, 32.81%) had an unjustified reason for absence (X^2 = 7.759, df = 1, p<0.01, Table 5).

TABLE 5

Global objective evaluation of reasons for absence

Justified	Boys (N=94)	Girls (N=64)	Total (N=158)
Yes	42 (44.68%)	43 (67.18%)	85 (53.79%)
No	52 (55.31%)	21 (32.81%)	73 (46.20%)

X^2 = 7.759, df = 1, p<0.01

PREVALENCE OF MALADJUSTMENT STUDY

Shen et al., in a separate study (1978), looked into the behavior problems of 2,035 children (1,047 boys and 988 girls) from the fourth to the sixth grades of the East-Gate Elementary School. The modified Chinese version of Bower's three instruments, Thinking about Yourself, Pupil Behavior Rating Scale, and A Class Play (Hsu 1970) were used to screen and score the behavior of the children. The findings showed that 157 boys (14.9%) were screened out as moderately and severely maladjusted while 111 girls (11.2%) were rated as such. The difference is statistically significant (X^2 = 6.28, df = 1, p<0.05, Table 6).

TABLE 6

Prevalence of maladjusted school children

Maladjusted	Boys (N=1047)	Girls (N=988)	Total (N=2035)
severely	29 (2.7%)	20 (2.0%)	49 (2.4%)
moderately	128 (12.2%)	91 (9.2%)	219 (10.7%)
Total	157 (14.9%)	111 (11.2%)	268 (13.1%)

X^2 = 6.28, df = 1, p<0.05

DISCUSSION

The above findings strongly suggest that Chinese boys are no better protected from school stresses than girls, in spite of their preferential treatment at home. In other words, Chinese boys fall into the same universal pattern as reported for other societies (Bentzen 1963; Werry and Quay 1971; Weinstein and Geisel 1960). Rutter (1970) attempted to explain sex difference in children in response to family stresses by the following major factors: conditionability, temperament, imitation and identification, conformity and suggestibility. According to the personal experiences of the authors, some of these factors, e.g., imitation and conformity, seem to be relevant in understanding the sex difference in school adjustment in Taiwan. However, each society also has its own set of factors operating to influence the sex difference in response to stress. The authors will address a few major ones in the current sociocultural and educational context of Taiwan.

THE TRADITIONAL EMPHASIS ON SCHOLARLY ACHIEVEMENT

For thousands of years, under the influence of Confucianism, the literati have always occupied high social status and been the most respected persons in Chinese society. It is widely accepted that scholarly achievement not only is a symbol of success and an honor for the family but actually leads to economic betterment. Hence, there are hundreds of stories in the Chinese literary classics about the struggle of people to become scholars in order to gain prestige and wealth. In contemporary Taiwan, even though industrialization and Westernization have brought about certain changes in the traditional social structure and life style of the people, the emphasis on scholarly achievement still prevails and a majority of people are convinced that going to school, especially going on to a higher education, is the best way to advance one's social status and to bring more wealth to the family. "A degree from college is a guaranty for better job and better life" is a common belief. Consequently, the competition within and among schools is extremely keen. Students, as early as elementary school, are constantly living and struggling under the pressure of serious academic competition. For example, from kindergarten on students are competing in placement examinations to get into the best schools which create an ever narrower funnel toward the very high status universities. Suicide of students who have failed placement examinations is not unknown, even as early as 12 years of age.

PARENTAL EXPECTATIONS

The preferential treatment of Chinese boys is not without its negative consequences. Boys have many duties to fulfill. They carry the family name and bear the burden of social and financial responsibilities. Thus, their every movement, achievement, or failure, and their careers are constantly under the watchful eyes of their family. For individual achievement is not just for the individual alone, but for the entire family. Similarly, shame is experienced not only by the individual but by the family as a whole. The high expectation on Chinese boys often is viewed by them as unbearable and certainly constitutes a profound stress. The pressure from parents about school achievement also applies to girls, but is relatively less when compared to that experienced by boys. The central concern seems to focus on girls' conduct and their finding a suitable partner for marriage. In modern Taiwan where equal opportunities for education are open to girls, graduation from a good school is also regarded as a passport to a satisfactory betrothal. This aspect seems to play an important role in girls' adjustment in school.

SEX-TYPING

In Chinese society, sex-stereotyped behavior used to be marked and well-defined. While perseverance, courage and a certain degree of independence are emphasized as the sanctioned virtues for boys, obedience, patience and conformity are the virtues reserved for girls. In the Nü-Fan (女範), an ancient teaching for women, it is clearly stated that girls should be gentle in touch, manner and voice. The most important life tasks for women were being a filial daughter in their childhood, a considerate wife after marriage and a loving mother to their children. Recently, because education is open to both sexes and many women have proved themselves successfully in many professional fields, the role of women in Taiwan and other Chinese societies has begun to change. Nonetheless, the basic virtues highly regarded in *Nü-Fan* are still the guidelines for parents in socializing their daughters. Such training, in fact, facilitates girls' initial adjustment in school and helps with their relationships with peers and teachers.

THE EDUCATIONAL MILIEU

In the past two to three decades, education in Taiwan has made great strides. For instance, compulsory education has been extended to 15 years of age, more vocational schools have been established, and many special classes have become available to help the needy and handicapped. However, the current elementary schools still have a great deal of room for improvement:

1. Size of class and school: Due to the baby boom in the 1950's and the drastic decrease of infant mortality rate, the population of school children has increased rapidly. In 1979, the attendance rate in elementary school reached 99.64%. Therefore, a school with three to five thousand students is the rule rather than the exception in cities and a classroom with more than 50 students is also very common. Under such circumstances, teachers' responsibilities become extremely heavy and individual guidance is almost impossible. The enormous class sizes have intensified the use of discipline by teachers, which also has been a culturally-sanctioned method of teaching in Chinese society. Again, boys tend to react to teachers' reliance on physical discipline more strongly than do girls, who are usually more compliant.

2. School curriculum and school tests: A well-planned school program which includes diverse and flexible activities for students can help a child's total development. In fact, this was emphasized by the Ministry of Education in its recent instruction on curriculum planning. Yet the aforementioned emphasis on children's entrance into higher educational institutions combined with a lack of facilities and opportunities for physical activities means that education is restricted to classroom didactic cramming. Girls, being more patient and being taught to be obedient to their superiors, seem to conform better to the rules and follow the curriculum more faithfully than boys, who more often become restless and bored in such educational settings.

School tests in recent years have been designed in such a way that better grades are positively correlated with good memory and cramming. Since girls sit longer and concentrate better in memorizing details in textbooks, their academic performance is usually better on the whole. Hence today's school tests put more pressure on boys than on girls.

CONCLUSION

The above observations help explain our research findings that boys have more adjustment problems in elementary schools in Taiwan. For educators and mental health professionals, the differential influence of pressures from family, school, and society on the sexes should not be overlooked. Schools should provide more and sufficient space for boys' physical activities, limit the class size to 30 students to allow more individual interaction and guidance, and offer a flexible curriculum to meet different needs of children. In other words, it is essential that school education in Taiwan should shift its focus from a rigid, test-oriented, performance-dominated, teacher-centered approach to one which is flexible, growth-oriented and child-centered.

ACKNOWLEDGEMENT

The authors would like to thank Professors Tsung-yi Lin, Chen-chin Hsu and Mrs. Mei-chen Lin, who initiated and developed the school mental health program in Taiwan, for their constant help, support and valuable criticism to make this paper possible.

REFERENCES

Bentzen, F.
  1963 Sex ratios in learning and behavior disorders. American Journal of Orthopsychiatry 33:92–98.
Chen, C. C.
  1979 Group therapy with Chinese school children. Paper presented in Regional W.F.M.H. Conference, Taipei, Taiwan.
Hsu, C. C., Lin, T. Y., Ko, Y. H. and Lee, S. C.
  1968 Special education for mentally subnormal children in Taiwan. American Journal of Orthopsychiatry 38:615–621.
Hsu, C. C. and Lin, T. Y.
  1969 Mental health program at the elementary school level in Taiwan. In Mental Health Research in Asia and the Pacific. W. Caudill and T. Y. Lin, eds. Honolulu: East-West Center Press, pp. 178–194.
Hsu, C. C.
  1970 Early Identification of Maladjusted Students. Taipei: Ioushi Publication.
Hsu, C. C., See, R., Lin, C. C. and Yang, S. K.
  1976 Sex and intellectual development in Chinese children as measured by Raven's Progressive Matrices: A six-year longitudinal study. Psychiatria et Neurologia Paediatrica Japonica 18:81–88.
Hsu, C. C., Su, S., Shiao, S. T., Lin, C. C., Soong, W. T., and Chang, C.
  1978 Chinese child development inventory: A tentative normative data. Acta Paediatrica Sinica 19:142–157.
Rutter, M.
  1970 Sex differences in children's responses to family stress. In The Child in his Family. E. J. Anthony and C. Koupernik, eds. New York: Wiley-Interscience; pp. 165–196.
Shen, C., Wong, S. J., Chen, K. M., Yang, Z. K., Soong, W. T., Hsu, C. C. and Lin, C. C.
  1978 The prevalence of maladjustment among the urban elementary and junior high school population. In Proceedings of the Conference on the Youth in the Changing Society. T. I. Wen and K. S. Yang, eds. Taipei: Academia Sinica Press; pp. 117–140.

Soong, W. T.
1977 A clinical-epidemiological study of enuresis, 1st report. The age trend of and factors associated with bladder control among urban Chinese children. Acta Pediatrica Sinica 18:11–23.
Soong, W. T., Hsu, C. C., Chen, C. J. and Lin, C. C.
1978 A clinico-epidemiological study of and the effects of immediate home visits on absenteeism among elementary and junior high school students. *In* Proceedings of the Conference on the Youth in the Changing Society. T. I. Wen and K. S. Yang, eds. Taipei: Academic Sinica Press; pp. 83–115.
Weinstein, E. A. and Geisel, P. N.
1960 An Analysis of sex differences in adjustment. Child Development 31:721–728.
Werry, J. S. and Quay, H. C.
1971 The prevalence of behavior symptoms in younger elementary school children. American Journal of Orthopsychiatry 41:136–143.

SECTION III

FAMILY STUDIES

INTRODUCTION TO SECTION III

In his article, McGough, an anthropologist, presents an extremely comprehensive review of deviant marriage patterns in Chinese society based on his ethnographic field work along with his detailed research on collections of Chinese customary laws. He first summarizes the standard Chinese marriage form and demonstrates how it differs from Western conceptualizations of marriage and accordingly is distorted when viewed from a Western perspective. Then he reviews such deviant marriage forms as adopted daughter-in-law marriage and uxorilocal marriage. He sheds new light on several other deviant forms of marriage, as well as homosexual unions. McGough doesn't only describe these relationships and suggest how prevalent they were and still are. He goes on to analyze their function within particular Chinese cultural systems of meanings, norms and power. For example, he discusses how China's power elite helped generate these deviant marriage patterns, gives reasons for why participants entered into them, and, what is most important, reviews their politico-economic function in terms of "group recruitment" to the family viewed as a production unit. Along the way, McGough offers a compelling account of the organization of domination and control in the Chinese family in terms of sanctioned transactions between *yin* and *yang* social roles. His article represents a major contribution to the historical anthropology of marriage and the family in Chinese society that goes beyond the traditional sinological bias that deals only with elite class patterns and life styles. McGough outlines the cultural code of non-elite marriage. His article presents a classification of deviant marriage types that could be used by other investigators both to better document their frequency and prevalence in particular Chinese communities and to make cross-cultural comparisons.

Parish, a sociologist particularly concerned with recent developments in the People's Republic of China, reviews continuities and changes in the family's functions and problems. Based on his interview survey of refugees in Hong Kong, he argues that the family still is the primary unit of rural life. In rural China, in spite of the now dominant ideology and real attempts at bringing about basic changes, Parish demonstrates the persistence of key domestic roles, relationships, and practices, such as the continued dominance of men in family decision-making and the practice of demanding a "bride price." He does show distinct changes in ritual practices, but concludes that ancestor worship persists, albeit in disguised forms. In urban areas, Parish suggests that the family may have undergone more change, though it still maintains its distinctiveness in communal living arrangements. But even in Chinese cities, Parish outlines key continuities such as the structural conflict between daughter-in-law and mother-in-law and the rarity of divorce. His article fills out our picture of crucial social develop-

169

A. Kleinman and T.-Y. Lin (eds.), Normal and Abnormal Behavior in Chinese Culture, 169–170.
Copyright © 1980 by D. Reidel Publishing Company.

ments in the People's Republic that affect both group and individual behavior; he suggests what may be the major contemporary stressors, such as some of the difficult problems facing youth that will determine future patterns of personal and social deviance.

In the last article in this section, Rin, a psychiatrist with extensive clinical experience in Taiwan, presents empirical findings from a study he conducted investigating the extent, types, and effects of family pathology on juvenile delinquents entering the court system in Taipei. He shows that such pathology appears to function as a major determinant of this form of social deviance, and that much of it is indigenous to Chinese families and not a direct result of modernization per se, which, however, may contribute by worsening already existing problems. Rin's work documents the negative consequences on families and their children of poverty, chronic physical or psychological impairment of family members, absent or ineffective parents, and maladaptive cultural attitudes concerning parenting. He illustrates these problems with case examples. His work should help dispel the myth that Chinese families are problem-free utopias, and should advance our understanding of both their traditional and current problems. Rin also shows that the effects of family pathology on delinquents are often mediated via work and school failure, and that delinquency in Taiwan is associated with a higher rate of violent crime than in the past was expected in Chinese communities. Clearly these findings suggest interventions that can be applied by planners, clinicians, and members of legal, social service and other relevant agencies to help identify families under stress before they disintegrate and turn out delinquent youth. One would like to know more about similar problems in the People's Republic of China and other Chinese communities. Again Rin's data, like McGough's, can be compared cross-culturally to derive a more adequate assessment of family problems, social deviance, and their relation to established and changing socioeconomic and cultural patterns.

Readers of this section will have already noted that many questions relevant to the family in Chinese culture are touched upon in earlier sections of the book, and these and other family-based questions receive additional coverage in some of the articles in the section that follows. For culturally constituted family patterns, and the socioeconomic and other forces that influence them, obviously play as central a role in the development of psychiatric disorders as in the genesis of normal behavior and social deviance.

JAMES McGOUGH

10. DEVIANT MARRIAGE PATTERNS IN CHINESE SOCIETY

INTRODUCTION

The basic concerns of anthropology are cross-cultural understanding of other peoples, analyzing other societies and investigating other ways of life. One of the things which confuses attempts to do these things is that as cultural beings we take so many things for granted; we unconsciously assume so very much in every social situation. The things that people take for granted, the assumptions that they make, vary, of course, from society to society. One becomes painfully aware of this when thrown into a new society, or a completely new situation. This is an occupational hazard in anthropology, though anthropologists of course have no monopoly over it. Culture-shock, the disoriented feelings, the sense of free-floating anxiety, that comes of trying to deal day-in and day-out with an unfamiliar language, unfamiliar society, and unfamiliar patterns of social interaction, is a favorite topic of anthropologists who have done field research.

Anthropologists usually live for a year or so in the society they are studying and confront this problem in everyday life. When they return home, and sit in an office or library writing up their findings, the problem persists in another form. It is dangerously easy to uncritically and unconsciously rely upon assumptions taken from one's own familiar society when trying to analyze other, relatively unfamiliar, societies. This is the anthropological sin of ethnocentrism; taking, consciously or unconsciously, one's own society's ways of doing things for granted as natural and right, and judging other societies and other ways of doing things, by those standards.

Perhaps an illustration is in order. I did research in a rural, rice-growing village in Northeastern Taiwan on family, marriage, and adoption. A colleague of mine did research in Southern Taiwan, in a sugar-cane growing region, touching also on family and marriage. He found that most first children were born far fewer than nine months after the marriage of the parents, and in many cases were born before the marriage. "Ah-ha! Pre-marital sex!" he exclaimed. Tongue-in-cheek, he devised an "ecological" explanation: sugar-cane grows tall and dense, and offers more hiding-places for amorous unmarried couples than does, say, rice.

My own research did not support his hypothesis. I found the same evidence for what seemed to be pre-marital sex in the North, where sugar-cane is not grown, and where the omnipresent rice offers little cover. An alternative argument might link pre-marital sex with the modernization of Taiwan, and the breakdown of traditional customs and morals that is often said by theorists of "social pathology" to accompany such social change.

My own explanation is rather different. My friend made too many assumptions

171

A. Kleinman and T.-Y. Lin (eds.), Normal and Abnormal Behavior in Chinese Culture, 171–201
Copyright © 1980 by D. Reidel Publishing Company.

in his tongue-in-check analysis that turned out to be false when applied to rural Taiwanese society. He assumed that the Taiwanese term *kiet-hun* (Mandarin *chieh-hun*) should be translated into English as "marriage," and he assumed that this ceremony, this social transaction, made sex "OK," just as "marriage" makes sex "OK" for most Americans. The error lies in both assumptions. Taiwanese marriage is more usefully conceptualized as a process involving a number of steps, none of which can be correctly translated as "marriage." In any society "marriage" causes a number of changes, only one of which has to do with making it permissible to go to bed together. In rural Taiwan, at least, this latter change takes place more often at *ting-hun,* or "betrothal," not at *kiet-hun,* which is more literally translated as "completing the marriage." Thus the "problem" of explaining pre-marital sex vanished. There was none (or at least we couldn't prove that there was any. The couples weren't jumping the gun; the anthropologists had sounded the gun at the wrong juncture).

What I have tried to do in this paper is to avoid some of the problems of ethnocentrism in cross-cultural analysis by *not* starting out with a specific assumption of what "marriage" is, or ought to be, in Chinese society. The standard, officially approved, form of marriage in China is often described in great detail. It is often taken for granted that this was the most common form of marriage. If alternate forms are mentioned at all, they are listed rather mechanically and are described as vulgar or despised forms found occasionally only among uneducated peasants.

I found this simple listing of exceptions unsatisfactory. My research in Taiwan showed that the exceptions were often very common, and not despised by the majority. I found, for example, that 10 to 20 percent of marriages in the village where I lived in Taiwan had been initially uxorilocal; that is, a deviant form in which, contrary to the standard form, the couple moved to live with the wife's family (the husband sometimes taking the wife's surname instead of vice-versa). The mayor of this village was, in fact, an uxorilocal husband, and took no pains to hide the fact. Arthur Wolf has found that as many as eighty or ninety percent of marriages in the last century in the village in North Taiwan where he did research were of the "little daughter-in-law" type (see below).

Some have suggested that these and other assumed peculiarities of Taiwanese society were due to its own history, particularly its fifty years as part of the Japanese Empire. I began, then, to look into what data I could find about real marriage patterns in traditional mainland China, as distinct from the ideal patterns. In order to minimize my own assumptions, I resolved to pay attention to all types of marriage, "deviant" as well as "regular," and to a number of marriage-like forms as well, not just those that looked most like "marriage" to Europeans.

In this paper I will briefly describe the deviant forms of marriage practiced in traditional Chinese society and then discuss the motivations for entering into such unions, and why they were considered deviant.

Marriage in China

The Chinese Empire was an agrarian state. These two factors, agriculture and state organization, are crucial for understanding traditional Chinese society. The ultimate source of wealth was agriculture, carried out in many millions of domestic units scattered across the face of China. Agricultural "surplus" produced above and beyond the basic needs of peasant domestic units moved upward through the social and political hierarchy in the form of rent, taxes, and interest. At the same time successful upward mobility was measured by power. Elites were powerful people with direct or indirect connection to political status. Wealth, a counterpart to elite status, could be safeguarded from greedy officials only through political connections and power, and was safeguarded from theft, loss, or destruction through investment in land, an investment with a low rate of return, but with relatively high security. Family and kinship ties came to be important both to elite family enterprises and to peasant family agricultural enterprises. In the former case family and kin ties helped to extend and expand political and economic ties, while in the latter they functioned to provide the family production unit with its labor supply.

The socio-economic supports for the family system that are mentioned in the *Taiwan Min-shih Hsi-kuan Tiao-ch'a Pao-kao* are as follows:

1. China has long been an agrarian country, and common, cooperative labor is profitable in agriculture. The common saying, "have many sons and you'll get lots of money" indicates that only through coresident cooperation can one bring prosperity to the family.
2. Because China was so large, the government was usually unable to ensure peace and order in local areas, and because self-protection was necessary, there naturally developed large families and other self-protection organizations.
3. To maintain a family's power, influence, and capital, it is necessary to follow a large-family system.
4. Economy of scale: the ancient saying was "living together, many expenses are saved; divided, each person has expenses."
5. In order to support normal human relationships and develop morality, the government promoted coresidency and common property among families; honors were awarded to virtuous families, and sometimes they were made exempt from tax payment. The Code also prohibited brothers from living separately and dividing the property as long as the parents or grandparents were alive (*TMS:* 323).

Even non-agricultural pursuits like banking, for example, were often organized on the model of family and kinship. Frank H. H. King has pointed out that in indigenous banking (the so-called "native banks") in the 19th century managers of branch offices were adopted into the families of the head managers, thus providing legally sanctioned mechanisms of authority and compliance within the organization (King 1965:94).

I have found it most useful to view the family or household as a type of informal interest group, one which makes use of various kinship, ritual, and other forms of symbolic and practical activities to protect or develop power (in the broadest sense) for its members. The family is and was a particular kind of interest group in an on-going, ever-changing politico-economic field. In the Chinese case, certainly for any time period of interest to us, this politico-economic field does and did include the existence of a formally organized state polity.

The analysis of marriage and related social transactions, then, must be carried out in such a way that explicit reference is made to the state and to the general politico-economic setting (see Cohen 1974: 128–129). Marriage, no less than some other related forms, was traditionally a transaction between interest groups, between families, and not just individuals. Thus it is necessary to focus on power variables; on the legal and economic characteristics of such trans-actions. "Failure to take proper account of the transactional nature of social relationships — especially in their jural aspects, where rights and duties are involved — may well have contributed to anthropology's conceptual problems in defining marriage, family, and kinship" (Goodenough 1970: 22). My procedure, then, will be to examine the various deviant or irregular forms of marriage that existed in traditional Chinese society, particularly in their jural aspects, and particularly in the context of the political and economic systems.

This is not an easy thing to do. Traditional Chinese society was bipolar in its class structure. The power elite consisted of the so-called "gentry," or literati. What we know about traditional China from historical materials is usually heavily influenced by what this educated class thought and wrote about its own society. The elite, being literate, were almost the only ones whose accounts and descriptions made it into writing, to end up on our library shelves. It has also often been true that European observers and transmitters of Chinese culture knew best, listened to, and learned from the educated and elite classes. The elite in Imperial China often knew little about the life-style of rural peasants and urban poor. This paper explores a number of ways to reduce the problem of elite bias, and to discover through other sources what the non-elite life style was like in traditional China.

Though a good number of the marriage forms I will discuss are no longer practiced, it is possible to interview people who participated in them in one way or another in the past. The household registration materials collected first by the Japanese and later by the Nationalists in Taiwan are another rich source of information about marriage. Collections of customary laws are also very helpful. In particular, I have used the collection for mainland China done earlier in this century and titled *Chung-kuo Min-, Shang-shih Hsi-kuan Tiao-ch'a Pao-kao Lu* (*Report on Investigations into Chinese Civil and Commercial Customs*, ab-breviated *MSS*), the somewhat similar but later collection for Taiwan titled *Taiwan Min-shih Hsi-kuan Tiao-ch'a Pao-kao* (*Report on Investigations into Taiwanese Civil Customs*, abbreviated *TMS*), and the collection of contracts and other documents made originally by the Japanese but later reprinted by the Bank of Taiwan in their *Taiwan Szu-fa Jen-shih Pien* series (*Taiwanese Private Law: Civil Collection*). Finally, I have made some use of fictional works. Though these latter must be used with caution, they constitute an important source of material on both elite and non-elite social life. What follows is a discussion based on all of these sources of marriage forms in traditional Chinese society.

I. STANDARD MARRIAGE

Marriage, in the classical formulation, consisted of six stages, the so-called "six rites" (*liu li*). These were "asking the name" (*wen ming*), "betrothal" (*ting-hun*), "exchange of goods" (*na ts'ai*), "exchange of wealth" (*na pi*), "setting the date" (*ch'ing ch'i*), and "welcoming the bride" (*ch'in ying*). These steps were not always followed in their entirety, but they did furnish a general pattern, a guideline, for the wedding ceremony (e.g., see Fei (1934) for an account of the geographical distribution of the last stage and its variants).

As Arthur Wolf puts it, "three things happen in a marriage of the patrilocal type [that is, virilocal, or standard marriage]. The bride leaves her natal home and relinquishes membership in her family of orientation; she steps over the threshold of the groom's home and becomes a member of his household; and she is presented to the groom's ancestors and thereby acquires the status of wife" (Wolf 1966: 883). The bride paid homage to her parents-in-law as well, and then afterwards repaired to the kitchen to cook a chicken and begin her service to the family.

Marriage was, of course, very important in traditional Chinese society. It was at the center of the development of one's status with respect to family and kinship. Thus its arrangement was more a matter of concern for the family than for the individual, in part because of the religious connotation that marriage carried. It was incumbent upon the younger generation to provide offspring to continue the sacrifices to the ancestors. These offspring had to be male, not female, as only males were thought to be capable of offering effective sacrifices.

This distinction is important because it underscores the fact that (as I am prepared to argue) all social transactions and relationships in Chinese society were traditionally between parties of unequal standing. One of the basic and most important sources of this inequality is the social distinction between sex roles. Women, of course, played an absolutely indispensable role in the social system, but it was a role which was distinctly different and distinctly inferior to that of men. The rights and duties of children in a family differed sharply depending on sex, and the rights and duties of the husband and wife were likewise differentiated.

The existence of this clear inequality in the husband-wife relationship did not mean, of course, that there were no mutual obligations; though a hierarchical relationship, it was not completely one-sided. Mutual obligations, followed and enforced in varying degrees, were those of mutual support, cohabitation, and maintenance of sexual fidelity. Mutual support was not defined in the Ch'ing Code, but according to customary law, the husband was bound to support the wife and the concubine as well; if he was unable to do so, the wife then had a duty to support him (*TMS*:85).

Still, the woman took her basic social position from that of her husband, and had no real independent existence; she was expected to be subordinate and submissive in relation to her husband (see, for example, Tai 1966:233). In fact, the relationship between husband and wife was in many ways comparable to that between elder and junior within a kin line, and was at times likened to the relationship between ruler and subject, heaven and earth. The husband had the right, in customary law, to issue orders to the wife and it was her duty to obey. The husband's ill treatment or punishment of the wife was not actionable in court, no matter how arbitrary or unreasonable it might have been, unless it went as far as serious injury or death. On the other hand, in the event of injury or death caused to the husband by the wife, her punishment exceeded the norm because the wife had additionally violated the socially and legally defined relationship between herself and her husband. This was also true when a junior or inferior assaulted a senior, or superior. Indeed, a woman was traditionally thought subject to her father's authority while unmarried, to her husband's authority after marriage, and to her son's authority after her husband's death. (see, for example, *TMS*:86).

The officially approved or standard marriage system was in theory monogamous, but was in fact often polygamous. That is, under the Ch'ing Code, it was a crime to have more than one principal wife (*ch'i* or *cheng ch'i*). The only legal exception was that a man could marry a second principal wife as a "stand-in" for his deceased brother, to ensure that his brother's line would not die out (see Chiu n.d. (1966?):33–35).

Secondary wives, or concubines, were, however, permitted. Ostensibly these wives were taken only when the first wife proved barren, but in practice a man could take as many concubines as he wanted or could afford. The concubine, or secondary wife, had a definite and legally protected position in the household and family, but one which was inferior to that of the principal wife. The children she bore were not considered illegitimate, but their rights in the family estate were inferior to those of the children of the principal wife.

It is safe to assume that observance of the "six rites" and adherence to the standard marriage forms was a class-related phenomenon in China (see, for example, Kataoka Iwao's *Taiwan Fuzoku Shi* for data on marriage rites in Taiwan during the Japanese occupation). While the upper class attempted to follow the six rites, the lower classes often deviated from the standard form and included variants such as marriage by sale and the temporary marriage of one's wife to another man (Kataoka 1921:20).

The following sections will examine these and other "deviant" or non-standard marriage forms in China (a summary account of some of the deviant forms to be discussed can also be found in Ho 1951:57–68).

II. ADOPTED DAUGHTER-IN-LAW MARRIAGE

The "little daughter-in-law" (Taiwanese *simpua,* Mandarin *t'ung-yang-hsi* "daughter-in-law raised from youth") was a woman or girl who was "adopted" into a family with the idea in mind of later marrying her to one of the sons of this family.

This was a very widespread custom in Chinese society. It is sometimes said to be a peculiarity of, or to be particularly well-developed in, Taiwan (see *Taiwan Szu-fa Jen-shih Pien* II:188). But the *Chung-kuo Min-, Shang-shih Hsi-kuan Tiao-ch'a Pao-kao Lu* says that about 80 to 90 percent of households in Shun-ch'ang Hsien of Fukien Province had an adopted daughter-in-law (*MSS*:1578) and goes on to report it for the old Chih-li, for Honan, Shantung, Shansi, Anhwei, Kiangsi, Chekiang, Fukien, Hupei, Hunan, Shensi, Kansu, etc. Far from being peculiar to Taiwan, I think it is safe to assume that it existed wherever there were Chinese populations, and was often, in fact, tailored to meet local conditions.

The *Taiwan Min-shih Hsi-kuan Tiao-ch'a Pao-kao* says of the adoption of daughters in the Ch'ing that:

> The flourishing custom of adopting daughters in Taiwan, apart from the so-called T. *chio-ti* [an adoption intended to stimulate the birth of a child], was because one could take advantage of their labor. If a family had no children, they could adopt a daughter; if they already had a daughter, they could adopt another, and even if they already had an adopted daughter, they could adopt in yet another one. If there was no male among the relatives who could be adopted as an heir, a girl could be, and could be made to inherit.
>
> Taiwan also had the system of the adopted daughter-in-law, colloquially called *simpua*. The adopted daughter and the adopted daughter-in-law were different as far as the motivation for the adoption was concerned. The latter was a young girl of another surname adopted with the intention of later making her one's daughter-in-law. It did not matter whether or not it was yet determined to whom she should be married; she added the adoptive family's surname to her own just the same as if she had already married in, and a "quasi-affinal relationship" was created between her and the relatives of the adoptive family.
>
> The adopted daughter was different from this. The motivation for the adoption was not the same as the above, she took the adoptive family's surname as her own, and a kinship relation was created, just as if she were born to that family.
>
> However, in the northern part of Taiwan, the people usually mixed up the two terminologically, calling both "little daughter-in-law" (Taiwanese *simpua*; *TMS*:154).

This quote mentions phenomena that I observed during my field research in Taiwan; most adoptions were of females, and often families adopted several young girls, or in some cases adopted out their own daughters, then turned around and adopted in the daughters of others. Furthermore, it was often unclear until later whether these girls would become "daughters" or "daughters-in-law." It was this that originally piqued my interest in the custom; it was obvious that there were motivations involved that went beyond just "getting rid of" excess children.

Given cultural values which made females less important than males, and a system of customary law which offered many alternative forms of transactions involving rights over persons, females could be "used" much more flexibly than could males. A female was cheaper to raise than was a male, since her intrinsic value was seen as lower, and she could begin to contribute labor to the household earlier than a male child. Even today in Taiwan, in my experience, female children, whether adopted or not, begin to work much earlier for the family than do the male children. Girls of nine or ten can and do contribute much valuable labor in looking after younger siblings, preparing food, cleaning up the house, and so on, usually while their older brothers are out playing.

Thus one can get eight or ten years of increasingly productive labor out of a girl before she is of an age to marry. If she is one's own daughter, then she will marry out and be lost to the family (unless, of course, an uxorilocal husband is married in for her; as is noted in the section on that form of marriage, however, one must "sweeten the pot" to get such a man). One will, of course, get the brideprice in return, but this may not amount to much in the balance, and in general the alternatives available in the "disposal" of a daughter are not as many as in the case of an adopted daughter.

One can get more labor out of an adopted girl than out of one's own daughter; it is commonly felt that since such a girl is not one's own, it is easy to work her hard, and spend less on her. When she is of marriageable age, one is not restricted to arranging a marriage out or an uxorilocal marriage in, but one could also marry her to one's own son (or adopted son).

A Taiwanese folk-song puts it well:

> Bring a basket of rice to feed the rooster;
> If you raise a rooster, it can crow the time.
> If you raise a dog, it can bark at the ghosts.
> If you raise a pig, you can butcher it.
> If you raise a sister's son, it's all expense and no return.
> If you raise a daughter-in-law, she'll support the family.
> If you raise a daughter, she becomes someone else's.
>
> (Li 1936:240)

III. UXORILOCAL MARRIAGE AND POLYANDRY

As I have mentioned, the standard, officially approved, form of marriage was viri-patrilocal. The married couple was expected to live with the husband's father. Uxorilocal marriage, though negatively valued in the eyes of the elite, has had great temporal and geographical distribution. In the *Han Shu*, in the biography of Chia I is a passage which says "In the state of Ch'in if a family is rich and the sons vigorous, then they divide the estate and leave. If the family is poor and the sons vigorous, then they marry uxorilocally and leave." This passage occurs in a memorial presented by Chia I to the Emperor in 174 B.C. to illustrate to what depths the state of Ch'in had sunk because the Lord of Shang had abandoned propriety and benevolence, and it shows that even then the custom of uxorilocal marriage was associated, rightly or wrongly, with poverty (*HS*:48, 15a).

The uxorilocal husband was often called *chui-hsü* or *chao-hsü*. The former term emphasizes the man, the husband himself; one meaning of the term *chui* is "an excrescence," something unnecessary. But it is also sometimes identified with another character which looks a little similar, *chih* "to pawn": a man too poor to manage a betrothal gift would, in effect, offer himself to the bride's family as a pledge, or in bride service. The other term, *chao* (*hsü* in both instances means "son-in-law"), puts more emphasis on the bride's family; meaning "to call, to invite," it can be used in *chao-hsü* "invited son-in-law" or in *chao-fu* "invited (second) husband."

The following is an account of uxorilocal son-in-law marriage as practiced in Hupei earlier in this century:

> In Chu-hsi there are three types of uxorilocal marriage; that in which the man obtains rights in property but not in the sons (*yu ch'an wu tzu*), that in which he obtains rights in both property and sons (*yu ch'an yu tzu*), and that in which he obtains rights in neither (*wu ch'an wu tzu*). In the first case the son-in-law continues his wife's family line and inherits her family property. He must change his surname to that of the wife's family. The second type occurs when the woman's family loves her very much, and this sentiment is extended to the son-in-law. He later receives a portion of the property, and need not change his name. In the last case, the son-in-law usually changes his name, but at times he does not. (*MSS*:1630)

Other variants included "inviting a son-in-law for support (of his parents-in-law) in old age" (*chao-hsü yang-lao*), "property-managing uxorilocal husband" (*tso-ch'an chao-fu, tso-shan chao-fu*, etc.), "uxorilocal husband for the support of the (first husband's) children" (*chao-fu yang-tzu*), "uxorilocal husband for the provision of heirs" (*chao-fu sheng-tzu*), and "temporary uxorilocal husband while the first husband is missing" (*shih-tsung chao-fu*).

This last, particularly, may sound far-fetched, but it was practiced in a number of areas. Here is an account from what is now Liao-ning:

> In Sui-chung Hsien there is the custom of *ta-huo*, which means to marry a husband in to live uxorilocally for support. If a woman's husband has died or has been gone for several years without any trace, and the family circumstances are poor, so she cannot support herself, then she can establish this relationship with another man. Their relationship is the same as in ordinary remarriage, but a contract must be written up and in the contract it must clearly state that this is because of poverty, and that the second husband will assume a certain number of her debts. If the first husband happens to return, then the money will be returned to the second husband, who must then return the wife (and any children she may have taken with her). This kind of custom is found only too often in both urban and rural areas, each case for its own reasons (the relatives of the first husband, for instance, may be desirous of the money, or may oust her from the estate). In lawsuits the contract becomes very important. In the minds of rural people, this is a perfectly proper custom (*MSS*:1308).

The next logical step would be to invite in a second, uxorilocal, husband despite the continued presence of the first one. This would be a form of polyandry, and decidedly deviant with respect to traditional elite values. In fact, however, it seems to have been fairly widespread, though its incidence is hard to gauge. In parts of Shensi,

There are women, already with husbands, who invite in another husband to come and live with them, in order to support the family. This is called *chao-fu yang-fu* ["uxorilocal husband for the support of the (first) husband"]. This sort of custom is frequent in the Hsiens south of the Han River. In seeking reasons for this, one finds that in most cases it is because the first husband is disabled and cannot make a living. The couple, after consultation, is forced to do this. There are also those, however, who are not disabled, but through the profligacy of youth have expended the family property, and so endure humiliation, swallow their pride, and allow the wife to marry in another husband (*MSS*:1702).

Uxorilocal marriage seems to have been reinvented in contemporary China. According to an article in the March 16th, 1976 issue of the Hong Kong newspaper *Man Wui Po,* there were then 205 uxorilocal couples in Ch'ing-lan Commune in Wen-ch'ang Hsien on Hainan Island. The article mentions that these couples moved to live uxorilocally in order to attack the old, traditional, patrivirilocal customs as part of the campaign to criticize Lin Piao and Confucius. There was no mention of the fact that uxorilocal marriage was an old and widespread custom in China, at least among the masses.

IV. DOUBLE GENERATION MARRIAGE

When a man died leaving a number of children and little to support them, we have seen that one way of dealing with the situation was through uxorilocal marriage. A second husband was married in for his widow, to support her and her children. In certain circumstances she might instead marry out of her dead husband's family and take her children with her. This was, in fact, a common enough practice that it was associated with particular terminologies in a variety of local areas:

When a widow brings along her former husband's children when she remarries, they are colloquially divided into *huo-tai* and *szu-tai*. No matter how long she has been widowed, those children who do not change their surnames, and for whom it is clearly stated in the marriage contract that they will later return to their original kinship line, are called *huo-tai*. The *szu-tai* are those children whose surnames are changed to that of the second husband. Their given names remain the same, and they inherit equally with the step-father's own children. If he has no such children, then they can succeed him (*MSS*: 1436–37; see also 1447, 1450, 1454, 1723).

In a society in which parental arrangement of marriages was taken for granted, it is not surprising that a common variant on the above pattern was that of "double generation marriage," that is, the marriage of a man and a woman, and, simultaneously, the marriage of one of the man's children to one of the woman's.

In Shansi and some other areas, this was called, with tongue in cheek, "brother-sister marriage" (*hsiung-mei hun; MSS*:1436).

When a woman's husband dies she commonly takes her children with her when she remarries. Sometimes her son might marry a daughter of her second husband by his former wife, or her daughter might marry a son of the second husband by a former wife, so that the parents and the children, respectively, marry each other. This is colloquially called *t'ao-hua chia-chu* "grafting a peach blossom onto bamboo" (*MSS*:1603).

This last phrase is the one used in contemporary Taiwan; the peach blossom is a common symbol for the female, and the bamboo represents the male (see, for instance, Wu 1970:142–3).

V. THE LEVIRATE, SORORATE, AND COUSIN MARRIAGE

Thus far, a number of alternative solutions have been considered for the problem of what to do when a woman with young children is widowed. A logically possible solution which has not yet been discussed is that the dead husband be replaced by his brother in what is called the levirate. This solution has many advantages. Because the sociological relationship between the two affinally linked families does not change, no money or new presents need change hands. The brother of the original husband gets a "free" wife, and neither family has the problem of how to support the woman. The children would be kept in the first husband's family, and his kin line would be in no danger of dying out. The popularity and acceptability of *kuo-fang* adoption, that is, adoption within the patrilineal kin group, meant that it was quite natural for the second husband, the original husband's brother, to care for and support his dead brother's children and have them share in the division of his estate upon his own death.

The levirate, however, was seen, at least in the value system of the elite classes, and in the written classics, as an alarming sort of incest. It was not the worst form, to be sure, but it was nevertheless abhorrent. One writer deplored the custom of keeping slave girls on the basis that such girls might find themselves being pursued by two brothers (see *Taiwan Szu-fa, Jen-shih Pien* I:155–156). The idea of two brothers having sexual intercourse with the same woman, even if serially, was considered disgusting, as was; to an even greater degree, the idea of father and son in the same situation.

The levirate did, however, exist, but doesn't seem to have been prevalent among the elite. In parts of Shansi:

If the older brother dies, and his younger brother has no wife, then the younger brother can take his sister-in-law as wife. If the younger brother dies and the older brother has no wife, then he also can take his sister-in-law as wife (*MSS*:1418).

The compiler's comment:

This marrying the wife or concubine of a relative is not permitted in the law. Moreover, in regard to right human relationships and public morals, this is truly an evil custom. (*MSS*:1418).

In another part of the same province,

When a family is poor, and among several brothers one who has married dies, then one of the brothers who has no wife can, after discussing it with the woman's family, marry her as his wife. This is called *t'e-pieh hsü-ch'in* ("special remarriage"; *MSS*:1455).

The compiler's comment:

> This custom was reported by the Hsien Magistrate Chang Liu-hsing, and is the same as that in . . . (other named Hsien). Marrying the wife or concubine of a relative is clearly prohibited in the current Code. These customs in these Hsien cannot be regarded as having a beneficial effect on public morality (*MSS*:1455).

The levirate was found in Anhwei, where the compiler's comment was that "no custom is worse than this" (*MSS*:1477–78). In parts of Kiangsi it was called *sheng-fang*, "elevating to the (next family) branch" when it was the younger brother who died, and his older brother married the widow. "But this kind of evil custom is found only among the poor" (*MSS*:1505). In Lin-hai Hsien, Chekiang, the levirate was said, again, to be found among people of poor families (*MSS*:1548), and there are also reports of its existence in Hu-nan (*MSS*:1679, 1681), Shensi (*MSS*:1744, 1745, 1756), Kansu (*MSS*:1775, 1801), and so on.

A discussion of the levirate logically brings to mind its companion, the sororate, the marriage of sisters serially to the same man. This was evidently much less common than the levirate was, which should occasion no great surprise. Still, the sororate did exist. In Yu-yü Hsien, Shansi,

> If A marries the oldest daughter of B, and then she becomes ill and dies, and B has a second daughter, he may marry her to A as A's second wife. This happens in those familes which have good and close relationships (*MSS*:1448).

The levirate and the sororate are only two examples of "preferential" marriage patterns. Other such patterns occured in Chinese society; various kinds of "cousin marriage", for example.

More has been written about these latter forms than about other forms of marriage, so I will refer readers to such works as those by Fei (1946), Hsü (1945), and Gallin (1966).

VI. SAME SURNAME MARRIAGES

The permissible cousin-marriage forms mentioned above all preserve the state-sanctioned surname exogamy, but even this was not inviolable. Intra-surname marriage is specifically mentioned as practiced in the Hopei-Tientsin region (and most of the provinces north of the Yangtze River; *MSS*:1292), various parts of Shansi (*MSS*:1430, 1449), parts of Kiangsu (*MSS*:1478, 1482), Fukien (*MSS*:1585), all of Hupei (*MSS*:1608, also see 1618, 1639), Shensi (*MSS*:1739), and all of Kansu (*MSS*:1768). In most, if not all, of these accounts, it was specified that such marriages were permitted and customary as long as the people involved were not actually of the same kin line, or were not too close genealogically.

VII. CONSENSUAL UNIONS

In addition to forms clearly labelled "marriage," there are also a number of marriage-like forms to consider. Because of their nature, it is no surprise that there is little information about them, historical or otherwise. These were temporary or "common-law" marriages that were recognized socially, and in customary law, though the partners had not been married in the "regular" way.

Hsü K'o reports on such a custom from the Shanghai area (or at least from the Wu dialect area) in his *Ch'ing Pai-lei Ch'ao*, the relationship called *cha p'ing-t'ou*, which is translated by Mathews' *Chinese-English Dictionary* as "to form an illicit connection, to live as man and wife without regular marriage." Hsü's account is as follows:

> *cha p'ing-t'ou* means a man and woman who form an irregular union, who act as man and wife, and who, moreover, live, eat, and drink together. It also applies to those who only form a liaison, but do not live together. As for this term *p'ing-t'ou*, it is used reciprocally by the man and the woman. After such a relationship has been established, and recognized by each side, it may also be recognized by a third party. For instance, one can say "He (she) is my *p'ing-t'ou*," or "He (she) is her (his) *p'ing-t'ou*." This term *p'ing-t'ou* particularly pleases those of a literary turn of mind. In the dialect of Peking we call it *wai-chia*, "house on the side" (this term, however, implies that there is a fixed house or apartment, while the term *p'ing-t'ou* does not necessarily imply that; this is the only, slight, difference in meaning).
>
> *che p'ing-t'ou* is the term that is used when, either because of some actual clash of opinion the two persons decide to part, or their interests become opposed, and they go their separate ways. This is just as in business, when there is a split in the stock of a joint-stock company. After such a split the two persons look upon each other as strangers (Hsü 1920: XVI;43).

Hsü's account establishes that this was an institutionalized form, recognized by society; the relationship has a clear beginning and a clear end, and it links two persons in socially recognized, named, roles. It is also clear that it is a deviant form, clearly distinguished from marriage proper.

Information is available about some other such relationships, but one becomes increasingly suspicious of their degree of institutionalization. Yao Ling-hsi, for example, discusses the "dew husband and wife" (*lu-shui fu-fu*):

> A temporary union is called a "dew marriage" (*lu-shui yin-yuan*). It is not a regular marriage because it is as temporary as the dew, which evaporates with the light of day. It means to conduct a temporary illicit relationship (Yao 1940:147).

VIII. SPIRIT OR GHOST MARRIAGE

Spirit marriage, or ghost marriage, is fairly well known from reports based on research done in Taiwan (see, for example, Jordan 1971; Jordan 1972; McGough 1976). It was also found in various parts of mainland China. In Honan, for example,

> If a son dies before marriage, usually a girl of another surname is selected who died young, before marriageable age, and a ghost marriage is conducted. This is colloquially called *ch'ü kuei ch'i*, "marrying a ghost wife." It is also called *p'ei ku*, "marrying the bones." After the marriage they are buried together (*MSS*:1379).

In P'ing-hu Hsien (Chekiang) in upper, middle, and lower class families, when a son dies before marriage, usually an appropriate, matching family is selected, with a deceased daughter of the right age, and the two are betrothed. Then her spirit tablet is brought into the house. The ceremony is like that for a living person. This is called *ming-hun,* "hell marriage." If this is not done, the soul will have nowhere to belong, cannot enter the ancestral temple for sacrifices, and moreover descendants cannot be instituted. Once the ghost marriage has taken place, the necessary qualifications have been fulfilled for having an heir, and one can then have a descendant instituted (*MSS*: 1557—8).

This form of marriage has existed from pre-Han days through the Northern Wei, T'ang, Sung, Yuan, Ming, and Ch'ing dynasties. In the Ch'ing

... it was still flourishing; in Shansi, for example, all those males or females who die young after being betrothed will go through a spirit marriage ceremony. If the girl dies, then she will be buried in the man's tomb; if the man dies, and the girl is re-betrothed, then another, deceased, girl will be sought to marry him, an auspicious day will be selected, and the two buried together.

Today in the Hopei, Shansi, Shantung, and Chekiang regions this custom still exists, and is called, "*yin* marriage" (Ch'en 1937:112).

IX. PURCHASE AND PAWN MARRIAGES

Quite a variety of terms are used for these types of unions, usually meaning "purchase," "pledge," "mortgage," "pawn," "rental," etc. A few illustrations will suffice. In Ching-ning Hsien, Chekiang, for instance,

In the lower clases there have been cases of mortgaging one's wife to someone else. The two parties discuss and set the amount of money and length of time of the mortgage, and a contract is drawn up, called a "mortgage marriage contract" (*tien-hun shu*). The mortgaged wife may move to the family of the one who bought the mortgage, or may remain in the family of the one who sold it; there is no fixed pattern. The children born during the specified time period belong to the one who bought the mortgage. As for the goal of this form, it is financial gain for the one mortgaging his wife. For the holder of the mortgage, there are two reasons for this: (1) Because he has not yet married, and can't afford to marry in a wife, and so accepts another man's wife for a temporary period, or (2) Though he has a wife, she has no children, so he takes in another, mortgaged, to provide heirs.

Sometimes men have been known to take two or more such wives at the same time. This kind of custom is also practiced in the upper and middle classes. The sale of a wife occurs when, due to poverty and inability to support her, she is sold to another as wife or concubine. The seller executes a contract, called a "contract of marriage by sale" (*mai-hun shu*) (*MSS*:1560—61).

Such arrangements were of course open to varying amounts of abuse, with outright slavery sometimes the result, though it is often difficult to distinguish these unions absolutely from more "ordinary" marriage. Feng Ho-fa says of Shensi in the 1930s that

Because of lack of food grains, and because all other possessions were already sold, persons were bought and sold, and there were even human markets. In Wu-ling and Fu-feng Hsiens, there were at least three of these, centers in trading in women, where the price was dependent on age and beauty. Attractive girls of around twenty brought eight *yuan* according to the January 1, 1930 edition of the *Shen Pao*. For the most beautiful, the highest price was no more than ten *yuan*. The majority was around eight *yuan*, the next most common price three or four *yuan*.

In Sui-yuan human markets were set up. When the local government stopped it, they were disguised as marriage brokerages. One could buy a marriage contract for four foreign dollars, and then could take the girl whose name was on it. One could then tell the government that it was a marriage, or taking a concubine. The government then set up a ten percent tax on this, and in a short time earned as much as 10,000 *yuan* (Feng 1933:142).

This association of servitude with marriage brokerage was not fortuitous; over 100 years earlier the same thing was recorded in Fukien (see *Taiwan Szu-fa Jen-shih Pien*; 1:154–55). Such trafficking in "wives" continues in some Chinese communities. It has been estimated that around a thousand such marriages are arranged each year in Hong Kong, mainly involving women from overseas Chinese communities. The price for such a bride is about U.S.$2,000, "but men of Chiu Chow and Fukienese descent are apparently quite prepared to part with this sort of sum provided they get the right type of girl. The 'wrong' type at the moment would seem to be the Cantonese girl. 'They spend too much time playing mahjong and wasting money. We want women who are frugal and will look after us in our old age' said one Chiu Chow bridegroom who appeared to be at least twenty years older than his bride" (*South China Morning Post* August 10, 1975).

X. SAME SEX UNIONS

There were few alternative life-styles for women in traditional Chinese Society. Apart from the officially endorsed role of wife and mother, there were few ways a woman could make a living. One way, of course, was that of prostitution, and we have seen how some forms of marriage, particularly pawn and purchase marriage, and "little daughter-in-law" marriage, approximated this, sometimes differing from it only in certain respects. One alternative was domestic service in another family. Women who worked as domestic servants sometimes renounced "normal" marriage and family life, and instead banded together for moral and other kinds of support.

Another alternative was made possible by other forms of wage labor; something that became much more prevalent with increased foreign investments in China in the last century. Once factory jobs were available in any numbers, women had greatly increased sources of income, and could be much more independent of the family system.

This happened, for instance, in the silk producing areas around Canton:

In P'an-yu the land is fertile, and the people mainly make their living from silk production. Whether rich or poor, the daughters of the families there all know how to pick mulberry leaves and how to reel off silk from cocoons. In one day they can earn as much as eight or nine *chiao*, but at the least three or four *chiao*. The standard of living in rural areas is of course not as high as in the cities, and this amount is enough for self-sufficiency, and even for a bit of surplus. Such girls, then, have a means of support, and regard marriage as the most shameful of human affairs. Thus they form pacts not to marry. If they are forced to marry by their parents, they do not move to reside with the husband. These latter, after marriage, do not have intercourse with the husband, and the next day return to their natal family, to be companions to their sisters and female cousins. This means that they are lost to the husband's family (Hu 1936: II; 7, 30).

It is in this context that we find transactional social forms that are similar to, or are, marriage. The nonmarrying pacts were in the form of groups, or associations, of girls. They all entered into a kind of sworn sisterhood, called a "golden orchid society," "mutual admiration society," or "workmates' society."

In some cases two individuals would establish such a bond, and unite as a pair:

> In the drawing up of the contract, both sides must agree, much as in the legal form of contracts. If both parties are interested, then one will prepare ... gifts of respect, to symbolize her sentiments. If the other side accepts them, this constitutes consent. If not then it is refusal. When the contract is written up and put into effect, and if they have any savings, they invite friends for a night's feast, and the friends all congratulate them. After this they are inseparable, day and night, and happier than any married couple. After the contract has been established, if there is any difference of opinion, and one of them wishes to go back on the agreement, then they must submit to the judgment of one of their sisterhood leaders. Usually the punishment is some kind of beating or disgrace. Thus it has become a kind of customary law.
>
> As far as their cohabitation is concerned, though they cannot completely live as man and wife, yet they can actually have the pleasure that men and women do, either through massage and caresses, or through using mechanical aids. This is not a refined account, and it is difficult for a gentleman to speak of it. These women even select descendants, instituting a daughter to succeed to their estate, and later their adopted daughter will also enter into one of these compacts, as though there were a daughter-in-law, and it is really just as in blood relationships. This is really strange (Hu 1936: II; 7, 34).

Ch'en Tung-yuan attributed the custom to the unsettled economic situation: "To refrain from marrying because of lesbianism is really unnatural, and very harmful to the woman's health, but after the great changes in the circumstances of earning a livelihood, women not getting married at the proper time, and falling into lesbianism, has become much more widespread, and is truly a big problem" (Ch'en 1933:300).

Institutionalized same-sex unions for men were evidently much less widespread, though these are precisely the kinds of unions that one would expect to be least talked about and written about. This is a general problem in the study of many aspects of social life in traditional China. Only a small portion of the people were literate, and the use and contents of literary works were heavily influenced by socio-political factors. It is no accident that the standard histories and other works tend to ignore non-standard social forms and processes, and have very little that is reliable to say about non-elite social life.

This has been acknowledged by historians as a great pity, but not something about which anything could be done. More recently, however, more attention has been paid to the use of such things as short stories and plays as sources of historical material for the study of the "other side" of the traditional society (see, for example, Lo 1975). What little I have found on male-male marriages comes in part from a short story by Li Yü (1611–1679). For our purposes an important aspect of Li's literary philosophy is that he advocated a sort of "literature for the masses." Essays and other standard works were to be kept apart from stories and drama. The former were expected to be profound and even difficult; they were for the literate. The latter, on the contrary, were expected to be clear and simple, since they were intended for the illiterate as well as the literate. Furthermore, Li advocated a kind of realism; an author of plays and stories should stick to colloquial language and to realistic details, avoiding the fantastic and things outside of one's own experience and observation (Lo 1975:63–64).

One of the stories in Li's collection titled *The Silent Play* (*Wu-sheng Hsi*) is about a young, brilliant, and handsome scholar in P'u-t'ien Hsien, Hsing-hua Prefecture, Fukien, during the late Ming, named Wei Chi-fang, who married a young boy. Wei had earlier married a woman, who died after giving him a son. Having fulfilled his Confucian duty to provide offspring, he decided to remarry, this time to a young homosexual. The term for "remarriage" used here is *hsü-hsüan*, "to replace the string on one's lute," a common if somewhat literary term for remarriage. After a number of false starts, Wei finally managed to pay a brideprice of 500 taels, the two went through a marriage ceremony, and took up residence as man and "wife."

The background information provided by the author is very interesting. Fukien was said to be a center of homosexuality in China, and such marriages were said to be fairly common, with payment of brideprice:

In Fukien it happens that homosexuals pay a brideprice, but usually it's no more than symbolic; several tens of taels at most, but sometimes as little as several taels. It is a symbol of entreaty (Li 1969:377).

One must understand that with Fukien homosexuals, as in marrying women, first marriages are distinguished from later ones. For a virgin, men are prepared to pay a much higher brideprice, and to carry out a complete and proper wedding ceremony. If, then, one is not strict in controlling young boys, and they are seduced by someone, then they are called "fallen flowers." They do not become completely worthless, but a buyer will generally be interested only in a casual and temporary relationship, and will not enter into a permanent marriage relationship, and he will not select the boy to come to live with him (Li 1969:374).

What is of interest is the institutionalization and permanence of such relationships. There is some fragmentary information tending to support Li's claim that there were institutionalized, marriage-like, male homosexual unions in China. A much later writer, Yao Ling-hsi, says

The term "little brothers" (*hsiung-ti erh*) is the same as the Fukienese "bond younger brother" (*ch'i-ti*) ... Homosexuals raise them like younger brothers ... Fukienese homosexuals consider themselves as brothers (Yao 1940:154).

This term *ch'i,* "contract," "bond," shows up in many "deviant" social transactions. It is used for a kind of adoption found in many areas of China; it was used in connection with the consensual union described above under the term *p'ing-t'ou* (Hsu 1920:16:43;2). It indicated a kind of consensual union in Taiwan (Lien 1963:70), and Hsü K'o says that "bond brother," *ch'i-ti,* means male prostitute in Cantonese (Hsü 1920:16:43, 16). Indeed, this term (*kai-dai* in Cantonese) is common invective in Hong Kong today, used as a derogatory term for homosexuals.

It seems fairly clear to me, then, that there were at least in late Ming and Ch'ing China institutionalized relationships between males in some areas, and that these relationships were often expressed in terms of marriage and carried out in some the social forms connected with "regular" marriage.

CONCLUSION

In his influential work, *Totemism,* Claude Levi-Strauss argues that totemism is like hysteria, in that neither is an objective unitary entity. Once we regard these things with a critical eye, we find that the diagnostic signs, whether of the institution or the illness, dissolve or prove resistant to any unifying interpretation. He further suggests that the similarity between the two is due to a single underlying motivation, conscious or unconscious, to make *them,* whether "primitives" or mental patients, distinctly different from *us.* Thus, what at first seemed to be objective, "real," entities turn out to be mirror images of ourselves, images which have been reversed and objectified.

> The first lesson of Freud's critique of Charcot's theory of hysteria lay in convincing us that there is no essential difference between states of mental health and mental illness; that the passage from one to the other involves at most a modification in certain general operations which everyone may see in himself; and that consequently the mental patient is our brother, since he is distinguished from us in nothing more than by an involution – minor in nature, contingent in form, arbitrary in definition, and temporary – of a historical development which is fundamentally that of every individual existence (Levi-Strauss 1963:1–2).

Although Levi-Strauss uses the example of hysteria, at one time the paradigm of mental illness, the argument can, I suggest, be extended to include social deviance. There is no essential, intrinsic, difference between "deviant" and "normal" behavior, only that the one is distinguished from the other by an involution or transformation of common developments or processes, a transformation which is, as Levi-Strauss says, "minor in nature, contingent in form, arbitrary in definition, and temporary."

From the time of Charcot on, the dominant model of mental "illness" (which is a species of deviance) has been a medical one. Thomas Szasz is perhaps the best known proponent of another view, that mental illness is a "myth" (Szasz 1974). Szasz's argument is not that "mental illness" does not exist, but simply that it is misleading, and often dangerous, to assume that it fits a medical model, that it is really "illness." He distinguishes between a literal meaning and a metaphorical meaning of "illness." The former refers to the class of disorders associated with certain physical-chemical states of the body, a class which includes such things as syphilis, tuberculosis, typhoid fever, cancer, heart failure, fractures, other injuries, and so on. The metaphorical meaning of "illness," on the other hand, refers to the class of disorders associated not necessarily with physical-chemical states of the body, but with the disability and suffering of the person. This class contains such things as hysteria, hypochondriasis, obsessions, compulsions, depression, schizophrenia, homosexuality, etc., and according to many it can be broadened to include the various forms of social deviance such as, for instance, divorce or criminal behavior (Szasz 1974:40–41).

In other words, the medical model has become generally accepted in theories of social deviance, and all kinds of "irregular" behavior are assimilated to the model of disease, of pathology in both its literal and metaphorical meanings. A metaphorical interpretation of the medical model which is slightly different from that discussed by Szasz is to see deviance as "social pathology." Using a functionalist framework, proponents of this view take society, or some part of society, as the unit of analysis, and then apply a basically organismic analogy. By treating society as a kind of organism, they could look in it for signs of homeostasis (health) or of disruption (pathology). "Functional" features were those which promoted stability, and "dysfunctional" features were those which led to disruption or instability. The "social pathologists" of the Chicago School suggested that much deviance, such as juvenile delinquency, suicide, and mental illness, was the result of social disorganization, which in turn was the result of rapid immigration, industrialization, and urban growth, all of which had disrupted the commonly held and agreed-upon rules of conduct, standards, and patterns of life characterizing earlier, more rural, social life in America (Mills 1942).

In the 1960's and 1970's sociologists began increasingly to criticize the organismic model used in functionalist theory. Where the "social pathologists" tended to see deviance as the result of social disorganization caused by urbanization and "modernization," and structural functionalists tended to see it as "functional" in maintaining certain values and structures conceived as crucial to the stability of the society, a new group of writers argued for a "labeling" perspective, arguing that "deviants" are those who are so labeled by others. This latter approach brings out the important relativist point that deviance is not an objective quality, inherent in certain types of behavior, but is rather "the product of a process which involves responses of other people to the behavior" (Becker 1963:14). Social rules don't simply exist in a social vacuum, and aren't god-given. They are, instead, the creation of certain specific social groups. In any society which is not completely homogeneous we will find social groups organized along a variety of lines.

The next logical step is to incorporate the fact of power differentials among these groups. According to Alex Thio,

One may begin by defining deviance as conduct that is in violation of rules made largely by the power elite of a given society or group. The most important component in this definition is the concept of a power elite. It is based on the assumption that all societies . . . are founded upon unequal relations between powerful and powerless classes. The former consists of a small group of people with a disproportionately large quantum of power for protecting and enhancing their own interests more than, or at the expense of, those of the other class. (1973:1–2)

My task here is to explore the ways in which the Chinese power elite influenced the social-cultural (and I might add economic and political) structure so as to help generate deviant marriage patterns.

The Chinese peasant family farm was agriculturally quite productive. It is no accident that the co-resident family, and the cultural values that helped to support it, were endorsed and promulgated by the elite and the Imperial state. Agricultural productivity meant revenues for the state, since the majority of such revenues came from land taxes and other imposts connected with the peasantry. The state in effect operated a system of indirect, "colonial," rule, co-opting the head of the family and delegating authority to him. The head then found himself working for his own personal good (and, given the socio-political situation, for the good of the other members of the family) by serving the good of the state. The legal, and to a great degree the customary, powers of the head vis-à-vis the other family members were quite far-reaching. At the same time, however, he was also hostage to the state for the good behavior of the other members. Thus, to the degree that he pursued his own interests and the family's interests by increasing the domestic unit's productivity, he was also benefiting the state by ensuring revenues and ensuring social order by controlling, with his great powers, the other members of the family.

The Chinese family was characterized by relationships of generalized reciprocity and prescriptive altruism, reinforced by hierarchical relationships of an authoritarian nature, the latter in turn reinforced by the state political order. This is one of the reasons that families and households were able to function as domestic units of production. Mechanisms of authority and compliance were built into the structure and were supported and sanctioned by the wider social and political realm.

In situations in which there was a relative abundance of land, Chayanov (1966) has shown that one way that a domestic agricultural production unit can adjust itself to changing climatic and other environmental circumstances is to vary the area of land put under cultivation. In situations with severe restrictions on the amount of land available, different methods must be used to adjust levels of productivity. Chayanov acknowledged that "in cases where the land regime is not very flexible the relationship between land and family is regulated by a change in the amount of labor hired in or hired out" (1966:112). In the Chinese case the optimum balance between land, labor, and consumption was achieved not so much through labor hired in or out, as through "marrying" or "adopting" persons in or out, using the wide variety of transactional forms, both "normal" and "deviant," mentioned earlier in this paper.

Furthermore, these transactions occurred in a social situation dominated by a bipolar class structure. The statistical majority, the peasants, artisans, urban poor, etc., constituted the lower class, and the people who had, in one way or another, access to those in political office made up the power elite. One of the ways the elite justified and maintained its privileged position, and restricted entry to that rarefied stratum, was to label certain social forms, particularly those convenient or necessary to the masses, as deviant. I will comment briefly on the various "deviant" marriage forms that have been described above and how and why, in the context of two social classes, they have been so labeled.

A certain amount of ambivalence characterized the attitude of the elite towards the "little daughter-in-law" form of marriage. Such a girl would be socialized in her husband's family, and so would pose less of a threat than would a wife married in as an adult (Gallin 1966:163–166). The latter would tend more to identify herself with her husband and would tend to be protective of his interests and jealous of any perceived advantages held by his brothers. Bickering between sisters-in-law was often thought to be the cause of hostility and argument between brothers. If the "little daughter-in-law" identified her interests as the family's interests, such conflict could be minimized.

Another advantage is that one had many more alternatives to choose from when deciding what to "do with" such a girl than one did with one's own daughter, or with a wife married in in the standard way. This last is because the transferral of a girl in little daughter-in-law "adoption" was more complete than in standard marriage; a more comprehensive set of rights was involved. This meant that the adopting family had a greater amount of control over her than they did over a "standard" wife; the latter could always have appeal to her natal family in cases of maltreatment or other dissatisfaction, while the former, usually having been irrevocably transferred to the "adoptive" family, had no such rights. Thus the dominant/submissive relationship traditionally held to exist between husband and wife was in this case reinforced by the essentially father/daughter relationship (itself also, of course, one of dominance/submission) between the wife and her husband's father. It was this "double determination" which led to the very subservient position in which such a woman found herself.

For instance, such a girl could be kept permanently single in the household as a domestic slave or household drudge (Taiwanese *cha-bo-kan*, Cantonese *mui-tsai*), or she could be sold, rented, or pawned into prostitution. Thus, the terms "adopted daughters" and "adopted daughters-in-law" were often associated with prostitution. Barclay's "Supplement" to the *Dictionary of the Vernacular or Spoken Language of Amoy* lists as the meaning of the Taiwanese *iong-lu* "an adopted daughter; term for concubine or inmate of house of ill-fame in relation to owner," and Hu P'u-an says that rural prostitutes in Shantung were customarily called "little daughter-in-law" [*hsi-fu-erh*] (Hu 1936:II, 2, 12).

The "advantages" of greater flexibility, however, entailed, as the other side of the coin, two serious disadvantages. In the first place, this form of marriage amounted to a circumvention of the incest taboo upon brother-sister mating. Sociologically, one can say that a consequence of the existence of such a taboo is that families are led to, or are forced to, establish ties with other families in order to provide their own children with mates; ties which then become important for more general social, economic, and political functions (see Levi-Strauss 1969). Reliance on this form of marriage would tend to constrict a family's network of affinal ties, ties which often played an important role in the traditional society (see Gallin 1966).

Arthur Wolf has argued that marital relations tend to suffer in this kind of union. Following Westermarck's argument that the close childhood association of a boy and girl is inimical to the later establishment of a stable and enduring sexual union, he says that these marriages often had to be forced onto unwilling partners, that they tended to be less stable than standard marriages, and that they tended to be biologically less productive than standard marriages (Wolf has a series of articles on this marriage form; see Wolf 1966, 1968, 1970). It seems to me, however, that to the degree that such marriages were less "successful" (and my own research leads me to suspect that in fact they were), a more parsimonious explanation may simply be that a young man might be expected to be less than enthusiastic about marriage to a person with such a low status, a status associated with household drudgery and/or prostitution.

A second objection is related to the above. When a family "adopted" out a young girl in this manner, they lost almost all rights in her, and might well never see her again. Since such an "adoption" was often tantamount to sale into slavery or a brothel, the natal family, unable to say or do much about it, would lose face. Indeed, some domestic slaves and prostitutes were classed as "mean people" (*chien-jen*), not "freeborn" (*liang-jen*), and were legally and socially discriminated against.

The upper class attitude towards uxorilocal marriage was less ambivalent; it was usually scorned by the elite, and by the "high culture" system of ideals. Structurally, uxorilocal marriage is much the same as standard marriage; it is just that it is the biologically male actor who takes the sociologically "female" (or *yin*) role, and the biologically female actor who takes the sociologically "male" (or *yang*) role. At the level of abstract ideology, this is one of the reasons that the union is said to be negatively valued by the male and his family; the structure of the union is disharmonious with and an inversion of the structure of society generally.

Thus where "little daughter-in-law" marriage was perhaps rendered somewhat unstable because of an unfortunate coincidence of two substantively different but structurally similar relationship patterns, uxorilocal marriage found its instability in an unfortunate contradiction between two substantively similar but structurally different relationship patterns.

In more concrete terms, it is said by many informants in Taiwan that uxorilocal marriages are generally more likely to end in divorce than are standard marriages. This is because the woman's parents are likely to be critical and fault-finding with respect to the husband and his role within the family. Since by his marriage the husband has accepted a subordinate position, he can do little but endure such criticism, or else terminate the union. This fits in well with what Ira Buchler and Henry Selby, following Lloyd Fallers and Max Gluckman before them, have prompted as a general proposition; that "the degree to which the female or her group retains rights *in genetricem* [over a woman as bearer of children] and *in uxorum* [over a woman as wife] will be positively correlated with the degree of instability in the marriage" (Buchler and Selby 1968:29).

Since uxorilocal marriage put the man "under the thumb" of his father-in-law (or his wife's family generally), and since it was regarded as "deviant" by the elite-controlled cultural value system, men tended to avoid such unions. Why would any man then consent to such an arrangement? The reasons were primarily economic, or socio-economic. He often could set up a household and family this way without most of the usual expenses of a standard marriage. Since the wife's family was gaining a live-in, subordinate, provider of labor, management, and sons to continue that family line and had to overcome the man's reluctance to accept all of these conditions, they usually "sweetened the pot," whether with cash, guaranteed support, land and buildings, and/or some of the sons born to the union. Furthermore, if the parties reach an agreement that each views as an "equal exchange," the implication is that since the woman's family has the wherewithal to successfully recruit such a husband, it is of higher socio-economic standing than the man's. Thus, paradoxically, a "back-door" avenue to upward mobility, through the wife's family, may be opened if the man is willing to enter into this kind of relatively low-status union.

The levirate was prohibited in China. In his book on the Chinese kinship system, Feng Han-yi quotes a comment of P.G. von Möllendorf: "I have not been able to find the slightest trace of it (levirate), and it can never be of the same importance with the Chinese as with other people (e.g., to keep the family property), as posthumous adoption, the Chinese substitute for it, fully meets the object" (Feng 1967:51). According to George Jamieson, "In view of the severe penalty for it, it is scarcely possible that the levirate can be practiced in any part of China" (cited in Feng 1967:52). Feng's own conclusion is that "the junior levirate certainly exists in a few parts of modern China, at least among the poorer classes, but, even in the few places where it is practiced, it is not considered respectable. A man adopts this only as a last resort in getting a wife. If necessary, he can sell his brother's widow and use the 'brideprice' to marry another woman. Legally, marriage with the older brother's or younger brother's widow is stringently prohibited; the punishment is strangulation for both parties" (Feng 1967:51–52). Functionally, of course, such a prohibition helped maintain harmony within a household containing two or more resident married brothers and their families by unequivocally making the brother-in-law or sister-in-law forbidden fruit. Such a function was obviously more important in gentry, elite, circles where larger family size was possible, than among peasants and

other poor people, who had little chance to (and, perhaps, in some cases, little
desire to) develop and maintain such a large coresident kin group.

Structurally, one can also see this prohibition as an index of the degree to
which a woman was seen to be incorporated into the kin group of her husband.
The act of marriage quite clearly reduced the closeness of her kinship ties to her
natal family, and just as clearly established her within the husband's group. In a
sense, she was incorporated into his kin group to such a degree that her potential
sexual availability to the other males of the group became ambiguous.

Such a prohibition is not, however, common in other societies with patrilineally organized kin groupings. Robin Fox says:

> It is interesting that the exogamic ban in China extended to a widow of an agnate. Thus,
> if a man died his lineage had to marry his widow off to another lineage (if she was allowed
> to remarry). Usually, in patrilineal societies the opposite has been the case; once the lineage
> has obtained a woman it hangs onto her. Very often, for example, she is married to her dead
> husband's brother; a custom known as the levirate. China however was an exception to this,
> and I do not know the reason why this should be (Fox 1967:117).

I suggest that the levirate was, in fact, not absent. Fox says in another context of China, that "in such a complex society there was room for flexibility"
(1967:116). That was particularly true from the point of view of the class
system. China was able to have her cake and eat it too; despite a prohibition on
the levirate, it was practiced. There was far more variation and heterogeneity in
Chinese society than is sometimes reported. In the elite value system it was quite
easy to set up a rule which prohibited the practice of the levirate. If such a prohibition "helped" anyone at all, it was those in the elite class with large
corporate kin groups to maintain. The prohibition itself could then also be used
as a measure of elite status. Any family which, for economic or other reasons,
found it advantageous or necessary to practice the levirate defined itself as none-
lite by so doing.

The lower classes were generally left to go ahead and follow whatever
"disgusting" or "evil" customs they wished, so long as the social, political, and
economic status quo was not directly threatened. In fact, it was of course in the
interests of the elite to make sure that there would always be a lower class, one
defined as clearly different from their own.

Perhaps one of the reasons that there was a ban on marriage to widows of
agnates in China, while other societies with patrilineally organized kin groups
tend to follow the levirate, is precisely because China had an elite class and a
long and prestigious literary tradition which was shaped by, and helped support,
that elite class. In other societies, once a lineage obtains a woman, it holds onto
her because to do so makes good socio-economic sense; it is a rational use of
resources. To do otherwise is expensive, in a number of ways. One can argue,
then, that the ban on the levirate in China in part was a form of conspicuous
consumption. So, also, are some other customs, like the complete ban on remarriage of widows, footbinding of women, and so on. These things were all
expensive, and tended to be used as the criteria for membership in the elite class.

I think that it must be significant that out of perhaps 1,500 reports in over 500 pages, on kinship, marriage, and inheritance, the collection of customary laws I have been using, *Chung-kuo Min-, Shang-shih Hsi-kuan Tiao-ch'a Pao-kao Lu (MSS)*, has only a few notes on the sororate. Although they are few, it is significant that the rationale or explanation which receives emphasis is that of the existence and maintenance of good relationships between the two families. This factor is not mentioned in the many more reports on the levirate. The sororate, unsurprisingly, seems not to be a natural outcome of structural features of Chinese kinship organization, but is there to be used when other, particular, circumstances outweigh its disadvantages. Wolfram Eberhard, for instance, gives a number of reports of the custom in various areas at various time periods, but they seem to represent not highly institutionalized patterns, but more isolated and idiosyncratic cases (Eberhard 1968:181).

Double-generation marriage meets with one of the objections which was raised in connection with "little daughter-in-law" marriage. It too is a circumvention of the incest taboo on brother-sister mating, as is indicated by its appellation, "brother-sister marriage," and is thus "cheaper" than standard marriage. But, on the other hand, it constricts the potential circle of relatives gained through a standard marriage.

Another objection is that double-generation marriage works to disrupt the logical structure of the kinship system by confounding affinal and consanguineal kin. Much the same argument could also be raised in connection with same-surname marriages. People with the same surname were traditionally assumed to be related members of one patrilineal clan. Such clans were linked together in part through marriage relations. This implied the rule of exogamy; mates had to be obtained from other than one's own clan. An "inverted" expression of this rule is that members of the same clan (people with the same surname) should *not* marry. The crucial factor supporting the rule was, then, the importance of clan organization to the people involved. Such organization was more important to the elite than it was to those of the "poorer classes" both because they could better "afford" it and because they had more (wealth, land, political connections) to be protected by such an organization.

Purchase and pawn marriages were devalued because they involved the treatment of people as commodities to be bought and sold. The elite, of course, did not hesitate to exchange large amounts of wealth in their marriages, and indeed tried to outdo each other at it. Wealth in the form of presents, however, wealth which passed in both directions as prestation and counter prestation, expressed a relative equality of standing of the two families in the transaction, and a view of each as possessing some degree of automony and dignity. Cash, passing in one direction only, expressed instead a radical difference of standing between the two parties, and implied that the lower-status party lacked autonomy and dignity. Still, when one was poor, one often had to swallow one's pride and accept the loss of face for the tangible benefits to be derived.

Spirit marriages evidently did not arouse as much emotion as did most of the other "deviant" forms. This is perhaps in part because it was often simply a "ritual" action, with little tangible economic impact. It could, potentially, be used to forge links between families, but it seems most often to have been aimed at placating the angry spirits of those who had died unmarried. The objection to it that I have heard most frequently voiced in Taiwan is simply that the practice is "superstitious."

Consensual unions and same-sex marriages, on the other hand, constituted direct, if implicit, threats to the whole kinship and marriage system. Consensual unions threatened the very concept of "marriage"; they muddied the waters and made it painfully obvious that one could be "married yet not married." As for same-sex unions, it is obvious that they threaten the very foundations of marriage conceived as the union of male-female (or *yang-yin*) roles. This is well put by Li Yü:

> It isn't known when homosexuality began, or who started it, but it has been handed down to the present, and indeed, has become a challenge to the natural male-female relationship. How can this not be regarded as strange? How do we know that the male-female relationship is natural? Simply by noting that the male's body has a projection, while the female's body has an indentation. How was this kind of structure created? The male and the female embody the forms given by heaven and earth, that which is in abundance supplementing that which is lacking. When it has been supplemented to just the right point, then pleasure automatically results. How could this sort of process be forced? After intercourse, the male's semen and the female's blood congeal to form the fetus. After a full ten months a boy or a girl is born. How could such a result be by chance? This is simply a consequence of acting in accordance with the intercourse of *yin* and *yang* . . . . It resembles the molding of creation; it is natural and so can be taken for granted. Though this is all better left unmentioned, it is no threat to morality. Though it is dalliance, it is beneficial to propriety.
>
> As for homosexuality, in form there is no distinction between surfeit and lack. In emotions, there is no aspect of mutual pleasure and enjoyment. Under the circumstances, there is no procreation. I don't know where it gets its interest. Since its origin, it has caused suffering to people, and has brought no benefit. Of what use is it? (Li 1969:350–351).

One objection to the approach that I have adopted here is that I've talked about a lot of rather exotic and strange unions, but weren't they, after all, statistically very rare? Wasn't standard marriage always by far the most common, and these other things rare and fleeting? Standard or major marriage was probably in most times and places statistically most prevalent, but not always, and not everywhere. I found in the village where I did research that at times in recent history the adopted daughter-in-law marriage was just as common as "regular" marriage. Arthur Wolf, also working in Taiwan, found that in the last century in the village where he did research the vast majority of marriages were of the adopted-daughter-in-law type (approaching 80% or 90%; see Wolf 1966, 1968, 1970). This was so not only for Taiwan, which many researchers seem to think isn't really "Chinese," but areas on the mainland also have been reported to have such very high incidences (see *MSS*:1501 for Kiangsi). An important point is that we simply don't have the data to tell just how common these various "deviant" forms were. We do know that some of them were very common in some places, and that most of them were geographically very widespread, both of which considerations lead me to believe that they were probably much more common than most have supposed.

What do we have then? Just a jumble of miscellaneous customs, sometimes erotic, usually exotic? It would be a poor analysis if I could not offer some other, more useful approach. Let me offer some brief conclusions here and refer the reader interested in more complete documentation to another work (McGough 1976).

I think that there is in fact underlying order and unity to all these varied forms, "normal" and "deviant." The problem is that it is at a high level of abstraction. I have implied that our Western social-science analysis of marriage in China went wrong somewhere. Where was that? It was, I think, in giving an overly personal and sexual interpretation to "marriage." All of the data that I have collected, and all of the thought that I have invested in the matter have led me to the conclusion that in the Chinese case, considering all the social classes together, the overriding motivation is group recruitment. The goals involving sex and reproduction were obviously not absent, but they were subordinated to that of recruitment. The family, or domestic group, was a social, legal, political, economic, and, very importantly, a production unit. What was necessary for a complete and satisfactory life was a demographically complete family. Thus people had to be recruited in various ways to create and maintain a domestic structure. The biology of sex and reproduction offered one mechanism for recruitment, but it is a notoriously slow and unreliable mechanism, and came to be supplemented, and in many cases replaced, by the various social transactions outlined above. When Westerners arrived on the scene they saw a number of these transactions which looked much like their own "marriage," and automatically selected these and ignored others which did not fit their definition.

These were all transactions between parties of clearly unequal relative status in which control over individuals was transferred. I find it convenient to express the unequal standing of the parties in terms of *yin* and *yang*; the *yin/yang* dichotomy might be expressed in terms of female/male, passive/active, junior/senior, etc. The control that I mention refers to control over, most importantly, labor power and what might be called reproductive and sexual power or services.

Men and women in most societies have long had an interest in the labor, sexual, and reproductive potential of other people (particularly of women and children). The tendency has been to see control over people as a form of property, to be (in disguised form or not) sold, rented, pawned, traded, or used, according to the rules of property transfer that are allowed in any particular society.

Thus the basic pattern underlying all of these forms, I think, is that of a transaction between *yin* and *yang* social roles in which control over individuals is transferred. This general, abstract model can then be used to generate, in particular circumstances, all of the different marriage forms we've considered, both "standard" and "deviant." Thus we must look at the particular circumstances;

the social and economic standing of the two families, and the number, age, sex, etc., of the respective members will all determine the particular form of "marriage" that a transaction will take. When the individuals involved happen to be of approximately equal age, and of different sex, then we will see what looks to us like marriage. When they are of radically different age, and one is a child or infant, then it will look to us like adoption. If one or more of the individuals is dead, then we get "ghost marriage." What is of interest in the last case is that control over sexual and reproductive powers continue to exist in "ghost form." The goal was to provide the formal possibility of descendants, who would in turn sacrifice to the ghost.

The anthropologist Arthur Wolf noted a curious incident in his dissertation (Wolf 1964). This incident involved a prostitute who adopted an infant girl. In Taiwan after a woman has been a prostitute for a while, she may realize that she won't be able to get out of the business and marry a husband and settle down to a more normal life. When she comes to this realization and her earning powers start to diminish, the problem of support in old age comes immediately to mind. A common thing to do at this point is to adopt a young girl to raise to be a prostitute also, a daughter who will then support her in her old age.

In Wolf's description, the infant was wrapped in red cloth, a color associated with, among other things, marriage. The price that the woman paid for the child was called the brideprice. More usually it is called "milk money," and is said to be compensation to the natal family for giving birth to and raising the child. The woman took the baby away to her home, but returned it to its natal home three days later to "play the role of guest" (*tso k'e*), something which is done in ordinary marriage, symbolizing that the married woman is now a stranger in her own natal home.

The "adoption," then, if we call it that, was done in the language and symbolism of "marriage." Was this adoption or was it marriage? I suggest that it was, in a sense, both. That is, it was a transaction between two parties in which control over the sexual and reproductive potential of the baby were put in the prostitute's hands. She did not exactly "adopt" the child, because that would have implied that the adopted child would later have been married out to some man, and thus lost to the prostitute. She instead intended to actually use the girl's sexuality later, by renting it out piecemeal, so to speak. Thus the transaction had a family resemblance to both marriage and to adoption. Thus the language and symbolism used.

Finally, whether or not my analysis is right, or, more properly, useful, we must at least realize that there was in the social life of traditional China much more variability and complexity than has usually been assumed. Much of this variability was deemed deviant by the elite, and so was downplayed and under-reported. We should try, more than we have in the past, to understand these and similar things in terms of the ideas, categories, and realities of Chinese society — particularly lower-class Chinese society — and not in terms of the ideas and categories which arose in the context of the realities of our own society.

CHARACTERS

cha-bo-kan 查某嫺
cha-p'ing-t'ou 軋姘頭
chao 招
chao-fu 招夫
chao-fu sheng-tzu 招夫生子
chao-fu yang-fu 招夫養夫
chao-fu yang tzu 招夫養子
chao-hsü 招婿
chao-hsü yang-lao 招婿養老
che p'ing-t'ou 拆姘頭
cheng-ch'i 正妻
ch'i ("contract") 契
ch'i ("wife") 妻
ch'i-ti 契弟
chieh-hun 結婚
chien-jen 賤人
chih 質
ch'in-ying 親迎
ch'ing-ch'i 請期
chio-ti (Taiwanese) 招弟
ch'ü kuei-ch'i 娶鬼妻
chui 贅
chui-hsü 贅婿
hsi-fu-erh 媳婦兒
hsiung-mei hun 兄妹婚
hsiung-ti-erh 兄弟兒
hsü-hsüan 續絃
huo-tai 活帶
iong-lu (Taiwanese) 養女
kai-dai (Cantonese) 契弟
kiet-hun (Taiwanese) 結婚
kuo-fang 過房

liang-jen 良人
liu-li 六禮
lu-shui fu-fu 露水夫婦
lu-shui yin-yüan 露水姻緣
mai-hun shu 賣婚書
ming-hun 冥婚
mui-tsai (Cantonese) 妹子
na-pi 納幣
na-ts'ai 納財
p'ei-ku 配骨
p'ing-t'ou 姘頭
sheng-fang 升房
shih-tsung chao-fu 失踪招夫
simpua (Taiwanese) 媳婦仔
szu-tai 死帶
ta-huo 搭夥
t'ao-hua chia-chu 桃花夾竹
t'e-pieh hsü-ch'in 特別續親
tien-hun shu 典婚書
ting-hun 訂婚
tso-ch'an chao-fu 坐產招夫
tso-k'e 做客
tso-shan chao-fu 坐山招夫
t'ung-yang hsi 童養媳
wai-chia 外家
wen-ming 問名
wu ch'an wu tzu 無產無子
yang 陽
yin 陰
yu ch'an wu tzu 有產無子
yu ch'an yu tzu 有產有子

REFERENCES

Barclay, Thomas
  1923 Supplement to Dictionary of the Vernacular or Spoken Language of Amoy. Shanghai: Commercial Press.
Becker, Howard
  1963 Outsiders: Studies in the Sociology of Deviance. New York: Free Press.
Buchler, Ira, and Selby, H.
  1968 Kinship and Social Organization. New York: Macmillan.

Chayanov, A. V.
    1966 The Theory of Peasant Economy edited by Daniel Thorner, Basile Kerblay, and
        R. E. F. Smith. Homewood, Illnois: The American Economic Association.
Ch'en Ku-yuan 陳顧遠
    1937 Chung-kuo Hun-yin Shih (1966 Reprint) Taipei: Commercial Press. 中國婚姻史
Ch'en Tung-yuan
    1933 Chung-kuo Fu-nü Sheng-huo Shih Shanghai (1965 reprint) Taipei: Commercial
        Press. 陳東原 中國婦女生活史
Chiu, Vermier Y.
    1966(?) Marriage Laws and Customs of China Hong Kong: Chinese University of Hong
        Kong.
Chung-kuo Min-, Shang-shih Hsi-kuan Tiao-ch'a Pao-kao Lu (MSS)
    1930 Nanking (1969 reprint) Taipei: Ku-t'ing Bookstore. 中國民商事習慣調查報告錄
Cohen, Abner
    1974 Two Dimensional Man. Berkeley: University of California Press.
Eberhard, Wolfram
    1968 The Local Cultures of South and East China. Leiden: Brill.
Fei Hsiao-t'ung
    1934 Ch'in-ying hun-su chih yen-chiu. She-hui-hsüeh Chieh 8: 155–186.
        費孝通 親迎婚俗之研究 社會學界
    1946 Peasant Life in China. New York: Oxford University Press.
Feng Han-yi
    1967 The Chinese Kinship System. Cambridge, Mass.: Harvard University Press.
Feng Ho-fa
    1933 Chung-kuo Nung-ts'un Ching-chi Tzu-liao. Li ming shu chü: Shanghai.
        馮和法 中國農村經濟資料
Fox, Robin
    1967 Kinship and Marriage. Baltimore: Penguin.
Gallin, Bernard
    1966 Hsin-hsing, Taiwan: A Chinese Village in Change. Berkeley: University of
        California Press.
Goodenough, Ward
    1970 Description and Comparison in Cultural Anthropology. Chicago: Aldine.
HS: Han Shu, Pan Ku, Po-an ed. 漢書
Ho Lien-K'uei
    1951? Min-tsu Wen-hua Yen-chiu. Taipei. 何聯奎 民族文化研究
Hsu, F. L. K.
    1945 Observations on cross-cousin marriage. American Anthropologist 47, 1:83–103.
Hsü K'o
    1920 Ch'ing Pai-lei Ch'ao (1966 reprint) Taipei: Commercial Press. 徐珂 清卑類抄
Hu P'u-an
    1936 Chung-hua Ch'uan-kuo Feng-su Chih (1968 reprint) Taipei: Ch'i-hsin Press.
        胡樸安 中華全國風俗志
Jordan, D. K.
    1971 Two forms of spirit marriage from Taiwan Bijdragen tot de taal-, land- en volken-
        kunde van Nederlandische Indie 127, 1:181–189.
    1972 Gods, Ghosts and Ancestors. Berkeley: University of California Press.
Kataoki Iwao
    1921 Taiwan Fuzoku Shi. Taipei: 片岡巖 台灣風俗誌
King, Frank H. H.
    1965 Money and Monetary Policy in China 1845–1895. Cambridge: Harvard University
        Press.

Levi-Strauss, Claude
  1963 Totemism. Boston: Beacon Press.
  1969 The Elementary Structures of Kinship. Boston: Beacon Press.
Li Hsien-chang
  1936 *Taiwan Min-chien Wen-hsüeh* (1970 reprint) Taipei: Wen-kuang Press.
         李献章　台灣民間文學
Li Yü
  1969 *Wu Sheng Hsi.* Helmut Martin, ed. Taipei: Ku-t'ing Press. 李漁　無聲戲
Lien Heng
  1963 *Taiwan Yü Tien.* Taipei, Taiwan: Wen-shien Tsung K'an reprint #161.
         連橫　台灣語典
Lo Hsüeh-lun
  1975 *Li Yü Hsi-chü, Hsiao-shuo, so Fan-ying te Szu-hsiang yü Shih-tai. Tung-fang Tsa-
         chih* 50, 2:56−87. 駱雪倫　李漁戲劇小說所反映的思想與時代　大陸雜誌
MSS: See *Chung-kuo Min-, Shang-shih Hsi-kuan Tiao-cha Pao-kao Lu.*
Man Wui Po. Hong Kong. 文滙報
Mathews, R. H.
  1963 *Mathews' Chinese-English Dictionary.* Cambridge: Harvard University Press.
Mills, C. Wright
  1942 The professional ideology of social pathologists. American Journal of Sociology
         49: 165−80.
McGough, James
  1976 Marriage and Adoption in Chinese Society with Special Reference to Customary
         Law. Unpublished Ph.D. dissertation. Michigan State University.
South China Morning Post. Hong Kong.
Szasz, Thomas
  1974 The Myth of Mental Illness. New York: Harper and Row.
TMS: See *Taiwan Min-shih Hsi-kuan Tiao-ch'a Pao-kao*
Tai Yen-hui
  1966 *Chung-kuo Fa-chih Shih.* Taipei: San-min Shu-chu. 戴炎輝　中國法制史
Taiwan Min-shih Hsi-kuan Tiao-ch'a Pao-kao (TMS) 台灣民事習慣調查報告
  1969 Taipei: Szu-Fa Hsing-cheng Pu.
Taiwan Szu-fa Jen-shih Pien 台灣私法人事編
  1961 Five Volumes. Taipei: Bank of Taiwan.
Thio, Alex
  1973 Class bias in the sociology of deviance. The American Sociologist 8: 1−12.
Wolf, Arthur
  1964 Marriage and Adoption in a Hokkien Village. Unpublished Ph.D. dissertation.
         Cornell University.
  1966 Childhood association, sexual attraction, and the incest taboo: A Chinese case.
         American Anthropologist 68, 4:883−98.
  1968 Adopt a daughter-in-law, marry a sister: A Chinese solution to the problem of the
         incest taboo. American Anthropologist 70, 5:864−74.
  1970 Childhood association and sexual attraction: A further test of the Westermarck
         hypothesis. American Anthropologist 72, 3:503−515.
Wu Ying-t'ao
  1970 *Taiwan Min-su.* Taipei: Chen-wen Press. 吳瀛濤　台灣民俗
Yao Ling-hsi
  1940 *Ping-wai Wei-yen.* Tientsin Shu Chu. 姚靈犀　瓶外危言

WILLIAM L. PARISH

11. FAMILY AND COMMUNITY
IN THE PEOPLE'S REPUBLIC

In the West, we are still grasping for models to help disentangle Chinese fact
from fiction. Though abandoned in some circles, one model is that of the
authoritarian state which can produce organizational and behavioral change on
command. Even if the state consigns few people to labor camps, it has such a
monopoly of jobs and economic resources that everyone must comply. Another
model which tempts us is that of the ideologically-mobilized state with mass
consciousness transformed through study combined with group criticism and
self-criticism. So transformed, behavior moves in directions desired by official
ideals because people have already internalized these ideals in their own person.
We know that both these models are too simplistic. They are too monolithic,
assuming a uniformity of living conditions which are surely absent in China just
as they are absent in our own country. This absence of uniformity, and the need
to consider concrete living conditions, is no better illustrated than in comparisons between Chinese rural and urban life.

This essay summarizes findings from a 1973-74 study of sixty-three villages
of Kwangtung Province in south China and preliminary impressions from a
1977–78 study of 133 urban neighborhoods scattered throughout China. Both
studies are based on the methods of anthropology-at-a-distance, with refugees
and legal emigres in Hong Kong being asked to give concrete details on life in
their community and among their neighbors back in the village or city that they
lived in just before leaving China. Veracity is insured by probing for concrete
details, by controlling on background characteristics of informants, and by
comparing our sample results with official radio reports. Control on characteristics such as past political errors and negative class origins leads to no change
in results. Comparison on six dimensions – including grain yields, proportion of
villages with cooperative medical programs, and number of barefoot doctors per
village – shows virtually identical results for official and interview results in
1973 (see Parish and Whyte 1978, Appendix One). Other less systematic comparisons to press reports on topics such as marriage, urban services, and work
organization suggest that the interview information is close to the mark – as
well as being a far richer source of data than usually available.

Villages

In rural community life, the Russian experience provides a useful point of
contrast. Due to their large size, outside leadership, rigid central control, and a
negative history of low state prices and forced collectivization, Russian collective farms have had great difficulty inspiring peasant enthusiasm and cooperation.

203

A. Kleinman and T.-Y. Lin (eds.), Normal and Abnormal Behavior in Chinese Culture, 203–212.
Copyright © 1980 by D. Reidel Publishing Company.

Chinese collective units have been much more successful in this effort, not only by providing adequate prices and more flexible central direction but also by utilizing and strengthening natural solidarities. The effective unit of production and income sharing (the production team) remains small and is organized around a pre-existing small village or neighborhood of a larger village which at the same time may be part of a single kinship group. Leaders are chosen from their native village, are kinsmen and long-time neighbors of the people they lead, receive little or no extra-pay in their work, and can expect to spend the rest of their life in the same village, often retiring from office in just a few years. With the possible exception of brigade Party secretaries, there is then minimal differentiation between leader and led. This commonality of status and interests among villagers is further reinforced by strict migration laws keeping males in their home village and increasingly by intra-village marriage keeping females near home as well. As in Russia, while not eliminating all inequalities among families, collective payment systems have narrowed sharp income differentials which would separate one family from another while collectively held land has given all families in a production team a common set of economic interests. These commonalities plus cumulative years of experience in hammering out payment systems, grain distribution systems, work arrangements, and so on have given peasants a new sense of collective unity.

While providing excellent incentives for collective farming, this comparative unity of purpose need not support all government goals. Unity within small collective units can inhibit cooperation with larger collective units. Government attempts to enlarge collective units first in 1958–1959 and then in a few places in 1968–1969 have been resisted by small production units which saw their interests threatened, and the stories of conflict among collective units struggling to protect their own land, water, and animals or trying to usurp that of others sounds very much like conflicts between villages before 1949 (Parish 1976). Similarly, though model villages have leaders who identify with national goals and drag villagers along in pursuit of these goals (Meisner 1975), most southern village leaders are so captured by their village as to be unable to force unpopular programs on their neighbors, friends, and kinsmen. When forced by the government to do so, many will resign, thereby exposing a weak link in the system of authoritative control. Ideological control is weakened by the inability of most villages to sustain political study groups in the face of more practical concerns of peasant life. As a result of the internal unity of villages, the inability of leaders to identify totally with the bureaucracy above, and the difficulty of ideological penetration, social changes tend to be decided in terms of the collective interests of villages and villagers rather than according to some unified administrative or cultural norm.

In family and ritual realms this tendency towards selective adoption of new values and programs is further supported by the government's emphasis on persuasion in place of coercion as well as by the pro-family and pro-male incentives which present collective structures provide. Though deprived of major land holdings, families remain significant income, housing, child care, and welfare units. Rural families are paid neither equally nor according to need but according to how much their members — especially their men — work. Being physically stronger and uninhibited by child-care duties, men earn one-fourth to two-thirds more than women. And once they grow up, daughters marry out to other families while sons stay behind to help support their parents. This is critical, for there is no generalized old age assistance program in the countryside. Only those with no sons can rely on the collective, and then the level of support is minimal. Daughters are not obligated to provide support to their parents and usually don't. Since families with many laborers are two to three times better off than those with few laborers, and since parents have to rely on sons in old age, parents are understandably eager to have several sons.

Married sons also have reason to want their parents around. First, virtually all rural housing remains private. With no mortgage program for houses, the average family has to save ten years or more to build a house. Young men just beginning their married life initially must rely on their parents for housing, a favorite tactic being to simply wall off a room or build a new room abutting the old family home. Second, in south China and much of north China, virtually all younger mothers work in the fields during the day. With only a small minority of villages having child care facilities, grandmother's assistance in cooking, cleaning, and tending to children is most welcome. Third, both grandparents and young children can help cut grass off the hillsides, feed the family pig and chickens, weave mats, sell vegetables in the free market, and do other tasks in the private sector — the source of twenty to forty percent of every household's income. A large household with different members doing different tasks is far better off than an isolated nuclear household (see Parish 1975).

This set of conditions has led to some changes favored by the government. Though parents and aunts often provide the initial introduction to potential marriage partners, children now have a veto power over the final choice and some opportunity to get better acquainted before the marriage ceremony. New brides are less subservient vis-à-vis their in-laws, and the authority of family elders has generally softened. Young couples marry at later ages than formerly (even if not as late as the government would like). Even with the other virtues of a large household, working mothers find children a burden, and families are beginning to have distinctly fewer children (even if the rural population growth rate remains above the government ideal of 1.5 percent a year). Though still very rare, divorce initiated by women has increased.

Balanced against these kinds of changes are a number of areas of continuity. The family rather than the individual is still the primary unit of rural life. Newly married couples almost always live with the groom's family at first, rather than with the bride's parents or by themselves. Women still do the lion's share of domestic work in addition to their work in the fields, men dominate family decision-making, and women receive only token representation in the village power structure. The groom's family has to provide the bride's family with a very substantial bride price in order to seal the marriage agreement, and marriage finance today appears to represent the proscribed "marriage by purchase" even more than in the past, because the value of dowry the bride brings back with her has declined. In cases of divorce or death and remarriage the woman does not, in fact, achieve the equal rights to family property and child custody which official policy proclaims.

The pattern of mixed response to government appeals for social change is repeated in ritual realms. There has been a general retreat from community, lineage, and professionally led rituals to rituals centered around family life. Temples and religious specialists became inactive in the 1950s. Lineage halls were deprived of their ancestral plaques and converted to other usages in successive campaigns, culminating in a complete elimination of lineage hall activities in the Cultural Revolution. In contrast, though often simplified in form, family rituals connected with birth, marriage, and death continue very much in a traditional pattern. Many families continue to revere their ancestors as symbolized in domestic plaques, red strips of paper with the proper names written upon them, or simply by pictures placed in the main family hall. Weddings continue to be highly elaborate with many guests and multiple tables laden with food. New political rituals such as on National Liberation Day or International Women's Day continue to be pale images of the community rituals they were to replace, while annual festival celebrations in the home continue to be vigorously attended to. Collectivization, then, has narrowed the circle of ritual celebration but neither eliminated its traditional content nor diverted it to political paths.

Significantly for the study of interrelationships between ideology and social change, those changes in family and ritual which have occurred are related less to political and educational conditions than to structural conditions such as village prosperity, population, land, and the like. Villages with more Party members, political study groups, broadcast networks, and full school enrollments might be presumed to be more attuned to central values and programs of social change, but they are no more likely than other villages to have low bride prices, husband-wife equality, extensive birth control, simple rituals, or a host of other government sponsored social conditions. Instead, response to government ideals is predicated on more specific village conditions. Prosperous villages give low bride prices because, given the marriage market, families anxious to get their daughters into affluent villages must accept a smaller price. Populous villages are likely to use more egalitarian time as opposed to task-rate work point systems simply because it is too difficult to keep account of task-rates with a large work force. Villages with little land are more likely to restrict their birth rate. Response to government programs, then, is less in terms of broad political and cultural trends in the society than in terms of very local costs and benefits. Collectivization in the mid-1950s caused a major restructuring of these costs and benefits and some rapid changes in family and ritual life followed. Since that time, changes in costs and benefits and their associated social practices have been much slower.

Cities

In cities, both social practices and the structure of costs and benefits are strikingly different. Many of the features which favor village autonomy and family solidarity are absent. Work and residence are separated. Work organizations are large, highly bureaucratized, and led by officers with whom one has no personal ties. There is no private sector to speak of. Each working family member earns his or her income away from home, and men and women are paid equally for equal work, even if some people's work is more equal than others'. More and more old people are self-supporting, with pensions set at seventy percent of pre-retirement salaries. Few families have claim to private housing.

Many city conditions favor both administrative control and ideological appeals. Each city neighborhood of 30,000 to 50,000 residents is organized around a police station containing household registers for everyone in the neighborhood. The police and neighborhood units are backed up by smaller resident's committees which beat policemen help oversee and, then, by small groups. Small groups of thirty to fifty households are supervised by a small group head, typically an unemployed woman in her forties or fifties, who helps disseminate bulletins, call meetings, lead study, conduct household sanitation inspections, and report any suspicious activities. Her reports of suspicious activities may be followed by late-night, surprise household register checks in the company of the beat policeman. The neighborhood apparatus helps issue rations, issue travel permits, wedding permits, and many other necessities of life. One's work organization is equally vital for many of life's necessities, including housing, marriage permits, divorce permits, hardship allowances, purchase certificates for bicycles, watches, and sewing machines, and a host of other needs. One's life is bound up in a web of bureaucratic control supervised by outsiders.

Political study is not always more successful in cities than in the countryside. Unemployed old people in neighborhoods are notoriously difficult to organize. Skilled workers may ignore the call to come to factory meetings, or come late and then spend the time reading their newspaper. Yet in many organizations, especially schools and administrative bureaus, attentive study is a prerequisite for career advancement. Many people spend at least an hour a week in study meetings, learning the proper political slogans and behavioral cues of the moment regardless of how independent or compliant their inner thinking might be (see Whyte 1974). The higher the status, the more people are affected by this ritual, especially in recent campaigns directed largely at bureaucrats, intellectuals, and other "power holders." In the Cultural Revolution the web of administrative control and political study had a distinct impact on urban ritual and family life. Those temples and Christian churches which had remained open up until 1966 were permanently closed, their windows and other ornaments often being smashed by militant Red Guards in a sweeping attack on "the four olds" or feudal practices. Wedding ceremonies were drastically simplified. Families turned from restaurants for elaborate banquets to simple meals at home for one or two dozen closest kin and friends.

Nevertheless, much of the shape of urban family and ritual life defies explanation by administrative control and ideological appeal. Many of the injustices that the government was set against such as foot binding, child brides, and bride prices had disappeared from cities before the 1949 revolution. Many of the remaining problems such as mother-in-law/daughter-in-law conflict, equality in household chores, and an equal position for women outside the home were of lower priority and presumed amendable to gradual change through propaganda and the indirect effects of putting women to work. The great success of the urban birth control campaign and the attempt to delay urban marriages provides an example of how constraints other than administrative control and ideological appeal come into play. First, marriage is delayed when young teenagers are sent to the countryside for a stint of two, three, or four year's labor. Second, on returning to a city (not necessarily the city of origin), those destined for skilled manual jobs enter a two or three year apprentice program in which they continue to get only a subsistence wage which would prevent them from marrying even if there were no formal prohibition on apprentices marrying. Third, the urban housing crunch is so severe that it is very difficult for a prospective couple to get a room. Even if one has met the administrative requirements of a minimum age of 25 for the bride and 28 for the groom, one's work unit or one's neighborhood housing office frequently has no room to assign. Marriage will have to be delayed for a year or two unless one is willing to make do with a corner of a single-person dorm, a partitioned off section in one's parents' rooms, or some other make-shift arrangement. Fourth, just before and after marriage there are things to be purchased which the modern couple considers necessities – radio, watches, wooden furniture, bicycles. All but the radio are quite expensive, the bicycle alone costing almost five months' of a young worker's salary. The tendency then is to have one child as soon as married but to delay the birth of the second until more of the household's "necessities" can be accumulated. Fifth, the burdens of being a mother when virtually all women are working are so extreme that virtually none want a third child, even if the first two are girls. Housing tends to be assigned by the husband's work unit while creche and nursery care is by the mother's unit. Young mothers must get up early to shove their way onto an overburdened public transport system with the small child on their back. They face the same crush coming home, and unless there is a grand-parent at home they also have to stand in line to buy vegetables and meat for the evening meal. In a land without refrigerators, shopping is daily, and, as the People's Daily keeps reminding us, can be a hassle. Commuting, attending after-hours study meetings at least once a week, and generally having no annual vacation, the mother's one day off a week is taken up with shopping, cooking, cleaning, mending, and sewing. Finally, many of the positive incentives for having children are missing. Financially, children get jobs only in their twenties, and even then they need not turn all of their salary over to parents. Old age support depends on pensions, not children. Emotionally, some of the pleasure of having young children around is diminished by parents not being at home when their children are. To help alleviate congestion and even-out the demands on an inadequate electricity supply, many factories give their workers a day off only in the middle of the week, while children continue to get off from school only on Saturday and Sunday. (One's spouse may be off on yet another day of the week.) Except for the sending of urban youth to villages and the rotation of work days, this set of structural conditions appears in all communist societies, and the results are always the same — a drastically falling urban birth rate. In the Soviet Union this falling rate is found even in the face of ideological appeals and administrative rewards to have more children. In China, then, regardless of ideological appeals or threatened administrative sanctions for excess births, it is not surprising that very few people can recall any of their former neighbors or workmates having had a third pregnancy in the last decade.

This dynamic response to changed living conditions is repeated in other social realms. There is still such a degree of reserve in boy-girl relationships that third-party peers often have to provide the initial introductions, but virtually all parental intervention in urban marriages has disappeared. Though the groom may give small gifts to the bride's parents, bride prices are absent. The groom spends extra money to spice the wedding feast with meat, eggs, and vegetables from the rural free market on the outskirts of town and he hires a taxi to bring the bride to his house on the wedding day, but other expenditures are modest. Both wear new clothes, but only in a contemporary style that can be used over and over again. Both return to work after their officially allotted three day's wedding leave. After marriage husbands do the heavier chores about the house such as buying and hauling home bags of grain and loads of coal for cooking and heating. But, as in our own society, wives tend to get stuck with the more tedious day-to-day tasks of vegetable buying, cooking, dishwashing, clothes washing, sweeping, mending, and sewing. Some younger and more educated husbands help more, but by and large women are caught in the familiar double bind. Neither official propaganda nor equal work is sufficient to lead to equal responsibility for chores inside the home. Most women accept this division of responsibilities as their natural lot, and no conflict results. Conflict between husband and wife over money and other issues seems neither particularly common nor rare. But regardless of the frequency of conflict, there is little way of either husband or wife getting out of an unsatisfactory relationship. Out of every dozen divorces requested no more than one is ever granted, and then only after years of appeals. Most people are simply stuck with their original choice.

Some of the woman's burden is alleviated by shifting the responsibility for chores to growing children. By age seven or eight, many children have begun to help buy vegetables, cook, wash dishes, wash their own clothes, and sweep. Coming home in mid-afternoon, they often start the rice or other staple food cooking. To complete the meal, the mother only has to cook a single vegetable dish when she returns from work. Children have a lot of time at home by themselves, from mid to late afternoon and then on Sundays as well in some working class families. Prior to 1966 this caused little concern. But increasingly in the late 1960s and early 1970s, unsupervised youth became a problem in large Chinese cities. Youth sent to villages drifted back into cities illegally only to drift aimlessly among each others' houses and up and down the street. Younger siblings were infected as well. With a political climate critical of teachers and all other intellectuals, an absence of exams, and students despairing of having any career other than a life in the countryside, school morale and discipline dissolved. Students turned to smoking and breaking school windows. Pickpocketing, bicycle theft, and other petty theft increased. There were gang rumbles over girls and turf — the only saving grace being that it was sometimes done in style, the loser buying the winner drinks or a meal. Compared to American cities, the level of juvenile disorder was still minimal, but it was a great shock to Chinese parents who were accustomed to social order and an obedient teenage population. The situation began to improve in 1975 with urban youth being more systematically rotated back from the countryside after a labor stint of two or three years and again in 1977 with exams, teacher authority, and school discipline being restored. The degree to which the former order can be fully restored remains to be seen.

Grandparents continue to reside with at least one married child, and in most instances, that child continues to be a son even if there is a barely perceptible trend towards increasing residence with daughters. As in the countryside, the young working mother is grateful for help with chores and child care. Most grandmothers remain happy to give this assistance, even though they have lost their authority in the household and sometimes have pensions of their own which could make them independent. (Whether there will be more change in these attitudes once all grandmothers have pensions is uncertain.) Despite this willingness, tension between wife and mother-in-law remains not uncommon, leading some grandmothers to say that they would prefer to live not with their son's wife but with their own daughter. In large cities, all old people are cremated — a practice objected to by some old people but now accepted by all the young and middle aged. Worship of the ancestor's ashes are rare, and enough gravesites have been moved to make way for farming that worship at ancestral graves is increasingly impossible.

Not only ancestor worship but also most other traditional religious and festival activities have disappeared from the home. The traditional lunar new year continues to be the most important festival of the year, providing extra rations like sugar and peanuts as well as three days off from work during which time family and friends continue to visit back and forth, even if with fewer customary touches like ancestor worship and lucky money envelopes for children. The second biggest festival is the new National Day on October 1, which again provides special rations as well as two days off from work and special entertainment in public parks. The only other days off during the year are one day at the solar new year on January 1 and one day at international labor day on May 1. Since there is no annual leave time for most workers, often these public holidays provide the only relief from the continuous six day cycle of work. Accordingly, most emigrés report that the most important dissideratum for them was not whether a holiday was traditional or modern but simply whether it provided relief from the drone of work and something a little better to eat.

There is much, then, in the contemporary urban scene which denudes the family and community of their traditional meanings. Those tendencies and the harshness of the environment which induces them should not be overstated, however. Some of the same tendencies in the environment create a warmth and sharing among workmates, neighbors, friends, and family which emigrés often find wanting in foreign settings. Skilled factory workers are initially apprenticed to an older master who can remain their mentor and confidant for years to follow. One doesn't go looking for jobs on one's own and it is almost impossible to get fired, so most workers have spent their career with a single set of co-workers whose wants, needs, and personal quirks they know well. The work pace is moderate and interpersonal relationships often enjoyable (even though political campaigns can make things a bit tense). Similarly, in neighborhoods the housing crunch means that residential turnover is low and most neighbors know one another well from years of contact. Even when relationships are not intimate, there is a sharing of food, newspapers, and other minor conveniences as well as looking out after one another that can be comforting. The restriction of pay differentials and a forced, spartan uniformity of dress reduces status differentials among people, making social interaction and friendships easier for many. A core loyalty to one's immediate family remains. Even when they have moved away, and when parents have an adequate pension of their own, married children still send token amounts of money in continuing recognition of their loyalty and obligation to the parents who brought them up. On holidays and on days off, when visiting occurs, it is most often among siblings and between parents and children. The range of family obligations has shrunk drastically but is still very much there. The separate identity of the family is seen most clearly in the sharing of kitchens. Most families have to share a kitchen with two, three, or four other families in the same building. This sharing is the most frequent source of conflict among neighbors. To eliminate this conflict and eliminate congestion in what often is no more than a dingy cubicle, one might think that adjacent families would simply cook and eat together, especially when the meal is no more than rice or noodles and a dish or two of vegetables. Yet, there are no known instances of this sharing, and when queried about such a possible arrangement people think it is the most ludicrous idea they have ever heard of. The family still maintains its distinctness under almost communal living facilities. There is, then, an irreducible core of family loyalty which people find supportive even in this very special environment.

Overall, as we should have realized all along, neither Chinese peasants nor urbanities are automatons responding to simple commands or ideological appeals from above. The relationships between government appeal and popular response are much more dynamic, depending on the particular circumstances of each person's life. If we are to understand Chinese patterns of social change, we must understand the circumstances in which each sector of the population is involved. For peasants, the most salient circumstances are a highly solidary collective/ village community combined with a continuing central role for individual families. For urbanites, the salient circumstances include rural work stints for youth, cramped housing, long hours of work for women as well as men, minimal salaries relative to rising expectations, sparse and time consuming urban services, as well as stability of employment and residence — circumstances which require radical adaptations, but which leave intact and even support certain core family and broader friendship loyalties. It is only as we begin to understand these circumstances that we begin to grasp the full texture of Chinese social life and social change.

REFERENCES

Meisner, Mitch
    1975 Ideology and consciousness in Chinese material development. Politics and Society
          5:1–31.
Parish, William L.
    1975 Socialism and the Chinese peasant family. Journal of Asian Studies 34:613–30.
Parish, William L.
    1976 China — team, brigade, or commune? Problems of Communism 25:51–65.
Parish, William L. and Martin K. Whyte
    1978 Village and Family in Contemporary China. Chicago: University of Chicago Press.
Whyte, Martin K.
    1974 Small Groups and Political Rituals in China. Berkeley: University of California
          Press.

12. THE EFFECT OF FAMILY PATHOLOGY ON
TAIPEI'S JUVENILE DELINQUENTS

INTRODUCTION

In the past juvenile delinquency was not thought to be a serious social problem in Chinese communities. A study carried out by Murphy (1963) in Singapore, for example, demonstrated a low level of delinquency in Chinese as compared with Indian youths. Two decades ago, however, Lin (1958) reported a rapid increase of *t'ai-pau*, a nickname for juvenile delinquents, in Taiwan, and attributed this development to post World War II urbanization which spored, among other things, a modern subculture of uprooted youths. Lamson (1935), working in China prior to 1949, regarded this and other forms of social deviance as the result of social disintegration, including breakdown of traditional family structure. Murphy (1963), along with other behavioral scientists, held that Chinese familism protects children from developing deviant behavior. But he recognized that this same family system, when it came into specific conflicts with broader social interests, also could foster delinquency. Although increasing rates of juvenile delinquency have been reported in recent years for Chinese in Hong Kong and the United States (Allard 1975), according to reports of the Police Bureau, delinquency in Taiwan remains low, with annual rates of 3.3 to 4.0 offenders per 1,000 juvenile population (ages 12 to 18) throughout the past decade. Increased numbers of youths in the island's population are responsible for a rise in the total number of delinquents, however. In addition, a change has occurred to a slight extent in some types of delinquent behavior. For example, cases of robbery and drug abuse have increased.

The present study was carried out under the sponsorship of the Republic of China's National Science Council as part of its analysis of the problems faced by youth in Taiwan's rapidly changing society. We analyzed family backgrounds of juvenile delinquents to determine how family pathology affected their social deviance as well as their work and school performance. It was plausible to assume that disorganized family life could directly affect youth, leading them to break social norms, and it seemed equally plausible that family pathology might exert an indirect effect on deviant behavior of juveniles by contributing to school and work failure. These were the hypotheses we set out to examine.

Obviously, juvenile delinquency in Chinese communities, in spite of cultural continuities, must be interpreted within very different contexts of social development. The findings from Taiwan presented below need to be understood in relation to Taiwan's very rapid modernization, and may only be applicable to Chinese and other communities undergoing similar change.

Socio-familial background data on this sample of 494 juvenile offenders and

A. Kleinman and T.-Y. Lin (eds.), Normal and Abnormal Behavior in Chinese Culture, 213–229.

delinquents were obtained during the period June 1976 – March 1977 with the assistance of three probation officers and a social worker. A sampling was made taking one out of five cases from consecutive court referrals and institutional admissions of the Taipei Juvenile Court and Institute. During the nine month study period, 1,850 cases appeared in the Taipei Juvenile Court and 717 cases were admitted to the Taipei Juvenile Institute. Five hundred and ten cases were selected, and after screening out duplicate cases, 494 youths comprised the sample of the present study. The subjects were 461 boys (93%) and 33 girls (7%) with ages ranging from 6 to 19 years (mean, 15.9 years); 152 (31%) of the sample were ages 17–18, 128 (26%) were ages 16–17, and 85 (17%) were ages 15–16. Fathers' social classes as calculated using the method of Hollingshead and Redlich (1958) disclosed: Class I – 3 cases (1%); Class II – 23 cases (5%); Class III – 89 cases (20%); Class IV – 257 cases (58%), and Class V – 70 cases (16%). Seventy-four percent (327/442) of them were from lower socioeconomic class families. Three hundred and twenty-four cases (66%) came from nuclear families, while 117 cases (24%) came from extended families, and 49 cases (10%) came from households with a single member or were living with some other relatives. Except for 27 cases from farmer or fisherman families, the heads of the majority of families in the sample (71%) engaged in small family businesses or worked as industrial laborers. Hence we see that the sample represents offsprings of urban dwellers. Their residences extended over the entire city and the industrial suburban areas of Taipei as well.

DISORGANIZING FACTORS IN THE FAMILIES OF DELINQUENTS

By family pathology is meant any disorganizing factor such as disruption of relationship between family members, chronic impairment due to physical and mental diseases, criminality, poverty and illiteracy, and detrimental attitudes of parents toward children. Each of the above categories might occur independently in a family; however, in most instances, several factors usually take place simultaneously. In the following paragraphs, the author reports the appearance of family pathology among Taipei's delinquent youth.

The Incidence of Broken Homes:

Numerous studies have shown that broken homes and lower-class family background are common conditions promoting delinquency, and this relationship seems to hold cross-culturally. It was supported by Murphy's (1963) study in Singapore. In a study of family life and delinquency in Japan, DeVos and Wagatsuma (1972) found that the influence of family disruption was not limited to the immediate parental generation, there were many more disruptions reported in the grandparent generation of the delinquent subjects whom they examined.

There was evidence of association in the present sample of delinquent youth between social class and family structure variables, and between family structure and broken home variables. However, social class and broken home variables were shown to be independent of each other. The rate of broken homes was 28% (139/490) as shown in Table 1. Combinations and frequencies of loss or separation of a parent or both parents occurring among subjects' families are illustrated in this Table. The frequency of father's death appeared to be somewhat higher than that of mother's death, but otherwise there was no significant difference in the frequency of death and separation of parents. The rate of broken homes among the sample seemed to be quite high when compared to other samples of school students and clinical patients previously studied by the author.

TABLE 1

Frequencies of loss or separation of a parent or both parents occurring among juvenile delinquents

Father died	Father separated	Mother died	Mother separated	Other conditions	No. of study case
X					46
	X				19
		X			29
			X		20
X		X			6
	X		X		6
X			X		6
	X	X			1
				X	6
		No. within each category			
58	26	36	32	6	139

In early studies on delinquents in occidental societies, it had been observed that delinquents from broken homes were apt to be sent to the court, particularly to juvenile institutions, because of the absence of persons in their families who could be responsible for them. In our sample, the rate of broken homes among institutionalized subjects was found to be higher than that among court subjects, but the difference did not reach a significant level. In the statistics of Taipei Juvenile Court (Taipei District Court 1974), broken homes were one of the major family problems associated with delinquent behavior.

Criminality of Family Members

There were 44 families (9%) in the present sample with criminal members. Altogether, 55 family members had criminal records or had been imprisoned. As seen in Table 2, crimes were committed most frequently by elder brothers (27 cases), and next in order by fathers (14 cases). In three families two elder brothers were both criminals. Among the elder brothers 19 cases were the eldest brothers in the sibship. The types of crimes these family members committed were both predatory and non-predatory, but most were adult offenses. We could not document a direct relationship between the criminal acts of family members and those of the subjects. Thus, criminality in a family may be a manifestation of more general disturbances in interpersonal relationships among family members, while specific criminal acts themselves seem to occur on an individual basis. For the majority of delinquent subjects, when they participated in a group crime, their peers were always friends rather than family members.

TABLE 2

Forty-four families of juvenile delinquents in which criminal members were observed

		Criminal member			No. of study case	
Father	Mother	Elder brother	Younger brother	Elder sister		
X					8	
	X				2	
		X			21	(Eldest brother 16)
			X		4	
				X	2	
X	X				3	
X		X			1	(Eldest brother 1)
X				X	1	
	X	X			1	(Eldest brother 1)
X	X	X			1	(Eldest brother 1)
		No. within each category				
14	7	27*	4	3	44	

* Nineteen among 27 elder brothers were the eldest brothers. Two elder brothers were both criminals in 3 study cases.

Our data is too limited to explain the frequent appearance of criminal eldest brothers in the subjects' families. Nevertheless, we might speculate that elder brothers would be influential in providing masculine models of behavior that their younger brothers would identify with. Some questions naturally arise in this regard: Do more delinquents have elder brothers and not elder sisters when compared to their non-delinquent peers? And is the existence of elder sisters effective in preventing the deviant behavior of their younger brothers? Thus far we have not found any support for these hypotheses among our subjects' families.

Physical and Mental Illnesses among Family Members

In this section physical and mental illnesses of family members which were serious enough to contribute to the disruption of family life are analyzed. Altogether 45 family members in 42 subjects' families were found to be ill. The categories of illness and the members of families suffering them are illustrated in Table 3. Without presenting detailed diagnoses for each family member, these illnesses are classified into physical invalidism (mostly cerebrovascular accidents), psychoses, alcoholism, organic brain syndromes and pathological gambling. They constitute chronic problems which might exert a potentially negative effect on family functioning and relationships. Nine cases of alcohol abuse were found. These predominantly involved occasional but heavy drinkers with manifestations of pathological sprees and turmoil in the presence of family members. This rate is notably high for a society with an extremely low rate of alcoholism in the general population (Rin 1978). The cases of gambling did not necessarily involve criminal behavior, but they presented family problems owing to their frequent absence from home. All ill members listed in Table 3 are limited to family members or relatives residing in the same home. Physical invalids were predominantly fathers of the subjects as were alcoholics. Psychoses were distributed among a wide range of family members. In the category of pathological gambling, four fathers and mothers each were found. Organic brain syndromes occurred in two sibs of subjects, one was post-traumatic and the other was epileptic. Only one case of mental retardation, a younger brother of a case, was recorded in family histories. This case was also deaf so he might more easily have come to the attention of probation officers. Milder degrees of mental retardation were not regarded serious problems of these families, either by family members of the subjects or probation officers.

TABLE 3

Invalid or mentally ill family members of 42 juvenile delinquents

Category of illness	Father	Step-father	Mother	Elder brother	Elder sister	Grand-mother	Uncle	Aunt	Total
Physical invalidism	8	1	2		1				12
Psychoses	3		3	2	1	1	2	2	14
Alcoholic	8		1						9
Brain syndromes				1	1				2
Gambling	4		4						8
Total	23	1	10	3	3	1	2	2	45*

* The total number exceeded the number of study cases because there were two family members who were suffering from the same or different category of illness in 3 study cases. All family members listed above were living together.

Since most family members with illness were suffering from chronic disorders but were not receiving on-going medical care, their conditions had created long-term crises for their families. Except for two cases of psychosis who were in mental hospitals for deterioration of their chronic mental illnesses, most other cases were found not to be receiving current medical treatment. This reflects the limited rehabilitation services available in Taiwan.

If factors such as the existence of one or more criminal members in the family and major chronic physical or mental diseases of any family members are added to the 139 cases (28%) from broken homes, a total of 187 cases or 38% (187/490) of the sample come from, in this broader sense, disrupted homes. This rate in my view is probably much higher than that for the general population in Taipei for whom no comparable statistics are available.

Poverty, Illiteracy of Parents, Hardness of Life, and Economic Hazard

All poverty-related factors are dealt here with respect to the effect they have on the disorganization of family relationships and the deprivation of children. General poverty closely relates to Class V socioeconomic status. We based our estimation of poverty conditions on the assessment of probation officers. Illiteracy of parents of subjects is a consequence of poverty in the parental generation, and also might be expected to exert a negative influence on children, especially in regard to educational achievement. Hardness of life does not mean only true poverty, but extreme prolongation of work hours of both parents and other adult members of the family which results not only in their being frequently away from home but also in chronic fatigue and absence from family functions even while in the home. Mothers in our sample who were working in family businesses or in outside jobs did so purely because of the need for additional family income, not because they desired to practice special skills or achieve personal goals. Therefore, they do not correspond to the contemporary Western ideal of "working mothers." Recent failure by the principal wage earner in family business, mostly small family business, constitutes yet another type of family disorganization (Table 4).

Among subjects' families, 83 were in a condition of general poverty; in families of 93 cases, there were one or two parents who were illiterate; parents of 144 cases were so extremely occupied in their work, they could be labeled hardness of life cases; and 28 families had met recent economic breakdown through business failure. With much overlap, as shown in Table 4, it was determined that 240 subjects' families had been experiencing one or more poverty-related factors. This number constituted nearly half of our sample, indicating a high correlation of social deviancy among adolescents with malfunctioning family systems under the stress of substantially insufficient resources.

Pathological Attitudes and Behavior of Family Members

All detrimental attitudes and behavior recorded in the case histories were analyzed, and types of pathological attitudes and behavior of particular family members are presented in Table 5. Only those attitudes or actions toward the juvenile subjects which were considered to exert a definitely negative effect are considered. These fell into three categories: (1) strict and overly authoritative parenting, or disciplining with excessive corporal punishment; (2) rejecting,

TABLE 4

Poverty, illiteracy of parents, hardness of life, and recent economic breakdown reported among 240 juvenile delinquents

General poverty	Illiteracy of a parent or both parents	Hardness of life, too busy	Recent economic breakdown	No. of study case
X				27
	X			38
		X		79
			X	7
X	X			11
X		X		23
X			X	4
	X	X		23
	X		X	4
		X	X	6
X	X	X		11
X	X		X	5
X		X	X	1
X	X	X	X	1
	No. within each category			
83	93	144	28	240

neglecting, emotionally cold, or deserting behavior; and (3) extreme over-protection. Sibling's running-away from the home was considered as one of the pathological family behaviors. In the first category, fathers were found to pre-dominate. Such maladaptive parenting attitudes were recorded in the histories of 42 cases. In a smaller number of families, i.e., 19 cases, inappropriate emotional detachment of parents or other family members were reported. This attitude was occasionally expressed as complete desertion of children by one or both parents. In 45 cases marked over-protection by family members, especially mothers and grandmothers, was observed. The combination of excessively strict father and extremely over-protecting mother was noted on occasion. In many cases, there was over-protection by all older family members. There were three instances in which sisters ran away from the home. These four categories of detrimental family attitude and behavior, again with some overlap, we found in 103 subjects' families.

As has frequently been observed among Taiwan Chinese, many families are authoritarian and use excessive corporal punishment, but no data are available on the actual prevalence of these parenting styles. It is our impression, however, that in most families, strict fathers and over-protecting mothers are the two stereotypic parental forms. But these patterns seem to be gradually disappearing in middle-class families, particularily among young parents. Whereas among older parents, less influenced by modern values, strict father and over-protecting mother are viewed as the social norm. This change in parental approaches,

TABLE 5

Pathological attitudes of family members reported in the histories of 103 juvenile delinquents

Member of family	Overly strict, authoritative, using excessive corporal punishment	Rejecting, neglecting, emotionally-cold deserting	Over-protecting	Running-away from home	Total
Father	31	4	3		38
Mother		6	11		17
Both parents	9	7	13		29
Parents and elder sibs			3		3
Parents and elder brothers			1		1
Father and elder brothers	1				1
Grandmother			9		9
Grandparents			3		3
Grandparents and parents			1		1
Elder sister				2	2
Younger sister				1	1
Other relatives	1	2	1		4
Total	42	19	45	3	109*

* Total frequencies exceeded the number of study cases because there were more than two kinds of family attitudes per family for some cases.

therefore, makes it particularily difficult to assess contemporary Chinese norms concerning child rearing. Generally speaking, children in Chinese families are not submitted to strict discipline during their childhood, but experience this after entering school. Rejecting or neglecting attitudes of parents or other family members, including lack of discipline or time spent with children, occur much less frequently. When they occur, these attitudes usually are associated with critical family conditions such as broken homes and grossly inadequate resources. Harsh treatment, including the use of corporal punishment by parents, especially fathers, occurs when children are disorderly or shirk their studies. Hence these attitudes are mostly expressed toward children older than preschool age, and more frequently to boys than girls. In my experience excessive authoritarian and over-protective parental attitudes can have and often do have negative consequences for child rearing. The fact that they occur in families in our sample seems to be consistent with their presence in Taiwan's culture, but we do not know if these attitudes differ significantly in degree or kind from the general population. In general, modernization itself does not seem to have greatly affected this attitude. Its chief effect has been indirect via economic and occupational influence on the structure of the family and the resources it can tap. This may change in the future, however, because corporal punishment especially by teachers is now strongly criticized in the public media, though punishment by parents has not been so criticized. The following examples illustrate some of these points:

Case 1. A 17-year old boy, eldest son and the third child among four siblings, was rearrested for theft of a motorbike. He had committed motorbike theft once before a year ago, and was sent to a reformatory for a period of eight months. His father, a primary school graduate, had devoted himself excessively to building up a company which had become successful. His mother, who was illiterate, had been overly protective of her sons. The boy was an average student in primary and middle schools, but his scholastic record started to decline during the third year of middle school. He disliked studying, and was often severely blamed by his father who wanted him to advance to higher levels of schools as a means toward future socioeconomic success. His mother was unhappy about his father's strict attitude toward her son and often quarreled with him. After the son's graduation from middle school, he began to help in his father's business. He strongly disliked his work of delivering goods via crowded buses. He stole a motorbike for the first time following his mother's objection to his desire to own a motorbike. After returning from the reformatory, his father was at first extremely hostile and eventually showed an indifferent attitude toward him. The boy said his family's attitude was unfair, because most of his friends owned their own motorbikes. He claimed he stole one again owing to his wish to obtain equal status with his friends. His father was angry and expressed great shame because he lost "face" when he appeared in the Juvenile Institute. As a result his father openly wished that the court would give his son a severe penalty for his repeated theft. His mother, on the contrary, begged for diminution of the sentence, mentioning that her son had been quite obedient at home since his return from the jail. This case illustrates the negative consequences of the relationship of *overly* strict father and *overly* protective mother.

Case 2. A 16-year old youth, second son among four male siblings, was arrested for burglary. He stole 10,000 NT$ cash (equivalent to $260 U.S.) from a house. His father, a primary school graduate and a truck driver, had been extremely busy in his work, hence spent little time with his family, and was excessively authoritarian. His mother, who is illiterate, was recently employed in a small restaurant so that she too spent little time with the family. She was notably incapable of disciplining her children. The boy was obedient as a primary school child, even helped with cooking and cleaning of their house, and had average school records. In middle school, however, he began to exhibit dislike for study and often failed in English and math exams. In response, his father frequently beat him, often severely. During the second year of middle school, the boy was found smoking in the school, which can be grounds for severe punishment by school authorities. When she was called by the school authority to appear in the school, his mother was very upset and told him that she would ask his father to hit him. He ran away from home immediately because of his fear of his father, and worked for awhile in a bamboo arts shop until he was brought back home. He gave up studying and started to work as a house painter. He sometimes participated in gambling with peers. After he stole money, he hid in his friend's homes and spent all the money before he was arrested. He later expressed regret for his lawbreaking behavior but he claimed he committed burglary to fulfill his wish to fit the model of an achieving, ambitious boy his father had transmitted to him. He believed that successful businesses were always based on some form of aggrandizement against others, and saw his own behavior within this light. His mother expressed at the Juvenile Court her view that he was an obedient boy who had never shown reckless behavior, and that he must have been taught by someone else to do such bad things. She attempted to protect him and put the blame for his behavior on others. This case again illustrates negative consequences of overly strict father, but rather than overly protecting mother, this boy's mother represents incapability in parenting owing both to her personality and time commitments outside the family.

EFFECT OF DISORGANIZING FACTORS ON SCHOOL
AND JOB ADJUSTMENT OF DELINQUENTS

When the five major disorganizing factors discussed above are combined, 188 cases are found to be affected by any one of them, and 164 cases were affected by two or more kinds of family problems. Notably, family disorganization appears in 352 cases, or 72% (352/490) of the sample subjects. All five factors – broken homes, criminality, chronic physical or psychological impairment, poverty and pathological attitudes and behaviors – we believe to be long-standing, "traditional" problems within the Chinese family and not the result of rapid socioeconomic change. However, social development is seen to play a role inasmuch as the family life circumstances within which our subjects have been reared are exclusively urban, the occupations of their fathers are predominantly commerce and industrial labor, and the structure of their families is largely nuclear. Hence modernization may be seen to augment or heighten family disorganization in Taiwan and to reduce the resources the family has available for coping with external and internal stress. The subjects are required, furthermore, to meet modern social values through nine years of compulsory education. The path to a higher education in Taiwan is still very narrow. Youngsters are engaged in serious competition and yearly entrance examinations. This pressured push toward modernity undoubtedly has added further burdens to the socialization of these adolescents. When the family is broken, or disrupted, or disorganized, the children are not well supported, prepared or motivated to meet these educational stressors and as a result are more likely to fail in school and later perhaps enter a deviant social role.

Table 6 shows the relationship between the disorganizing factors in families and school dropout rates of our subjects. We found that dropout rates are generally higher among the subjects in any one of the five categories of disorganization as compared with the rates among subjects whose families are free from these disorganizing factors. In Table 6, three conditions (*broken homes; disrupted homes* including broken homes, criminality of family members, and chronically physically and mentally ill family members; and *disorganized homes* including all five categories) are arbitrarily named, and for each condition, the school dropout rates are compared. Dropouts were consistently over-represented in the children of disorganized families.

The next section of the paper deals with the working status of the subjects in relation to family disorganization factors. The disorganizing conditions are again divided in the same three ways as in Table 6. As seen in Table 7, among the subjects whose families do not suffer from any of the disorganizing factors, the numbers of students (49–59%) always exceed those of each corresponding disorganized groups (31–38%). The most prominent findings are the rates of unemployment and unstable working status. These appeared in subjects from disorganized families at 32–37%, whereas in subjects of non-disorganized families they were only 13–22%, which is a statistically significant difference.

TABLE 6

Differences in dropout rates between two groups of juvenile delinquent with or without disorganizing factors in their families

Disorganizing factors	Dropouts		Non-dropouts		Total		
	%		%		%		N = 483
Broken homes	81	(60)	53	(40)	134	(100)	X² = 15.36
							df = 1
Non-broken homes	130	(37)	219	(63)	349	(100)	P<.001
Disrupted homes (broken homes; criminal, physically or mentally ill members in family)	103	(57)	79	(43)	182	(100)	N = 483 X² = 19.78 df = 1
Non-disrupted homes	108	(36)	193	(64)	301	(100)	P<.001
Disorganized homes (broken homes; criminal, physically or mentally ill members in family; poverty; pathological attitudes)	178	(51)	169	(49)	347	(100)	N = 483 X² = 29.02 df = 1
Non-disorganized homes	33	(24)	103	(76)	136	(100)	P<.001

TABLE 7

Differences in working status between two groups of juvenile delinquent with or without disorganizing factors in their families

Disorganizing factors	Studying or at preschool age		Working, stable		Working, unstable or now unemployed		Total		
	%		%		%		%		N = 481
Broken homes	41	(31)	43	(32)	49	(37)	133	(100)	X² = 14.87
									df = 2
Non-broken homes	169	(49)	101	(29)	78	(22)	348	(100)	P<.001
Disrupted homes (broken homes; criminal, physically or mentally ill members in family)	59	(33)	57	(32)	64	(35)	180	(100)	N = 481 X² = 13.57 df = 2
Non-disrupted homes	151	(50)	87	(29)	63	(21)	301	(100)	P<.01
Disorganized homes (broken homes; criminal, physically or mentally ill members in family, poverty, pathological attitudes)	130	(38)	106	(31)	109	(32)	345	(101)	N = 481 X² = 22.69 df = 2
Non-disorganized homes	80	(59)	38	(28)	18	(13)	136	(100)	P<.001

The above findings permit us to examine the influence of family pathology on the achievement of delinquents in academic work and occupation. When each of the five different types of disorganizing factors was independently analyzed, its influence was consistently in the same direction. This suggests that there is a pathway leading from family pathology to the subjects' failure in achievement, and then from that failure to the subjects' access to socially deviant activities.

It has been generally believed that the extended family system functions to protect family members from stresses related to economic and other aspects of life event change. However, in the present sample this does not turn out to be so. The family structure of both disorganized and non-disorganized groups reveals that there were 217 (62%) disorganized families of nuclear type vs. 167 (78%) non-disorganized families of nuclear type; disorganized families of extended type were 95 (27%) vs. 22 (16%) in the non-disorganized group; and of subjects who live alone or who live with others — 40 (11%) belonged to the disorganized group vs. 9 (7%) in the non-disorganized group. Disorganizing factors appear to be proportionally more heavily distributed among the cases whose families are of the extended type or the cases who live alone. The significance of this difference in family structures between disorganized and non-disorganized group is at the level of one percent.

The mobility of families in our sample, for both urban and suburban areas, was fairly high. This might have contributed to the formation of nuclear families.[1] Among the sample, two-thirds of families were of the nuclear type, and this figure is higher than expected because our data from general patients' records shows that about one-half come from nuclear families. Many families of this type have an average of 4 to 5 (4.7 ± 1.9 for total sample) children, and most adult members work very hard and long hours without help from relatives or friends. Hence it is natural for this to cause loose family ties. There was evidence to support this tendency in the analysis of sibling rank of our subjects. At a significant level, lastborns in the group of broken home families were found to be over-represented, while the number of firstborns and lastborns in the groups of non-broken home families were equal. Generally, the number of offenders who were born in the last half of the birth rank exceeded those in the first half for larger families (sib size 4 or over), while the number of first half and last half of the birth rank were equal in smaller families (sib size 2 or 3). Lessening of parent-child affiliation and disruption of parent-child relations were found to be important factors, and tended to be more prevalent among children born in the latter part of birth order, who, as other studies of Chinese suggest, receive less affection from their parents. It is likely that family planning will help remedy this situation sooner than attempts to reform extended families.

In the following several case histories the process of failure in school and in occupational achievements are illustrated.

Case 3. A 17-year old boy, the second son and fourth among five siblings, was arrested for aggravated assault. He with six boys intentionally assaulted two other boys and broke windows of a factory in retaliation for the victims' assault on him. At age four he lost his father who died in a coal mine accident. His mother reared her children while working in factories or in nurseries. His school records were constantly poor. He disliked studying and dropped from middle school during the second year. He alleged that he was embarrassed to attend school after some of his classmates laughed at him for wearing new clothing. However, his poor record was the main reason for his school leaving. When he started to work, he could not hold a job in one place for more than four months at a time. He changed work frequently, including: printing shops, painter's shop, textile factory, sterile water factory, etc. He noted that none of the above jobs fit his interest, and never developed any interest in them. He joined a group of agemates who banded together to have good times.

His mother wanted to move to another town to separate him from them, because she felt they were teaching him bad habits. She also objected to his working at a restaurant where he might readily observe and participate in adults' bad behavior. Not only do we see in this case failure in school and occupation, but also a broken home background with early death of father and mother's inability to control her children.

Case 4. A 15-year old boy, the eldest son among three male siblings, was arrested for robbery. His father, who is a retired soldier, previously worked as a truck driver, and has been currently unemployed. His mother is a worker in an electronics factory. Since the sixth grade of primary school, this subject began to exhibit deviant behavior. He often played truant, joined peers outside the school, and frequently participated in group fights. He organized a gang (*pang*) named North-Airport Golden Leopard *pang* and became its leader. He was openly hostile and disobedient toward his parents, and often ran away from home. Two years ago he was arrested for theft. He studied in a middle school, but was transferred to another school by the school authorities during the first semester, because he repeatedly broke school regulations. In the next school, he again broke regulations and finally was dismissed a year ago. Recently he was arrested once again for glue sniffing and later was rearrested with other boys for successive robberies; they robbed taxi drivers mostly at night. Although the deviant behavior is more severe, the background is similar to other cases described above.

Case 5. A 15-year old boy, fourth son and the fourth among five siblings, was arrested for theft. His father is a farmer, and his mother sells vegetables. He was noted to be restless and had a poor school record. In the first year of middle school, he broke regulations, such as the prohibition on smoking, and often fought with other classmates. Because of his mother's complaints about him, he disliked staying in the home and spent most of his leisure time outside with peers, going to the movies, walking around town, and stealing fruit. His father arranged for him to change schools at the end of the first semester, but he stopped attending school altogether. He made two "sworn brothers," and put a tattoo on his left arm as the symbol of their brotherhood. Two tattooed characters on his arm stood for "wanderer." He began working in a painter's shop run by his cousin, but he discontinued work there after two months with the reason that he could not have enough hours free from his cousin's control. He was arrested for theft once about ten months ago. Now he was arrested for the second time after he and four other boys stole milk cartons and cash from a bus ticket stand. This case is one of deviance in the absence of broken home with deviant behavior supported by peer group.

Case 6. A 17-year old boy, youngest of four siblings and the second son, was arrested for intimidation. He had previously committed blackmail and aggravated assault, and for the last eight months was sentenced to imprisonment. His father is a manager of a trading company, and his family is well-to-do, except for a time several years before when his father was absent from home while living with a mistress. He gradually became antagonistic toward elders and increasingly irritable. During the first year of middle school, he fought with other boys in the school; and during the second year he was dismissed from the school owing to smoking and fighting. Then he studied machine shop work for three months, after which he was expected to work in a car repairing factory, but he quit his job in one and a half days. Soon, he committed blackmail and was put on probation. Then he worked in his friend's paint shop, but only briefly. He later started to help his elder brother's new iron factory, but worked only occasionally. He spent most of his time with a peer group, in which he engaged in glue sniffing, abuse of sleeping pills, and intravenous use of Sosegon (an analgesic). He carried a metal hand protector to threaten people and defend himself. Fighting and assault occurred regularly in the group. Although he was sentenced to imprisonment for aggravated assault, he seemed to be unwilling to modify his behavior. Recently this boy and his friends intimidated and blackmailed people on six occasions until the present arrest occurred. This case illustrates juvenile deviance associated with both family pathology and peer group behavior.

SOME OBSERVATIONS ON THE PATTERN OF DELINQUENT BEHAVIOR

Lin (1958) defined and contrasted two types of delinquent youths in Taiwan, *t'ai-pau* and *liu-mang*. *T'ai-pau*, who are of recent origin, mostly came from middle-class or upper-class families and are middle-school or unsuccessful students. They tend to play truant in small groups around modern amusement sections of cities. Their law-breaking behavior includes: stealing, blackmailing, assault, and occasionally robbery. Loyalty to the group is emphasized, and toughness is regarded a virtue. The toughest boy usually becomes the leader. Assaults are frequently caused by intra-group conflicts or conflicts with non-*t'ai-pau* students. They are usually distinguishable from other youths by their conspicuous (modern) appearance and attention seeking manners. The group tends to have poor cohesion. The majority of *liu-mang* in contrast, are residents of cities and small towns and come mostly from lower-class or lower-middle class families. Their education seldom is higher than primary school and their ages range 10 to 20 or more. The most organized public activities of these *liu-mangs* are involvement in ceremonies or festivals of temples in the areas where they live. They take pride in helping their elders plan, organize, prepare, and participate in activities of the temple. Sometimes several small groups have a common affiliation with a temple. Loyalty is above everything and group discipline is often strict, ranging from beating to lynching. They engage in the practice of "blood-bonding" which consists of an oath made in front of the god of a temple by drinking the blood of a cock and swearing eternal loyalty to the members of the group, to the extent of sacrificing their lives for one another. The leaders are professional criminals who have a strong voice in community affairs. They also have a strong grip on the economic affairs of their local areas and with the help of their subordinates they control prostitution, gambling, trading of stolen goods, black-marketing, narcotic peddling, and protection rackets. *Liu-mang* were effectively controlled by the government in the 1950's and 1960's.

Interviewing hundreds of juvenile offenders and delinquents, we have found in contemporary Taiwan neither typical *t'ai-pau* nor typical *liu-mang* as reported two decades ago. Although formation of gangs by delinquents is quite common, and many of them follow the fashion of naming their groups, e.g., Golden-dragon *pang* or Black-light *pang*, etc., we never found a leader among those we studied who fit the traditional *liu-mang* behavioral style. Rather, these gangs, which are becoming an important public concern, are more likely to follow the *t'ai-pau* life-style. In the past two decades, well-defined *t'ai-paus* are said no longer to exist, yet 57% (279/489) of our subjects participated in group delinquent activities either with named gangs or with much looser peer group ties that are close to, although not exactly the same as, the classical *t'ai-pau* pattern. Most frequent group deviant activities were fighting with other groups of youths, assault and burglary. The practice of sworn brothers was found occasionally, often through tattooing symbol marks or letters on arms or chests, but hardly ever through the practice of blood-bonds. These observations suggest that the pattern of delinquent behavior has changed over time in that the two types of delinquency are merging owing to social changes brought on by urbanization and modernization.

The most common crimes were theft and burglary. Among our subjects, 53% (261/490) were found to have records of arrest for these offenses. Unlike Western societies (Glasser 1970), auto theft has not become a predominantly adolescent felony, instead, motorbike and bicycle theft are common among our sample. The peak age for motorbike theft arrest is 16, and that for bicycle theft arrest is 15. In only a few cases were theft and burglary committed because of financial need. For the majority of offenders these crimes were motivated by immediate personal gratification, e.g., obtaining money to spend on night life, gambling, etc. The next most frequent offenses were murder and aggravated assault which occurred in 23% (113/491) of the sample. Glue sniffing and abuse of other drugs (mostly hypnotics), and drinking behavior were recorded in the history of 17% (83/491) of the subjects. None of the cases had abused heroin. Drinking usually occurred in a group situation, and only a few cases resulted in assaultive acts owing to intoxication. Intimidation was recorded in 15% of cases (74/490), robery in 2% (12/491), breaking and arson in 2% (12/491), and rape and other sexual misbehavior in 5% (25/485). Several subjects had been brought to the attention of the police by the parents of their girl friends for dating without parental permission.

If we examine types of criminal or deviant behavior through which the latest arrests occurred, a classification of three categories of predatory (victimizing acts), nonpredatory (victimless crimes) and delinquent behavior can be made. The distribution of subjects in these three categories is 371 (77%), 64 (13%), and 45 (9%), respectively. Table 8 illustrates the influence of disorganizing factors

TABLE 8

Differences in frequencies of three types of offenses between two groups of juvenile delinquent with and without disorganizing factors in their families

	Predatory crimes		Non-predatory crimes		Delinquent behaviors		Total	
	No.	%	No.	%	No.	%	No.	%
With disorganizing factors	281	82	35	10	27	8	343	100
Without disorganizing factors	90	66	29	21	18	13	137	100
Total	371	77	64	13	45	9	480*	99

X^2 = 15.06, df = 2, P<.001

* Types of offenses in fourteen cases were unclassified.

involved in subjects' families on the frequency of predatory, nonpredatory and delinquent offenses. There is a tendency for predatory crimes, which are more aggressive, to be committed more frequently by subjects who come from disorganized families than by subjects from non-disorganized families. Obversely, subjects of non-disorganized families are apt to show higher rates of nonpredatory crimes and delinquent behavior when compared to those from disorganized families.

CONCLUSION

In this study of 494 Taipei delinquents we have seen the influence of family pathology on school and work failure. This finding strongly supports a hypothesis that failure in academic work and occupation is an indirect pathway for producing deviant behavior of youths who come from pathological or disorganized families. The nature of family pathology of our sample subjects was analyzed in detail. The major pathologies were classified as five factors: broken homes, criminal members in the family, major chronic mental and physical impairment of family members, poverty, and maladaptive parenting of children. The effect of each pathological factor on the subjects' failure in school and work was found to be in the same direction. The rate of broken homes was 28%. In 49% of the sample, poverty-related factors were clearly shown, and this rate was certainly higher than that among the general population. The majority of the sample (74%) were from lower socioeconomic class families. The school dropout rate of the subjects was as high as 44%. Children in these families, like other children in Taiwan, are expected to achieve in schools and at work, and there is considerable family pressure to do so. Only 13% (62/490) of the present sample were found to be mentally retarded or mentally ill, and for these reasons untrained in academic and work abilities. It is particularly noteworthy that violent crimes (murder and aggravated assault) involved almost one-quarter of our subjects, suggesting that the contemporary pattern of delinquent behavior in Taiwan is associated with much more violence than in the past.

It has been generally believed that modernization brings with it certain negative effects, especially for adolescents. The elements of modernization are complex, but it is the author's impression that two important factors are related to the negative effect of modernization: one is too rapid modernization, and the other is breakdown of traditional value systems associated with radical value change. Chinese families in Taiwan are fairly conscious about these effects which threaten the traditional Chinese cultural emphasis on family ties. Our observations in the present study, and our clinical experiences as well, indicate that evidence that it is the effect of modernization itself that inflicts individual psychological and behavior problems is minimal; instead, other factors related to family pathology are more influential. It is important to emphasize that our findings do not support the usually held belief that the extended family system functions to protect its members from stresses related to economic and other aspects of life event change. We are fully aware that these statements may not be applicable to other Chinese communities.

The family pathology of the subjects disclosed in this study is by no means unique to Chinese society, that is to say, broken homes, criminality of family members, mental and physical diseases of family members, and the problems of poverty are not unusual problems. All these factors, moreover, have been described in the past as indigenous to Chinese families, and hence cannot be regarded as the result of modernization per se, though it may augment certain of them. Attitudes toward parenting of the families we studied are obviously most strongly influenced by cultural background. Modernization worsens some and ameliorates others of these factors so that it exerts a complex effect that cannot be reduced to a simplistic and tautological formula equating social development with delinquency and explaining the latter by the former.

NOTE

1. We do not possess the data to evaluate the effect of migration from rural to urban areas in causing family disorganization and delinquency.

REFERENCES

Allard, W. A.
 1975 Chinatown, the guilded ghetto. National Geographic 148 (5): 627–643.
DeVos, G. and Wagastama, H.
 1972 Family life and delinquency. Some perspectives from Japanese research. *In* Transcultural Research in Mental Health. W. P. Lebra, ed. Hawaii: University Press of Hawaii.
Glaser, D.
 1970 Strategic Criminal Justice Planning. Crime and Delinquency Issues. A Monograph Series. Bethesda: National Institute of Mental Health.
Hollingshead, A. B. and Redlich, F. C.
 1958 Social Class and Mental Illness: A Community Study. New York: John Wiley & Sons.
Lamson, H.
 1935 Social Pathology in China. Shanghai: Commercial Press.
Lin T.
 1958 *Tai-pau* and *liu-mang*: Two types of delinquent youths in Chinese society. British Journal of Delinquency 8: 244–256.
Murphy, H. B. M.
 1963 Juvenile delinquency in Singapore. Journal of Social Psychology 61:201–231.
Rin H.
 1978 Psychiatry and the Society. Taipei: Buffalo Publishing Co. (In Chinese).
Taipei District Court
 1974 Three Years Report on Juvenile Delinquency. Taipei: Taipei District Court. (In Chinese)

SECTION IV

PSYCHIATRIC STUDIES: EPIDEMIOLOGICAL
AND CLINICAL

INTRODUCTION TO SECTION IV

The first article in this section by Lin, Kleinman, and Lin reviews both epidemiological and clinical studies. The authors note the limited findings from China proper, and then review epidemiological studies of mental illness in Chinese populations in Taiwan, Hong Kong, Singapore, Malaysia, and North America. They also discuss clinical epidemiological assessments of symptomatology, illness behavior, and help seeking. The second part of their chapter describes salient Chinese cultural influences on psychopathology, including somatization and culture-bound syndromes. It is an attempt to integrate anthropology with clinical and epidemiological approaches in order to forge a more powerful framework for analyzing and comparing cross-culturally the influence of culture on psychopathology. Although anthropological studies have been faulted for being clinically uninformed, this chapter points out that epidemiological and clinical studies all too frequently are anthropologically uninformed and therefore culturally naive. That is to say, they fail to come to grips with the meaning context of sickness and hence with the ways that cultural beliefs and value orientations shape illness behavior. Lin, Kleinman, and Lin call for ethnomedical (or anthropological) epidemiology and clinical studies that deal directly with these questions.

Lee's chapter examines the influence of sex role and social class on psychiatric symptoms. After reviewing relevant studies among Chinese and other societies, he presents findings from a survey in Hong Kong of the prevalence of psychiatric symptoms in a stratified sample of urban households. Using Langner's scale, and assessing potentially confounding variables, he found that as in previous studies both sex role and family's socioeconomic status exerted significant effects on psychiatric symptoms. In interpreting these findings, Lee reviews the major soicological arguments and then anchors his own explanation in a detailed assessment of findings from research on the social and cultural situation of contemporary Hong Kong, especially regarding the role of women and the effects of class.

The article by Tsai, Teng and Sue reviews what limited information is presently available concerning rates of mental disorders among Chinese-Americans. They discuss the erroneous assumption that the low utilization rates of mental health facilities by Chinese-Americans signifies that they have low rates of mental illness, presenting major social and cultural factors that confound this judgment. They conclude that rates of mental illness most likely have been severely underestimated for Chinese-Americans. Thereafter, the authors review research on personality and social stressors encountered by this American ethnic group, and cultural factors that may bias against recognition of the mental

A. Kleinman and T.-Y. Lin (eds.), Normal and Abnormal Behavior in Chinese Culture, 233–235.
Copyright © 1980 by D. Reidel Publishing Company.

health problems they experience. Among the key social stressors examined are culture conflict, social change, prejudice and discrimination. Tsai, Teng, and Sue also discuss juvenile delinquency, suicide, drug abuse, and alcoholism. They call for more culturally appropriate research to answer the many important questions raised.

In their article, Klein, Miller and Alexander review studies of Chinese students in the United States. Certain of these studies were conducted in collaboration with investigators in Taiwan, so that the authors can address both predeparture and acculturation experiences. They examine different patterns of student adaptation to American culture, and present findings from their analyses of maladaptation, including psychological and physical illness. Since substantial numbers of Chinese students have entered and continue to come to American society, this research is of practical value in better understanding and responding to the problems they face. The authors summarize some of their experiences in providing culturally appropriate therapy that may be useful not only in developing psychological and psychiatric services for this group, but also in planning mental health services for Chinese generally. The recent influx of Southeast Asians into North America suggests another relevant application for this research.

The next article is a report on mental illness and psychosocial problems associated with physical illness in the People's Republic of China based on the authors' visit in 1978 to medical and psychiatric facilities in China. It complements the article by Lin, Kleinman, and Lin by discussing the epidemiology of mental illness, somatization and related psychiatric issues in contemporary China. This article also delves into clinical themes covered by chapters that follow, e.g., cultural influences on psychopathology, illness behavior and psychiatric and medical care. The authors of this article discuss both achievements and current problems, and thereby present a somewhat more balanced account than many earlier reports on medicine and psychiatry in China. They also draw parallels with psychiatric issues in other Chinese societies and present a cultural framework for assessing what is specific to the People's Republic and what is universal for Chinese communities. This article outlines key questions for future visits and collaborative cross-cultural research, especially now that psychiatry and psychology in China are becoming less marginal to that nation's health and health care systems.

The next three articles deal with clinical problems. Drs. Wen and Wang, a psychiatrist and a urologist from National Taiwan University Hospital, present data from an empirical study of a Chinese culture-specific sexual neurosis, *shen-k'uei* (kidney deficiency or weakness) syndrome. The authors relate this problem to other culture-specific neuroses in Taiwan, *koro* and frigophobia, show how it is based on Chinese illness beliefs, review its clinical phenomenology, and compare it with culture-specific sexual neuroses reported for South Asian culture. They conclude that this syndrome represents culture-specific *illness behavior* for universal psychiatric *diseases*. Their chapter represents one of the most detailed clinical assessments of a culture-bound syndrome to date and describes an important problem among Chinese that heretofore has not been systematically analyzed in detail.

Tan, a psychiatrist who formerly headed the Department of Psychiatry at the University of Malaya and who has had extensive clinical experience in Southeast Asia, contributes an article that reviews culture-bound syndromes generally among overseas Chinese. The reader should compare his discussion with the review of the same subject in the first article of the section, which presents an alternative (anthropological) formulation of cultural effects on psychopathology that contrasts with Tan's rather traditional psychiatric inter-pretation. It is the feeling of the editors that there are at present several distinc-tive approaches to the culture-bound syndromes that readers need to be informed about. It is also our view that an adequate assessment of these clinical prob-lems requires an integration of models from psychiatry, anthropology, and psychology.

In the final article in this section, Lin and Lin draw on extensive experiences with the families of Chinese suffering mental illness to describe how such families cope with mental illness and the consequences of these coping styles for patients and care-givers. They outline a commonly repeated cycle of love, denial, and rejection that presents a major challenge for the planning and delivery of mental health services to Chinese patients. This chapter illustrates some of the practical implications for clinical services of the Chinese cultural meanings and social institutions reviewed earlier in the book. The editors wish to encourage future research to focus on the kinds of basic treatment issues dealt with by Lin and Lin in Chapter 20. Clinically-relevant themes are covered elsewhere in this volume, especially in Chapters 8, 12, 13, 15, 16, 17 and 18.

KEH-MING LIN, ARTHUR KLEINMAN, AND TSUNG-YI LIN

13. OVERVIEW OF MENTAL DISORDERS IN CHINESE CULTURES: REVIEW OF EPIDEMIOLOGICAL AND CLINICAL STUDIES

INTRODUCTION

Psychiatric epidemiology, a relatively new branch of psychiatry, has witnessed tremendous growth since the end of World War II (cf. Leighton 1959; Hughes et al. 1960; Leighton et al. 1963; Srole et al. 1962; Langner and Michael 1963; Lemkau et al. 1964; Lin 1953; Lin et al. 1969; Hollingshead and Redlich 1958; Gurin et al. 1960). The information derived from epidemiological studies of mental disorders not only serves the practical purpose of providing a rational basis for planning mental health care services, but also helps us better understand the causes and distribution of various mental illnesses (Cooper and Morgan 1973; Robins 1978).

Recently, epidemiology has increasingly involved cross-national and cross-cultural comparisons in order to assess sociocultural influences on the etiology and natural history of diseases (Alexander 1977). This development has held particular importance for the field of psychiatry, where one would expect social and cultural factors to exert an especially extensive effect (Cassel 1974; Beiser 1978; Marsella 1979). Seen in this context, the importance and relevance of epidemiological studies of psychiatric problems in Chinese cultures cannot be overemphasized. At the present time, the Chinese probably comprise one-fourth of the world's population, making them the planet's largest ethnic group. Chinese communities, frequently with abiding attachment to core indigenous cultural beliefs and behavioral norms, exist in almost every corner of the world. Hence any serious understanding of psychiatric disorders which seeks to make universal statements needs to take the Chinese case into account, along with other non-Western societies that together comprise more than three-fourths of the world's population. The distribution and phenomenology of mental disorders in Chinese culture, of course, is of special interest to those who wish to determine how Chinese culture influences psychopathology as well as to those concerned with providing Chinese populations with culturally appropriate mental health services.

PSYCHIATRIC EPIDEMIOLOGICAL STUDIES IN CHINA

Psychiatry was largely neglected in the China mainland prior to 1949 (Lyman 1947; Wong 1950; Bermann 1968). Consequently, no reliable community based studies on the distribution of mental disorders were conducted. The few reports concerning the prevalence of psychiatric problems were extremely crude estimations extrapolated from clinical experience (Kasamatu 1942; Lin 1953, 1963).

A. Kleinman and T.-Y. Lin (eds.), Normal and Abnormal Behavior in Chinese Culture, 237–272.
Copyright © 1980 by D. Reidel Publishing Company.

In 1960, Chu and Lin reported 1,716 cases of mental disease admitted to Peking Municipal Psychopathic Hospital during the years 1933–1943. Since the establishment of the People's Republic of China (PRC), there have been several large-scale descriptive studies of hospitalized cases of schizophrenia (T'ao et al. 1957; Hsia et al. 1958; Wang and Tuan 1957; Yu and Li 1958), and of manic-depressive psychosis, organic psychosis, epilepsy and neurosis (Wang and Tuan 1957). In 'Guideline for the prevention and treatment of psychiatric illness,' The Department of Health of the PRC (1958) estimated that there were more than one million psychotic patients nationwide (or 0.1% of the population). Cerny (1965), in his review of psychiatry in China, mentioned an epidemiological survey involving 2,200,000 subjects in Shanghai and Nanking, without citing a specific reference. Taipale and Taipale (1973) also mentioned this large-scale survey and attributed it to the Cultural Revolution, but again did not cite a specific reference. Similar large-scale surveys were mentioned by Chin and Chin (1969). No epidemiological data on the prevalence of psychiatric problems in the PRC has been published subsequently, however. As noted by Chin and Chin (1969), the socio-political atmosphere in the PRC during the Cultural Revolution was anti-intellectual and prohibitive of academic pursuits in psychology and psychiatry. There is recent evidence suggesting a gradual improvement. In May 1978, a national conference on psychology was held in the People's Republic, and since that time developmental and educational psychology have been discussed in the press (*Kuang-ming jih-pao* 1978–1979).

Recently, Xia et al. (mimeographed report) reported that 4 million inhabitants in Shanghai were surveyed during the period of 1972 to 1978, which revealed an overall prevalence rate of mental disorder of 0.728%, and that of schizophrenia of 0.42%. Urban districts had a slightly higher rate for both the overall mental disorder and for schizophrenia. Case finding was accomplished through reports from paramedical health personnel (barefoot doctors, nurses and health workers in factories) who had received short courses of psychiatric training by psychiatrists from the municipal and district mental hospitals. Persons suspected of mental disorders were recorded and the list was also submitted by lay persons serving in regional committees, who also had received similar kinds of training, to the paramedical group and the neighborhood cadres. The diagnosis of these cases was then ascertained by psychiatrists through home visits. The same report also indicated that through an intensive occupational therapy program of 3–5 years duration, a group of chronic schizophrenic patients improved dramatically, the majority of them being able to hold regular jobs, and very few of them needing readmission. Other recent communications from Hunan (Young and Li 1979; Teaching and Research Group of Psychiatry mimeographed report) and Nanking (Tao, Lin and Zheng mimeographed report) indicate a continuous interest in clinical research involving epidemiological principles among psychiatrists in different locations.

During a visit to America of a group of eight psychiatrists from the PRC in May and June 1979, it was unofficially announced that the aforementioned epidemiological studies as well as others had yielded an urban prevalence rate for schizophrenia in China of 3 cases/1000 population and that the rural rate was less, reputedly closer to 2 cases/1000 population, while the urban prevalence rate for all psychoses ranged between 5 to 7 cases/1000 population in several as yet unpublished studies. It is greatly to be hoped that data from these and other epidemiological studies in the People's Republic will soon be officially reported and the studies published in full, since they are essential for understanding the true prevalence of mental illness among Chinese (see Chapter 17). In their absence we are forced to lean heavily on findings from studies of mental illness in other Chinese societies.

MAJOR STUDIES IN TAIWAN

From 1946 to 1963, a series of major epidemiological studies on mental disorders were conducted in Taiwan (Formosa) by a team of psychiatrists at the National Taiwan University Hospital, led by T. Y. Lin. Their findings, cautiously interpreted, provide us with a basis for making rational estimates about mental illness among Chinese (Rin 1970). For a better understanding of the background and significance of these studies, a brief description of Taiwan and its people is presented here.

Taiwan is an island about the size of the Netherlands, located 100 miles off the South China coast, currently with an estimated population of 17 million. Owing to racial and sociohistorical factors, the population can be divided into three distinct groups:

(1) "Aborigines," who presently constitute only 2% of the total population, are Malayo-Polynesian in origin, divided into 9 large tribes, with varying degrees of contact with Chinese culture.

(2) "Taiwanese," 70%–80% of the current population, are the descendants of Chinese immigrants who came to the island from Fukien and, to a lesser extent, Kwangtung Provinces, between the seventeenth and nineteenth centuries. From 1895 to 1945, Taiwan was ruled by the Japanese and was largely cut off from Chinese influences. Relatively few Chinese continued to emigrate to Taiwan in this period. Thus at the end of World War II, when Taiwan was returned to Chinese control, Taiwanese had been living on the island for generations, had established a local variant of Chinese culture, but in urban areas especially had been influenced to some extent by Japanese culture.

(3) "Mainland Chinese," from various parts of China, started to arrive in Taiwan after retrocession in 1945. Most of them probably did not intend to stay for a long time, but the subsequent coming to power on the Mainland of the Chinese Communist Party made return impossible. In addition, from 1948–50, about two million Chinese (most of them members of the military) fled China and migrated to Taiwan. These migrants, although they came from different parts of China, have gone through more or less similar refugee experiences and are usually lumped together and classified as Mainland Chinese in contrast to the "native" Taiwanese.

In addition to the impact of political change and large scale migration, Taiwan has also witnessed dramatic social and economic changes in the last thirty years owing to rapid industrialization and urbanization. This process of modernization, on the one hand brought about economic prosperity and improvement of the standard of living, while on the other hand it helped create stressful conflicts between modern and traditional, Western and Chinese value-orientations and demanded constant adaptation to continuously changing lifestyles and social structural arrangements (Gallin 1966; Lin 1959; Yeh and Tseng 1971).

Retrospectively, it was not unreasonable to expect that, provided with this rich social and cultural matrix, a series of cross-sectional and longitudinal community-wide surveys would result in some important contributions to our understanding of mental illness and deviance in Chinese culture. Two other factors made these surveys additionally valuable:

(1) All the studies were conducted by a cohesive group of psychiatrists from the same department trained in the same research techniques. The methodology used was the same, the conceptualization and definition of mental disorders comparable from study to study, and the inter-interviewer reliability high.

(2) The surveys were notably thorough: a census examination method was used which involved three steps: (a) survey of the census registers and information gathering from key figures in the communities to identify psychiatric cases, (b) detailed study of the identified cases, (c) visits to every household for interviews and brief psychiatric examination of every individual to ensure the completeness of the survey. The generally reliable census registration system in Taiwan and the cooperation of officials and community leaders contributed to the thoroughness of the surveys.

First Survey – 1946–48 (Lin 1953)

This was done sequentially in 3 communities: Baksa, Simpo, and Ampeng, representing village, small town and city, respectively. The ecological boundary of each community was demarcated and a total census performed. Total population surveyed was about 20,000. The overall prevalence rates for different diagnostic categories are as follows:

	rate/1,000
Schizophrenia	2.1
Manic-Depressive Psychosis	0.7
Senile Psychosis	0.3
Other Psychosis	0.7
Epilepsy	1.3
Mental Retardation	3.5
Personality Disorders	0.9
Neurosis	1.2
Alcoholism	0.1
Total	10.8

After correction for differences in age distribution of the population, the rate of schizophrenia was found to be comparable with the results from other cultures. The rate for manic-depressive psychosis was slightly higher and epilepsy slightly lower than in most previous studies. Contrary to general belief, the age-adjusted rate for senile psychosis was not lower than that reported from Western cultures. Cross-cultural comparison of the rates for mental retardation, personality disorder, and neurosis was deemed unreliable due to variation in diagnostic criteria practiced by different authors. However, the extremely low rates for alcoholism and obsessive-compulsive neurosis were emphasized.

The data were further analyzed with various socio-demographic variables. Schizophrenia, personality disorders, and neurosis were more prevalent in urban than in rural communities. Schizophrenia and neurosis were also more concentrated in the central parts (consisting largely of market districts and business facilities) of each community. In contrast, mental retardation, epilespy and senile psychosis were more prevalent in the rural community and also the more peripheral parts (farms, residential areas) of each community.

The influence of age, sex, occupation and sociocultural status were essentially in accord with previous survey findings and clinical impressions cross-culturally: namely, 1) the prevalence of manic-depressive psychosis and neurosis was greater in females, while that for personality disorder and mental retardation was greater in males; 2) rates for both psychosis and neurosis were highest in the socially responsible age range (20—59); 3) mental disorders in general were more prevalent in the unemployed and in unskilled and lower status occupations; 4) schizophrenia, organic psychosis, and alcoholism rates were inversely related to socioeconomic status.

Surveys Among the Aborigines – 1949–53 (Rin and Lin 1962)

The same methodology was used in this community-wide survey of 11,442 people in 4 tribes. Compared to the Taiwanese of the previous study, the prevalence rate of schizophrenia was significantly lower among the aborigines, while the rates of alcoholism, personality disorders and organic psychosis were all much higher than those for the Taiwanese. The increased prevalence of organic psychosis was readily understandable in terms of the poor environmental hygiene and the endemic condition of various infectious diseases (especially malaria). Both alcoholism and personality disorder were found to be more prevalent among the two tribes with higher contacts with the Taiwanese, suggesting an association with social disorganization accompanying accelerated acculturation.

The relative rarity of schizophrenia among the aborigines represented an unexpected finding. What was even more surprising was the benign course of the majority of the cases: among the 10 identified cases, there was no relapse, and only one exhibited chronic deterioration. Although the possibility of the "survival of the fit" could not be completely ruled out, i.e., chronically psychotic cases may have failed to survive, a more plausible explanation seemed to be that, for unclear reasons, the sociocultural environment of these "simpler" societies was more favorable for the recovery of schizophrenic patients. This finding takes on added importance in light of the recent report from the nine cultures International Pilot Study of Schizophrenia of the WHO that recovery from schizophrenia varies inversely with the level of social development of the societies studied (Cooper and Sartorius 1977).

Follow-up Survey of the 3 Communities – 1961–63 (Lin, Rin, Yeh, Hsu and Chu 1969)

The 3 communities – Baksa, Simpo, and Ampeng – were surveyed again, with the same design and methodology, by the same research team 15 years later. The population of the Taiwanese in these communities had nearly doubled. In addition, there was a significant number of Mainland Chinese who migrated into all 3 communities, especially Baksa. The three communities had witnessed rapid urbanization, and Baksa in particular was becoming a modernized suburban annex of metropolitan Taipei.

The most significant finding in comparing the prevalence rates of the two surveys 15 years apart lay in the fact that while there was no apparent change in the rates of psychosis, the prevalence of neurosis had risen sharply from 1.2 to 7.8 per thousand among the Taiwanese. When Taiwanese were further divided into the original inhabitants who had established their residence there prior to the first survey and recent migrants who moved in between the two surveys, the most dramatic difference was again in the rate of neurosis (6.9 per thousand for the former group and 12.1 per thousand for the latter). Among Mainland Chinese, the rate was even higher (16.1 per thousand). The increase of the rate of neurosis in non-migrant Taiwanese over time indicated the effect of rapid and far reaching urbanization, while the marked difference between migrants and non-migrants testified to the potentially adverse effects of uprooting and adaptation on mental health status, which appeared also to be "dose-related." Neither one of these two trends was observed in the rate of psychosis. A finding in support of the central role genetically-determined biological processes are presently believed to play in predisposition to psychosis.

Other findings regarding the influences of key socio-demographic variables on mental disorder rates were similar to those found in the first survey: namely, neurosis was more prevalent in females, in middle-aged people, in more urban areas; personality disorder and mental retardation were more prevalent in males; mental retardation and schizophrenia were negatively related to socioeconomic status and education.

Studies of Psychophysiologic Disorders (Rin, Chu, and Lin 1966)

Although in the previously mentioned studies, psychophysiological reactions were largely neglected, the role of somatization in Chinese culture has long been recognized. In 1963–64, a study of an age-stratified, random sample of the previously studied Baksa population was conducted by detailed interview, questionnaire administration and physical and psychiatric examinations. An overall prevalence rate of 42% for psychophysiological reactions was reported. Age distribution was similar to that of neurosis: highest in the middle-age group. Significantly higher rates were also found in the following groups:

1) younger married males and females; males more than females;
2) lower-class males;
3) upper-class females;
4) oldest sons and youngest daughters.

While lower class males and individuals who married young were thought to be subjected to greater economic stresses, the upper-class Chinese women were held to be more confined by cultural restrictions. Chinese families usually place high expectations, and consequently more pressure, on the oldest sons; conversely the youngest daughters are often neglected or even overtly rejected.

The other two factors associated with the rates of psychophysiological reactions were 1) modernity-traditional value identification; and 2) migration.

The complex influence of modernity-traditional value identification is well-illustrated by Chance's (Chance, Rin and Chu 1966) observations among an Eskimo group that higher contact with modern lifestyles together with strong traditional value identification favor better health status, and conversely, lower contact with modern lifestyles coupled with modern value identification are conducive to ill-health. The results from the Taiwan study, clearly substantiated this finding.

The adverse effect of migration, furthermore, was again confirmed in this study: migrant Taiwanese and Mainland Chinese with refugee experiences showed higher rates of psychophysiological problems than others. The impact of migration appeared to be more severe in older females and in those from lower social class, indicating that passive migration and migration with inadequate resources pose more danger to the health of migrants (also see Chu 1972).

College Student Mental Health

1) *Studies in Taiwan 1963–67 (Yeh et al. 1972).* This prospective, longitudinal study commenced by interviewing a sample of the entire freshman class of a college upon entrance, which revealed an overall rate of mental illness of 5.1% (including psychophysiological reactions) for "definite" cases, and a rate of 30.7% when cases in the "highly probable" category were also included. This is lower than the rate for the comparable age group in the general community. This overall rate was found to be essentially the same 3–4 years later when the same group of students were interviewed again in their senior year, but by that time many cases carrying diagnoses of neurosis replaced those earlier diagnosed as having psychophysiological reactions.

These students came from 3 different ethnic groups: Taiwanese, Mainland

Chinese and Overseas Chinese. Higher overall rates were found in females, but not in males, in the latter two groups. Older students and those who came from small towns were also more prone to develop psychiatric problems.

2) *Studies in Transcultural Adaptation of Chinese Students in the U.S.* (*Miller et al. 1971*). Cooperating with the University of Wisconsin, a series of studies were carried out by investigators from National Taiwan University on the adaptation of Chinese students who had come to the United States for their studies. A high level of distress was found in these students, and among those who developed psychotic breakdown, a preponderance of paranoid manifestations was found (Yeh 1972; see also Chapter 16 in this volume).

Genetic Studies

Several studies (Tsuang 1972) in this area have been conducted by reviewing hospital clinical material. High risk ratios for the close relatives of schizophrenics (7.8–10.8) and affective disorder patients (19.5–33.0) were calculated. Analysis of family history using Slater's method revealed that those schizophrenics with heavy genetic loading disclose simple, dominant, major gene inheritance.

Other Studies

Analysis of symptom content in hospitalized psychiatric patients revealed a relative preponderance of paranoid symptom manifestations (Rin, Wu and Lin 1962). When compared to Japanese patients, more paranoid, projection-type symptoms were found in Taiwanese patients, and more depression, introjection-type symptoms were found in the Japanese patients (Rin, Schooler and Caudill 1973).

Yeh et al (1979) reported their statistical analysis of 1,561 discharged patients from the Taipei City Psychiatric Center during 1969–1978. The results are in general similar to those found in previous epidemiological and clinical studies.

Cheng et al. (1979) reported a dramatic improvement of global functioning of chronic psychotic patients after being transferred from chronic custodial care facilities to an intensive treatment center. The study indicated that the detrimental effect of long-term institutionalization ("social breakdown syndrome," Gruenberg 1974) is found among Chinese too and is partially reversible through similar kinds of intensive rehabilitation. The degree of improvement of these patients was also found to be positively correlated with the availability and attitude of their family members.

Taipei was also one of the 9 centers of the International Pilot Study of Schizophrenia (1966–72) (World Health Organization 1973). One hundred carefully screened chronic schizophrenic patients and 25 patients with other psychoses were evaluated in each center and follow-up was done one year, two years, and five years later. Preliminary results showed that the phenomenology of these schizophrenic cases resembled closely those found in the other centers, the only significant differences being that there were relatively more diagnoses of the subtypes paranoid and hebephrenic schizophrenia in Taipei. At the two year follow-up, there were more rehabilitated cases than in the more industrialized countries (Denmark, United States, Great Britain and the Soviet Union). At the five year follow-up the outcome fell between that of developed and developing countries (Chen 1978; Sartorius, Jablinsky and Shapiro 1978).

STUDIES IN OTHER CHINESE SOCIETIES

In a study of first admission rates of psychosis in Singapore, Murphy (1959) reported that the rate for Chinese was lower than that for Indians, but higher than that for Malays. Similar to the community studies in Taiwan, he found an age distribution (age not adjusted) with the middle-age range showing the highest rate, and a preference for first born males. A possible adverse effect of migration and minority status was revealed in the fact that the rates for functional psychosis in females and for suicide in males were inversely related to the size of the several Chinese dialectical minorities: the smaller the size of the community, the higher the rates.

Tan (1969) studied 111 patients with a diagnosis of anxiety neurosis, comparing them to other psychiatric patients as well as non-psychiatric patients treated at a university hospital in Kuala Lumpur in a 12-month period. He found that anxiety neurosis was more common among the Chinese than other ethnic groups. The diagnosis is more often seen in men than in women. Somatic symptoms were found in 88% of these patients. In contrast psychological symptoms were present in only 60% of them. A prominent feature deserving special attention was the prevalence of sexual complaints (44%) in male patients. Spermatorrhoea, in particular, was complained of frequently by the Chinese (and also by the Indians) but never by the Malays.

In a study on the mental health of the students of the University of Malaya, Teoh (1974) reported that Chinese students had significantly more severe acculturation gap differences from their parents than Malay students. They also showed higher rates of personality and family problems. The overall treated rates of psychiatric problems among the two ethnic groups, however, were proportional to the total student population.

In Hong Kong, Yap (1965) reported a retrospective and follow-up study of 130 inpatients with affective disorder. Depression was found more common than mania, and only 34% were biphasic or of mixed type. There were more females in those age 20 or younger, and again, during the involutional period. Recurrent depression appeared more often in women, and recurrent mania in men. Clinical picture was found similar to that described in the West, with the exception of the rarity and mildness of ideas of guilt and feelings of unworthiness. Sixty-two cases were traced successfully 10 to 14 years after the first admission. Among these, 3 died, 43 recovered completely, 8 were currently in treatment and 4 were chronically hospitalized.

Lo and Lo (1977) conducted a 10 year follow-up study of schizophrenics in Hong Kong. With 133 subjects identified as the cohort, 82 were contacted and re-evaluated. Sixty-five per cent of these fully evaluated subjects had full and lasting remission or showed only mild deterioration. This is considerably different than the poor prognosis of schizophrenia in the West. Factors associated with good prognosis included: being female, having a short duration of illness, and having an acute onset.

Mitchell (1969), in a large-scale sociological survey of the urban areas of Singapore, Malaysia, Bangkok, Hong Kong, and Taipei in 1967—68, revealed that his Hong Kong sample was economically and psychologically most distressed among the 5 areas surveyed. He also found that in all the areas, women were consistently more likely than men to be disturbed by emotional illness.

Lee (see the next article) examined interview records of 3,983 household heads in the urban areas of Hong Kong in 1974. The 22 item Langner Scale (1962) was used, which revealed a higher rate of psychiatric symptoms among women than men, and among members of lower socioeconomic groups. Degree of life satisfaction also correlated positively with mental health, and partially explained the correlation between socioeconomic status and mental well-being, but not the predilection for mental health problems in women.

In the United States, the utilization rates (treated prevalence) of Chinese-Americans were repeatedly reported as much lower than those of other ethnic groups (see the article by Tsai, Teng and Sue). Jew and Brody (1967) examined the first admission rate of male patients in the state hospitals of California between 1854—1961. They found that although the hospitalization rate of the Chinese has gradually increased over the past 100 years, the discrepancy between the rates of the Chinese and non-Chinese has persisted. Brown et al. (1973) reported that the Chinese in Los Angeles were seeking services at less than half the expected rate according to their population. When 23 Chinese in-patients were compared to a matched Caucasian control group, the Chinese patients were rated significantly more disturbed than their Caucasian counterparts. Similar findings were reported by Berk and Hirata (1973) and True (1975) in California. In an out-patient population, Sue and McKinney (1975) found that in 17 community mental health facilities in King County, Washington State, only 0.1% of the patients were Chinese, whereas the population served contained 0.6% Chinese. They also noted that these Chinese patients were more severely disturbed than other out-patients. Although these findings are highly suggestive of underutilization of mental health facilities rather than low susceptibility to mental illness, the absence of community-wide prevalence studies makes any definitive conclusion impossible.

STUDIES OF SUICIDE

Yap (1958) studied the suicide and attempted suicide rates in Hong Kong between June 1953 and December 1954, using data from the Registry of Birth and Deaths, the Criminal Investigation Department, and Queen Mary Hospital records (all reported suicide attempt cases were sent to this hospital for evaluation). Population data from several governmental sources were used for comparison.

This thorough study found a crude suicide rate of 12 per 100,000 for the total population and 23.5 per 100,000 for population aged 15 and over. This rate is in the medium range when compared to that found in other countries.

Males and older individuals had significantly higher rates. The female/male ratio was more than 1/2, which is higher than that of Western countries, but similar to Ceylon and Japan. The higher rate in the aged was also in accord with that observed in Western countries, and contradicted the earlier impression that suicide was rare in older Chinese and more prevalent in the younger age group.

Suicides were significantly more prevalent among the widowed/divorced, concubines, and those who were subjected to economic insecurity and uncertainty.

Urban dwelling and migrant status were also found to be important factors associated with suicide. The urban suicide rate was higher than the rural rate. "Native" born had the lowest rate, while post-war immigrants (largely refugees) had the highest, with pre-war immigrants in between.

Also similar to the findings from other cultures was the age-sex distribution of the attempted suicides, which was more prevalent in females and in younger age groups.

Economic stress and somatic illness were associated more frequently with suicide cases, interpersonal conflict more with attempted suicides.

In Singapore, Murphy (1954) studied the suicide rates between 1925 and 1952 with the data recorded in the register of the Coroner's Court. He observed that over a quarter of a century the suicide rate for persons aged 15 and above had remained fairly steady around 20 per 100,000. A striking low rate was found in Malays as compared to other ethnic groups, mainly Chinese, who showed overall rates similar to those reported in other countries. When the rate was broken down by sexes, the Chinese male rate remained similar to that of the Europeans, but the female rate appeared much higher than their European counterpart. Singapore-born Chinese showed a much lower rate than that of immigrants. Among the immigrants, the first 10 years after arrival appeared to place them at greater risk than the subsequent years. The suicide rate varied closely and indirectly with the size of the dialect group: the smaller the group, the higher the rate. This "minority effect" could also be demonstrated when comparing different geographic areas, those with more ethnic admixture of population having significantly higher rates than those with less.

Among other factors tested, security of employment and the existence of a social support system appeared to be most important in reducing the rate of suicide; and the presence of chronic diseases, especially tuberculosis, appeared to be significantly associated with a higher rate of suicide. Chen (1969) studied the suicide rates in Singapore between 1961 and 1965, and found very similar results as compared to those in the earlier decades studied by Murphy.

Rin (1978) studied the suicide rate between 1946–1971 in Taiwan and found that the annual crude rate varied between 10 and 19.0/100,000. The 4 peaks corresponded respectively to different periods of rapid social change and large-scale migration of the population. The age-sex distribution of the suicide cases in this series resembled that reported by Yap (1958). Rin (1978) also studied 2,105 cases of attempted suicide, and again found a predilection for this condition in young women.

Bourne (1973) studied suicide among Chinese in San Francisco between 1952 and 1968, and found a crude annual suicide rate of 27.9/100,000, similar to that of the rest of the San Francisco population which is much higher than the rest of the nation. The rate showed a possible downward trend over the 17 year period. Suicide was again more frequently found in males, in older people (age 55 and over), and in the widowed/divorced. Male suicide cases were mostly either single or just nominally married (wife and/or family left in China for decades, a prevalent condition among older Chinese males due to previous restriction of immigration). Suicide was highest among the elderly, the unemployed or retired, the isolated, and those suffering chronic physical disorders. More than half of the female suicide cases were psychotic patients. For both men and women, the suicide rate in first generation Chinese (born in China) was significantly higher than Chinese-Americans born in the United States.

OBSESSIVE-COMPULSIVE NEUROSIS

LaBarre (1946) was impressed with the rarity of obsessive-compulsive neurosis among Chinese, and attributed this to the pragmatism and lack of compulsion in Chinese culture, and also to the fact that Chinese in general were not very concerned about toilet training in their child-rearing practices. Lin (1953) did not find any case of obsessive-compulsive neurosis in his original survey in 3 communities in Taiwan. Rin (1959) also reported that obsessive-compulsive neurosis was rarely seen at the outpatient clinic of the Department of Neurology and Psychiatry, National Taiwan University Hospital. However, he was able to observe 6 such cases and reported that the symptomatology and treatment courses were not different from those reported for Western culture. Tseng (1973) observed 10 such cases, and agreed that toilet training was not important in them, but he indicated that these individuals all had extremely strong ties with a domineering, perfectionistic mother, which he thought might be specific to Chinese culture.

ALCOHOLISM

The rarity of alcoholism among Chinese has been observed and reported frequently for different Chinese societies: China proper, Taiwan, Hong Kong,

Singapore, Southeast Asia, Chinese communities in the United States (Singer 1974; Cerny 1965; Lin 1953; Teoh and Dass n.d.; Khoo and Jernandez 1971; Barnett 1955; Wang 1968; Chu 1972). However, most of these reports have been anecdotal and impressionistic. Lin's (1953) survey as described previously is the only exception to this generalization. In that study, only 2 cases of alcoholism were identified, giving the astonishingly low rate of 0.1/1,000. Lin further commented that in the subsequent 17 years only 10 cases of alcoholism were seen at the National Taiwan University Hospital (Chafetz 1964). Wolff (1972) and Ewing et al. (1974) have suggested there may be a physiological reason contributing to this immunity. They discovered that some Chinese are extremely sensitive to alcohol, and experience vasodilatation which manifests in discomforting facial flushing. However, other Asians and also American Indians appear to share this constitutional response which does not seem to prevent them from alcoholic indulgence (Chafetz 1964; Westermeyer 1974). Among the American Indians, conversely, this observed intolerance to alcohol has been implicated as one of the reasons for their high rate of alcoholism (Wolff 1973).

Possible sociocultural factors contributing to the rarity of alcoholism in Chinese have been discussed by Hsu (1955), Lin (1953), Wang (1968), Singer (1974), Rin (1978), and in the article by Harrell in this volume. They point out that (1) Chinese mostly drink only with meals and on ceremonial occasions; and (2) Confucianism and Taoism are the two main life philosophies guiding the behavior of Chinese. While Confucian ideology stresses self-control and moderation, Taoism teaches harmony with the environment. Both are strongly opposed to the impulse-releasing effect of alcohol. (3) The absence of drinking-centered institutions and groups (e.g., taverns and bars) discourages regular, excessive consumption of alcohol. In addition, among Chinese-Americans it has been speculated that gambling, which is very wide-spread, may be a symptom substitute for alcoholic indulgence (Alder and Goleman 1969; Chu 1972). However, this hypothesis has not been tested empirically. In a study of the attitude of Chinese towards alcohol during a random sample community-wide survey in Taiwan, Rin (1978) found that only 18% liked the taste of alcohol, and 33% believed that alcohol promotes health. In contrast, 48% had experienced uncomfortable intoxicating episodes, 84% indicated that alcohol could cause severe physical damage, 88% reported that his/her family frowned upon excessive drinking, and 96% were opposed to alcohol indulgence leading to embarrassing behaviors.

Another survey conducted by Chu (1972) in Chinatown in San Francisco compared the responses of 33 single Chinese with 180 comparable Caucasian subjects and found very similar results. Chinese consistently regarded drunkeness more as a condition to frown upon in friends, to be avoided in oneself and to prevent from happening even occasionally. Thus, these surveys support the above mentioned strong Chinese cultural sanctioning against alcohol indulgence.

In Hong Kong, Singer (1972) recently reported a low, but not rare, first admission rate of alcoholic psychosis; this rate also showed a trend of steady increase over the last 2 decades. The fact that a similar trend has not been observed in either Taiwan or the PRC suggests that it is determined by the unique sociocultural milieu of the Chinese in Hong Kong. Hong Kong was ceded to Great Britain and has been under British control for the last one hundred years. The Chinese living there have long been especially heavily influenced by Western cultural values and behavioral norms, and at the same time subjected to rapid social change and marked inequality in the context of social and political control by foreigners. These combined forces might negate the positive influence of the Chinese cultural heritage and lead to an increase in alcoholic problems. It is of interest to note that a rapid increase in alcoholism in Japan was also observed after World War II when it was occupied temporarily by the Americans. A similar explanation involving sociocultural changes was offered by Chafetz (1964) in the Japanese case. However, since in Singer's report alcoholic psychosis rather than alcoholism was addressed, and the definition of alcoholic psychosis was also not clearly specified, further evidence is required to substantiate this finding.

A recent study conducted in Vancouver, Canada, provided data contrary to Singer's. Lin (personal communication) reviewed medical, psychiatric and criminal records of individuals of Chinese origin for the years 1961–62 and 1971–72. Except for a few cases of drunk driving involved in traffic accident reports, there were virtually no Chinese alcoholic cases recorded in these documents. Since the Chinese population in Vancouver includes not only recent immigrants but also sizable second and third generations of Chinese-Canadians who have been generally successful in adapting to their new environment, this finding most probably indicates that alcoholic drinking pattern and rate of alcoholosm have remained the same for Chinese even after extensive acculturation.

NARCOTIC ADDICTION

This has been a haunting problem for the Chinese since the eighteenth century. The prevalence rate of opium addiction in Chinese up to 1949 was estimated as being around 10% (Merry 1975). Comparable prevalence rates existed in other overseas Chinese communities until recently (Leong 1974). As late as 1973, 6–10% of the population in Hong Kong were still estimated as addicted to opium or heroin (Singer 1974). Opium and heroin addictions have also been found to be prevalent in Chinese-Americans in the past. Bell and Lau (1966) found that 137 Chinese narcotic addiction patients were admitted to the Public Health Service Hospital, Lexington Kentucky from July 1957 through June 1962, a gross over-representation when adjusted for the total Chinese population in the United States. The Chinese addicts were found to be distinctly different from those of other ethnic backgrounds. They were mostly in their middle fifties, were foreign born, and were markedly alienated from American culture. They were mostly employed, and showed no violent criminal record. They admitted themselves to the hospital seeking abstinence, but were not interested in any psychological treatment, and often left against advice a few weeks later.

For unclear reasons, the prevalence of narcotic addiction among Chinese-Americans has declined rapidly since the early 1960's. The Federal Bureau of Narcotics reported a ten-fold decline of new Oriental addicts from 1955 to 1964. A similar trend also can be seen in the Lexington first admission data.

In Taiwan, narcotic addiction became less of a problem after it was ceded to the Japanese when it was cut off from narcotic traffic, and active eradication was enforced with heavy penalty for both drug dealers and users (Chen 1978). The PRC claims that they have eradicated narcotic addiction. Political indoctrination, popular campaigns, harsh penalties and tight social control of deviance appear to have been instrumental in their success in this area (Cerny 1965; Koran 1972).[1]

HOMOSEXUALITY

Although reliable epidemiological data have not been available, it has been the impression of psychiatrists working with Chinese patients that homosexuality is not often seen clinically. Lin (personal communication) indicated that in his 18-year tenure as Chairman of the Psychiatry Department at National Taiwan University, he was only aware of 3 such cases, and none received hospital treatment. Homosexual practices also appear to have a very low prevalence in China (Dr. Young Der-son personal communication). The majority of Chinese are apparently unaware and unconcerned about the existence of homosexuals in their population. In strong contrast with other countries in Southeast Asia, there is in Taiwan no publicly known quarters for homosexuals and no organized prostitution involving homosexual or transvestite prostitutes.

However, in classical as well as contemporary Chinese literature, homosexual practices appear not infrequently. The sexual preference of several prominent homosexual artists in Taiwan and Hong Kong is also well known to the public, and is talked about, joked about, but well tolerated.

The most plausible explanation for these two contradictory views seems to be that while homosexuality is regarded as a form of deviance by Chinese, it is not as highly stigmatized and feared as in many other cultures. As a result, there is no strong emotional attachment to the issue of homosexuality, and homosexual practices are mostly ignored and left alone. Wen's (1973, 1978) data from Taiwan appear to support such an argument. Wen (1973) interviewed 200 college students in Taipei about their experiences and attitudes towards homosexuality. He found that the rate of homosexual experiences and/or inclination was extremely low (4% in males and less than 1% in females). At the same time, these students were highly tolerant, sympathetic or indifferent towards homosexuals, and much less discriminating than American students. However, in another survey conducted 5 years later by the same investigator (Wen 1978), among 243 college students, 14% of the male respondents (n = 147) and 1% of the female respondents (n = 96) reported having pleasurable homosexual experiences. These data suggest that homosexuality may be as prevalent among Chinese as in other cultures, but because the society is less sensitive and generally indifferent or tolerant toward such a sexual orientation, people with this tendency may be less likely to develop psychological problems and consequently less often are seen by psychiatrists. Further research is indicated to test this hypothesis and also to determine the actual occurrence of homosexuality among Chinese.

The incidence of other sexual problems in Chinese populations, such as fetishism, transexualism, transvestism, is unknown. Teoh (1972) reported a case of transvestism in Malaysia successfully treated with behavior therapy, and Wen (1979, personal communication) has seen 10 cases of transexualism in Taipei within one year. Similar to homosexuality, the real incidence of these sexual deviances may not be as rare as it appears, but they may be less often encountered by psychiatrists because of the relative indifference and tolerance of Chinese culture. This possibility offers an important cross-cultural test of the social labeling theory that medicalized deviance is a function of societal response to primary deviance and therefore deserves serious study.

CULTURE-BOUND SYNDROMES AND SOMATIZATION

Although these problems are covered elsewhere in this book (see the articles by Kleinman and Mechanic, and Wen and Wang), we believe they need to be discussed here with regard to the questions they raise about comparative psychiatric epidemiology. To begin with, it may seem odd to readers to discuss them in this chapter, when there are virtually no epidemiological studies of culture-bound syndromes or somatization. But that is why we should discuss them. For these are precisely the disorders that are most extensively affected by cultural categories and behavioral norms (Kleinman 1978). Hence it is culture-bound syndromes and somatization that comparative psychiatric epidemiology needs to assess if it is to achieve a discriminating understanding of how Chinese culture influences deviance and psychopathology (Kleinman 1979: 119–179). That, in sharp contrast, quantitative epidemiological surveys have avoided these very problems goes a long way to informing us why these studies strike students of Chinese and other non-Western societies as so superficial and culturally naive, and also why they have had so miniscule an effect in psychiatry. Psychiatric epidemiology simply has failed to tackle the toughest cross-cultural questions.

The difficulty is part and parcel of the ethnocentric, medicocentric, psychocentric bias of psychiatrists and psychologists. This bias is built into the textbooks of psychiatry and psychology, the training of researchers, and the instruments and techniques used to survey populations. The bias is not removed when questionnaires are translated (and back translated) or when interviewers are bilingual, because the difficulty is not simply translating between different languages, important as that is. Instead the problem lies in translating between distinctive, often divergent, conceptual systems which differentially construe normal and deviant behavior.

For example, the Western psychocentric orientation of contemporary psychiatry conceives of depression and other neurotic problems as intrapsychic, existential experiences, whereas in Chinese and many other non-Western societies (and among lower class ethnic minorities in the West) these problems are most frequently experienced somatically and in terms of interpersonal dysfunction (see Kleinman 1977; Leff 1977; Marsella, Kinzie and Gordon 1973; Marsella 1978; Tseng 1975). Furthermore, somatization is the chief idiom through which Chinese culture articulates not just neurotic disorders but many other personal and social problems (Kleinman 1979: 119–179). Finally, the somatized complaints sometimes are unique to Chinese cultural beliefs and language (Kleinman 1979: 119–146). Hence psychiatric epidemiology is triply affected. By focusing on psychological symptoms it misses somatized ones. When eliciting the latter it misinterprets both symptom expressions which are unique to Chinese culture and others which, though similar in surface meaning to ones in the West, convey special significance among Chinese. Even when the right somatic complaints are used, the epidemiological net closes around many life problems that have little if anything to do with mental illness.

Similarly, the culture-bound syndromes — which are inseparable from the web of culturally-constituted meanings, social relationships, and behavioral trajectories that make up the very "stuff" of Chinese culture — are either missed altogether or mis-diagnosed when analyzed by conceptual frameworks and diagnostic categories based entirely on research with Western populations. It is not surprising then that psychiatric epidemiology has contributed not at all to sorting out which of the current major views of the culture-bound syndromes is correct — namely, that they represent culturally-specific variants of universally-occurring psychiatric diseases (Manschreck 1978), that they are unique psychiatric disorders specific to particular cultures, that they are culturally-constituted final common behavioral pathways along which many kinds of deviant behavior (only some of which represent psychopathology) are channelled (Carr 1978), or that they are symbolic representations of marginal status in society that have anthropological, not psychiatric, significance (Kenny 1978).

Ironically, as anthropologists have long argued and cross-cultural psychiatrists and psychologists are increasingly becoming aware, when confronted with somatization and the culture-bound disorders, modern psychiatric terminology and categories themselves appear hopelessly culture-bound (Carr 1978; Kleinman 1977; Marsella 1977; and see Chapter 19 below). Yet there is in principle no compelling reason why the qualitative accounts of these disorders found in anthropologists' ethnographies and clinicians' case reports cannot be supplemented by quantitative epidemiological determinations of their prevalence and statistically rigorous assessments of their determinants and natural history. That is to say, what we first need are epidemiological accounts of the distribution of these problems in Chinese and other non-Western populations that utilize indigenous illness concepts and symptom terms in order to accurately describe how prevalent these culturally-defined phenomena are and whom they affect, and then later to analyze what are the contingencies and risk factors associated with their onset and what are their various outcomes. The tools for such determinations are available; the chief difficulty is interesting the appropriate investigators to apply them to this subject. Such an application would represent the creation of a new interdisciplinary field: anthropological (or ethnomedical) epidemiology or epidemiological anthropology.

It should be clear from what we have said that there simply cannot be a comparative cross-cultural epidemiology of mental illness worthy of the name that does not regard culture-bound syndromes and somatization, and the vexing question of which of their aspects represent social deviance and which psychopathology, as legitimate avenues for quantitative field studies, but ones that demand culture-centered anthropological as well as psychiatry-centered epidemiological methods. To state this proposition, however, is to underscore the present limitations of psychiatric epidemiology, which is neither anthropologically informed nor truly comparative.

In the following few pages, we will draw a skeletal outline of findings from studies of culture-bound disorders and somatization in Chinese culture. Our intent is to describe what is known that suggests issues worth examining in future research, and in so doing to attract the interest of epidemiologists, and epidemiologically-oriented anthropologists and clinicians, to these subjects.

Traditionally, the "culture-bound syndromes" have referred to sickness concepts and experiences specific to a particular culture or culture area (almost always non-Western). The actual occurence of the "culture-bound syndromes" appears to be relatively infrequent (see, for example, *amok*: Tan and Carr 1976; *latah*: Kenny 1978; *koro*: Yap 1965). In a review of the literature on 7 culture-bound disorders, Neutra, Levy and Parker (1977) noted that there were no epidemiological surveys and that many cases which were inadequately described anecdotes were subsequently repeated in later series, so that the literature was filled with hearsay evidence and many competing theories unsupported by empirical findings. Indeed, they went so far as to suggest that some of the disorders may not in fact exist. In the same paper, the authors showed that culture-specific beliefs about epilepsy among the Navaho were not associated with actual culture-specific behavioral syndromes (Neutra, Levy and Parker 1977). This piece of research is the only example we are aware of that tested a hypothesis about culture-bound syndromes. Furthermore, Yap (1969) demonstrated that for certain culture-bound syndromes similar features are occasionally documented for individuals in other cultures. Hence the data base that supports this sickness category is just as controversial as are the theoretical frameworks used to interpret it.

Koro (*suk-yeong* in Cantonese, *so-yang* in Mandarin) is the best known of the Chinese culture-bound syndromes. Patients suffering from this syndrome are convinced that their penis is shrinking and are terrified that this may lead to death if the shrinkage is not reversed. Originally observed among Chinese in Indonesia, it has been reported only sporadically by Westerners among overseas

Chinese in Southeast Asia. At least one case has been described among Chinese in the United States (Albert Gaw unpublished manuscript). The largest series of cases was reported by Yap (1965) in Hong Kong. The 19 cases he described were collected over a 15 year period in a population of 3 million. Yap found that *koro* cases were usually young men of poor education who were characterized by immaturity, dependent personality with lack of confidence in their own virility, and conflict concerning the expression of genital impulses. Apparently all 19 patients understood and believed in the *koro* concept, while the onset of 4 cases was triggered by stories about its serious consequences. All patients in Yap's sample came from South China or the lower Yangtze River valley. In Taiwan, Rin (1965) reported 2 cases of *koro* in Chinese who originally came from central China. The clinical picture was similar to Yap's description, but Rin demonstrated how the *koro* illness concept was determined by traditional Chinese medical beliefs. No data on *koro*, or for that matter other culture-bound syndromes, have been forthcoming from the PRC.

In Singapore, a *koro* "epidemic" was observed concurrent with a rumor identifying eating flu-vaccinated pork as the cause for *koro* (Ngui 1969; *Koro* Study Team 1969). Within a few weeks more than 200 cases appeared in two local hospitals presenting themselves with *koro* symptoms. At the peak 100 cases were seen in a single day. The majority of them were Chinese. The incidence among the Malays and Indians was comparatively negligible. Of interest to note was that although *koro* is usually regarded as an illness affecting males, during this epidemic, 8 female cases were also observed. The "epidemic" subsided within one month. The majority of the cases responded to reassurance and patient education, and showed no recurrence of symptoms.

Closely related to *koro* are 5 cases of "frigophobia" among Chinese in Taiwan reported by Chang, Rin and Chen (1975). These patients had a profound fear of "cold." They bundled up in multiple layers of clothing and used numerous blankets even in warm weather, and they remained indoors in stifling conditions with windows tightly shut to prevent drafts and exposure to cold temperature. They also avoided symbolically "cold" foods, while consuming "hot" items, owing to their strikingly compelling belief that the "hot"/"cold" balance of their bodies was upset and that they were suffering from an excess of cold (*yin* qualities) which predisposed them to serious disease. Most of these patients suffered from obsessive-compulsive personality disorders and hypochondriasis. There is a close similarity with *koro*, inasmuch as *koro* represents the morbid fear of loosing *yang* (male element), whereas frigophobia, as we have noted, stems from the equally morbid fear of an excess of *yin* (female element). Venkoba Rao (1978) notes that in India, where a similar "hot"/"cold" cultural code exists, *koro*-like cases have been reported. But we are not aware of cases in the many other cultural areas of the world that share a hot/cold belief system. The prevalence of *koro* and frigophobia is unknown. Judging from the very limited number of case reports, these problems seem to occur infrequently. More detailed phenomenological descriptions are required to provide a better understanding of their morphology and natural history; epidemiological studies are needed to determine their prevalence; sociological inquiry should give us a more detailed picture of their psychosocial determinants and precipitants; and cross-cultural comparisons would help to decide if these are truly culture-specific disorders or if they are universal "diseases" (biological or psychological mal-functioning) in which only the "illness" behavior (the way cultural categories shape the individual's and the group's perception, experience and expression of symptoms) is culture-specific.

Another clinical state, *hsieh-ping,* has uncertain status as a "culture-bound syndrome." It is described as a transient possession state manifested by tremor, disorientation, clouding of consciousness or delirium, often accompanied by visual or auditory hallucinations. During the attack the patient is possessed by a "ghost" (usually a deceased relative or ancestor), who attempts to communicate with other family members through the patient. The contents of the attack express key family issues and may serve the coping function of manipulating interpersonal relationships and other aspects of the social environment asso-ciated with family discord. Patients with this disorder are mainly adult females from rural and traditional areas and impoverished backgrounds, with little or no education, who exhibit hysterical personality styles and who came from families heavily influenced by indigenous religious beliefs.

Lin (1953) reported 9 cases in Ampeng in his original community survey, which gave a rate of 0.9%, constituting two-thirds of the cases of psychoneurosis (14) found in that community. Yap (1960) reported 44 hospitalized cases with similar possession features in Hong Kong. Kleinman (1979) observed several cases during a year of field research in Taiwan, and noted similarities in their phenom-enology and course with cases of hysterical psychosis reported by Hollender and Hirsch (1964) and Martin (1971). It is questionable whether such "possession" behavior is culture-bound since it has been described for a large number of non-Western societies and for Puerto Rican and Black individuals from socially and culturally deprived backgrounds who recently migrated from rural to urban areas in the United States (see Crapanzano and Garrison 1977; Kleinman 1979; Ven-koba Rao 1978). Systematic clinical description and comparison with established psychiatric disorders should determine if these disorders are universally-occurring psychoses (e.g., reactive or psychogenic psychoses) with the same underlying psychopathological structure in which the content of delusions and hallucina-tions is shaped by cultural behavioral paradigms of trance and possession. Claus's (1979) ethnographic account of possession states in south India and many anthropological accounts of possession among shaman and laity in Taiwan (see relevant chapters in Kleinman et al. 1978; and Wolff 1974) argue persuasively that often such transient states are neither sickness nor deviance, but rather religiously sanctioned coping processes that are best interpreted in social and cultural terms. The ubiquity of trance states in non-Western societies, and the purported similarity of dissociation and hypnosis, make them a potentially important subject for comparative epidemiological research.

Shen-k'uei (kidney weakness or deficiency) is a widespread popular illness concept among Chinese that is based on traditional Chinese medical beliefs. It is believed to be caused by loss of *yang* (male element), leading to a "cold" imbalance in the body, owing to excessive masturbation and nocturnal emissions (Rin 1965). This is held to produce a physical illness characterized by weakness, easy fatiguability, insomnia, anxiety, and hypochondriasis. It is the most clearly delineated of a variety of related sexual neuroses among Chinese, based on the same traditional sickness categories. Such sexual neuroses are said by clinicians to be fairly frequent, but they have not yet received specific epidemiological evaluation. Obeyesekere (1976) and Venkoba Rao (1978) report a very similar clinical condition, associated with similar indigenous beliefs about masturbation and sexuality, among Ceylonese and Indians, respectively. See Chapter 18 for a detailed description of this culture-bound syndrome, including a comparison between its clinical features and those of related syndromes among South Asians.

Somatization is the most prevalent form of symptom manifestation in Chinese patients with neurotic disorders. For example, Rin et al. (1966) reported a higher percentage of psychophysiological complaints in the community he surveyed in sharp contrast to the relative paucity of psychological neurotic complaints. Tseng (1975) reported that 70% of patients seeking help in the psychiatric outpatient clinic of the National Taiwan University Hospital at least initially complained only of somatic complaints. Although somatization is more common among lower socioeconomic class patients and among those with traditional rather than Western value orientations and lower levels of education, Tseng and Hsu (1969) and Kleinman (1977, 1979) note that it is prevalent among all classes of Chinese patients, except the highly Westernized elite class including those who have acculturated fully to lifestyle and values in Western societies.[2] The consensus among investigators is that the socialization process teaches Chinese to suppress dysphoric emotions, and when they are experienced to channel them into a somatic idiom of communication (see Hsu 1971; Kleinman 1977, 1979: 119–179; Marsella 1978; Tseng and Hsu 1969; the Introduction and Chapters 15, 17, and 20 in this volume). Hence when they are suffering psychological or psychophysiological disorders, only the somatic symptoms associated with those problems are perceived, experienced, or communicated. This primarily occurs in patients suffering from neurotic disorders, but it is also found in normal individuals coping with life stresses of many kinds. Kleinman (1977) interviewed 25 depressed outpatients who presented consecutively to a psychiatric clinic in Taiwan, 22 of whom initially presented prominent somatic symptoms, and 10 of whom complained only of somatic symptoms and denied dysphoric affects even following treatment. In a comparison group of 25 Causcasian-American depressed patients, matched for age, sex, and socioeconomic class, only 4 primarily complained of somatic symptoms, and only one other patient completely denied dysphoric emotions. Marsella (1978) argues that the vegetative experience of depression among

Chinese and Japanese depressives is qualitatively different than the existentially-experienced psychological state of American depressives. Hence it raises the question as to whether these illness experiences should not be considered different diseases. Although Singer (1975) suggests that the somatization of depression is a worldwide phenomenon related to lower socioeconomic status, the Chinese example illustrates a cultural affect that appears to be substantially greater than the social class affect, which is nonetheless responsible for part of the variance (see Kleinman 1979: 119–179; Marsella 1978). For example, in Kleinman's (1977) study, the somatizing Taiwanese patients came from all socioeconomic classes and had both high and low educational backgrounds.

The most popular term for somatization used by Chinese in Taiwan and the PRC is "neurasthenia" (*shen-ching shuai-jo*). The term originated with European psychiatrists in the late 19th century who employed it to label neurotic conditions associated with weakness, lack of energy, sleep disturbance, vague physical symptoms in the absence of organic pathology, hypochondriacal fears, and a variety of psychological problems. One of its functions was to cover stigmatized mental illness (however minor) under the more respectable mantle of physical sickness. The same function is seen in Chinese communities. Lin (1953) mentioned that most of the neurotic cases he and his team identified in the communities they studied actually were labeled by others (family and physicians) and viewed themselves as suffering from "neurasthenia." Neurasthenia is still the most popular term used to label somatization in Taiwan (Kleinman 1979; Rin personal communication, based on a study of 1000 depressed Taiwanese out-patients). Kleinman discovered that roughly half of patients surveyed in Western-style doctors' clinics and shamans' shrines in Taipei were somatizers, and of these the great majority were either self-labeled or labeled by family or practitioners as neurasthenics (Kleinman 1979: 119–179).

In the 1950's there were efforts to study both the prevalence and treatment of this condition in the PRC, where it was reported as extremely common (Liu 1957; Chou et al. 1957; Chung 1957; Mo and Lian 1958; Chiang 1958; Li et al. 1958; Li 1958; Neurasthenia Study Unit 1958). Wang and Tuan (1957) studied 653 consecutive admissions to the psychiatric wards of the Peking Medical School from June 1951 to April 1955, and found that 16.4% carried a diagnosis of neurasthenia. According to this report, neurasthenia makes up two thirds of neurotic patients, and is only secondary to schizophrenia in this inpatient population. Patients suffering from neurasthenia were mostly in their mid-twenties. Although environmental stresses rather than genetic influence were cited as causes of this problem, it was viewed as a psychological disturbance involving higher cortical functions, according to Pavlovian theory, and was regarded as having an insidious onset, chronic course, and a prognosis even worse than schizophrenia in terms of recovery (Chin and Chin 1969). Li et al. (1958) mentioned that among the students in Peking University and Peking Medical School 10–15% suffered from neurasthenia. Several surveys further found that it had a preference for late adolescents and young adults (age 16–40), and was much more prevalent in "mind" workers and light manual workers as opposed to heavy laborers (Chin and Chin 1969). During the Great Leap Forward (1958—59), neurasthenia became the main target of mental health workers who searched for methods to treat this condition and vowed to eradicate it (Chin and Chin 1969). The prevalence of neurasthenia is not known since the Cultural Revolution, 1966—1969. Walls et al. (1975) during their visits to the PRC in 1973—74 noted that neurasthenia was still used by the psychiatrists there as a diagnostic category. In June 1978, Mechanic and Kleinman (1979) were told by psychiatrists at the No. 3 Hospital of Peking Medical School, the No. 2 Hospital of Hunan Medical School in Changsha, and the Neurology Clinic of Chung Shan Medical School in Canton that neurasthenia was the most common diagnosis among neurotic outpatients. Professor Young Der-son (personal communication) states that neurasthenia is the diagnosis carried by roughly half of all patients in the psychiatry outpatient clinic of the Hunan Medical School. Mechanic and Kleinman also learned that neurasthenia was the commonest diagnosis of patients with neurotic and psychophysiological complaints in the many county and commune hospitals they visited in 6 Chinese provinces (see the article by Kleinman & Mechanic). This diagnosis appeared frequently to lead to referral to traditional Chinese medicine clinics. Since most patients with neurasthenia in Chinese communities go to general (Western) medical clinics or traditional practitioners for treatment, it is likely that surveys limited to psychiatric clinics will significantly underestimate its prevalence and therefore the prevalence of somatization generally among Chinese.

Kleinman (1979: 133—146) has described a large number of lay symptom terms in Taiwan which are popularly labeled as physical sicknesses but which often express underlying psychological problems. For example, *huo-ch'i ta* (excessive internal hot energy) is a widely used patient complaint, based on traditional Chinese medical beliefs, to convey symptoms in the mouth and sometimes upper gastrointestinal system as well as irritability, anger, and anxiety. *Hsim tsap tsap* is a commonly heard Taiwanese term which expresses discomfort in the chest and palpitations, but which is most frequently meant to convey to the listener that the patient has anxious and depressed feelings. Psychiatric epidemiologies conducted in Chinese communities must focus on neurasthenia and these culturally-specific symptomatic expressions of somatization if they are to accurately determine the true extent of psychiatric morbidity. The examples we have cited should illustrate why such studies must incorporate ethnomedical accounts of indigenous illness beliefs and behaviors with epidemiological analysis and why they must focus on culture-bound syndromes and somatization if they are to determine the extent and distribution of psychopathology and deviance among Chinese as well as assess which of their aspects are culturally-specific and which universal.

SUMMARY AND CONCLUSIONS

A. Prevalence rates and their sociodemographic determinants:

The studies we have reviewed generally indicate that the overall prevalence rate of mental disorder as well as the rate for psychosis among Chinese are roughly similar to those reported from other cultures. In less economically developed and less modernized areas, the neurosis rate is lower, but the rate for organic psychosis is higher, due to unfavorable physical environment. The age-specific rate for senile psychosis is not lower than in other cultures, but patients seem to be better tolerated at home, resulting in a lower hospital admission rate. This also appears to be the case with psychotic patients in Chinese families, whose deviance is contained in the family, even in overseas Chinese communities, for much longer periods than among Western groups (Lin et al. 1978).

Alcoholism is very rare among Chinese, but may increase after long contact with Western culture. Narcotic addiction was a major problem in the past but has been well controlled and now apparently is no longer a problem in Taiwan or the PRC.

Most of the psychiatric disorders show a decided predilection for people in middle age, and in general, females have higher rates than males, with the exception of suicide, where males and older people predominate.

The higher rates in oldest sons and youngest daughters appear to be related to cultural patterns of stress and family structure.

Mental ill-health with its multiform manifestation is much more prevalent among people of lower social status who are under economic stress.

Urbanization and migration exhibit a dramatic impact on the prevalence of neurosis, suicide and psychophysiological reactions, but not psychosis. The adverse effect of migration is apparently "dose-related"; the more adaptation required, the higher the rate of psychiatric casualties. Migration also exerts a more severe impact on females and on people from lower social class. Although urbanization in general takes its toll on people's mental health status, the degree of modern life contact is positively associated with better mental health. Modern value identification without adequate modern life contact is deemed particularly detrimental.

B. Cultural Influences on the Symptom Manifestations of Mental Disorders in Chinese Population

In contrast to community survey studies which are based on Western psychiatric classification systems and tend to illumine the universal features of mental illness rather that societal differences, many clinical and anthropological studies in the past ten years have revealed striking particularities in the ways Chinese patients present their psychiatric problems.

Suppression of dysphoric emotion and somatization often drastically modify the clinical picture of many kinds of mental diseases, particularly depression and reactive psychosis. Instead of these disorders being experienced and expressed as psychological phenomena, illness terms derived from traditional Chinese medical concepts are used to label and interpret them as somatic experiences. In its most extreme form, Chinese cultural beliefs and norms construct so-called cultural-bound syndromes – e.g., *koro* and frigophobia – where the illness behavior is specific to this culture. Only anthropological psychiatry studies which investigate the meaning context of illness in different societies can supplement epidemiologies of psychiatric "disease" with descriptions of the natural history of psychiatric "illness" that will enable us to understand the psychosocial mechanisms by which culture shapes mental disorders.

C. Suggestions for Future Investigations:

1. Since past studies in communities in Taiwan have accumulated extensive, reliable background information for comparison, and since these communities are continuously subjected to social, economic, political and cultural changes, longitudinal follow-up surveys in the same areas in the future should provide us with additional valuable information on how these changes continue to affect psychiatric problems.

2. Because most Chinese communities, whether in Taiwan, the People's Republic of China, or in other countries, are undergoing varying degrees of modernization, it is important to determine how social development affects disease occurrence rates and symptom manifestation.

3. In addition, most overseas Chinese populations, e.g., Chinese-Americans and Chinese in Singapore, Malaysia, the Philippines, are constantly subjected to the pressure of acculturation and/or assimilation. This provides an especially important opportunity to examine in detail the effects of these phenomena on mental health. Also, marked differences between Chinese culture and the host cultures provide an appropriate occasion for interracial or interethnic comparisons.

4. The rarity of alcoholism among Chinese has been well established. A more in-depth search for reasons why might contribute to the prevention of alcoholism in other cultures.

5. Although drug addiction is no longer a threatening problem in most Chinese communities, a more careful historico-socio-psychological investigation into the reasons why it proliferated in China in the past and the conditions under which it was controlled might offer us an excellent chance to understand the control of deviance in Chinese societies and to relate this knowledge to drug abuse and related forms of deviance in other cultures.

6. We still know very little about mental illness in the PRC. One suspects that profound changes in political ideology, social structure, and cultural norms must exert a major impact on the mental health of its population, yet the information now available is very limited, fragmentary and at times even

contradictory. We are told from time to time that suicide is rare (Koran 1973), that neurosis is non-existent (Lin 1973), and that the prevalence rates of the major psychoses have decreased. Yet at the same time we are aware of stories of people coming under great stress and even committing suicide during the Cultural Revolution and other periods of political turmoil (Chen Jo-hsi 1978). Furthermore, visitors have queried psychiatrists and visited mental hospitals, and hence know that psychiatric disorders are not uncommon. And most recently, psychiatrists from the People's Republic have begun to correct romantic distortions and just plain lack of knowledge by sharing their clinical impressions and their limited research findings (see Chapter 17).

The importance of a closer understanding of the present status of mental health among the Chinese in the People's Republic of China cannot be underestimated. In order to accomplish this, better communication and more extensive exchange of information between the mental health professionals of Western countries and the PRC should be encouraged, and cooperative epidemiological and anthropological studies conducted if possible. Though the former is rapidly becoming feasible, the likelihood of the latter remains uncertain. Hence it is reasonable to assume that for some time our knowledge of psychiatric disorders among Chinese will continue to be derived from populations outside the China mainland. Nonetheless, it is essential that attempts be made to acquire all relevant statistics from the PRC which become available, and to vigorously pursue any opportunities for collaborative cross-cultural research.

7. Child rearing patterns, personality development, and coping styles are central to the issue of cultural influences on psychopathology. In order to further our knowledge in these areas in the future, cross-cultural psychological research needs to be fostered.

8. Finally, we have suggested that anthropological epidemiologies of culture-bound syndromes, somatization, and other salient cultural forms of mental illness in Chinese populations are needed if comparative cross-cultural research is to determine accurately the extent and nature of deviance and psychopathology in these populations and especially if it is to analyze how Chinese culture influences these problems. Rather than recapitulate these issues we refer readers to the suggestions we made for future research in our discussion of culture-bound syndromes and somatization. Only when we can supplement psychiatric epidemiologies of the natural history of mental disease with anthropological (or ethnomedical) epidemiologies of the natural history of the illness behaviors associated with these disorders will we break out of the ethnocentric and psychocentric confines of Western medical conceptualizations so as to widen our perspective to include the conceptualizations held by Chinese patients, families, and practitioner. This widening of perspective is essential for comparative (or anthropological) epidemiology for quite practical reasons if it is to be of use in the planning of mental health care services for Chinese populations (see Lin and Lin 1978). But it is equally important if psychiatric epidemiology is to become truly cross-cultural and therefore is to fashion a valid theoretical framework and

methodology. Without confronting the differing contexts of meanings and behavioral pathways within which mental disorders are coped with, psychiatric epidemiology is condemned to superficiality, irrelevance, and potentially dangerous cultural bias.

NOTES

1. With respect to abuse of hallucinogens: although several hallucinogens have been known and used by Chinese medicinally but principally for Taoist religious purposes for two millenia, there are no reports describing significant abuse of these agents either in the past or at present that we are aware of.
2. In a community attitudinal survey in 1963, Rin (1978) found that the majority of Chinese believe that sicknesses are always somatogenic, and are caused by weakening of some important physiological functions. They also tend to believe that psychosis is incurable and cases need to be isolated. Twelve years later, another community survey (Rin et al. 1977) revealed a strikingly similar tendency. People still tend to believe that the treatment of psychosis is difficult and expensive, that psychotic patients are not trustworthy and should be isolated or avoided. However, age and education were found to be negatively related to this stigmatizing tendency. Young subjects with greater exposure to education (more modernized sections of the population) tended to understand more accurately the nature of psychosis and be more tolerant and accepting, less fearful and critical of psychotic patients.

REFERENCES

Adler, N. and Goleman D.
    1969 Gambling and alcoholism: Symptoms substitution and functional equivalents. Quarterly Journal of Studies on Alcohol 30:733–736.
Alexander, E. R.
    1977 International Comparisons in Epidemiology. Seminar on Anthropological and Cross-Cultural Dimensions of Illness and Health Care, June 6. Division of Social and Cross-Cultural Psychiatry, University of Washington.
Ball, J. C. and Lau, M. P.
    1966 The Chinese narcotic addict in the U.S. Social Forces 45:68–72.
Barnett, M. D.
    1955 Alcoholism in the Cantonese of New York City, an anthropological study. In Etiology of Chronic Alcoholism. O. Dietheem, ed. Springfield, Illinois: Charles C. Thomas; pp. 179–227.
Bieser, M.
    1978 Psychiatric epidemiology. In The Harvard Guide to Modern Psychiatry. A. M. Nicholi, ed. Cambridge, Massachusetts: The Belknap Press of Harvard University Press; pp. 609–626.
Berk, B. B. and Hirata, L. C.
    1973 Mental illness among the Chinese: Myth or reality? In Asian Americans: A Success Story? S. Sue and H. Hitano, eds. J. Social Issues 299(2):146–166.
Bermann, G.
    1968 Mental health in China. In Psychiatry in the Communist World. A. Kiev, ed. New York: Science House; pp. 223–261.
Bourne, P. G.
    1973 Suicide among Chinese in San Francisco. American Journal of Public Health 63: 744–750.

Brown, T. R., Stein, K. M., Huang, K., and Harris, D. E.
		1973 Mental illness and the role of mental health facilities in Chinatown. *In* Asian-
		Americans: Psychological Perspectives. J. Sue and N. Wagner, eds. Palo Alto:
		Science and Behavior Books; pp. 212–231.
Carr, J. E.
		1978 Ethno-behaviorism and the culture-bound syndromes: The case of *amok*. Culture,
		Medicine and Psychiatry 2(3):269–293.
Carr, J. E. and Tan, E. K.
		1976 In search of the true *amok*. American Journal of Psychiatry 133: 1295–1299.
Cassel, J. C.
		1974 Psychiatric epidemiology. *In* American Handbook of Psychiatry (second edition),
		Vol. #2. New York: Basic Books; pp. 401–410.
Cerny, J.
		1965 Chinese psychiatry. International Journal of Psychiatry 1:229–239.
Chafetz, M. D.
		1964 Consumption of alcohol in the Far and Middle East. New England Journal of
		Medicine 271:297–301.
Chance, N. A., Rin, H., and Chu, H. M.
		1966 Modernization, value identification and mental health, a cross-cultural study.
		Anthropologica 8:197–216.
Chang, Y. H., Rin, H., and Chen, C. C.
		1975 Frigophobia: A report of five cases. Bulletin Chinese Society of Neurology and
		Psychiatry 1(2):9–13.
Chen, A. J.
		1969 Recent trend of deaths from unnatural causes (accidents, suicides and homicides)
		in Singapore, 1961–1965. Singapore Medical Journal 10:72–82.
Chen, C. C.
		1978 Personal communication, July.
Chen, J. H.
		1978 The Execution of Mayor Yin and Other Stories from the Great Proletarian
		Cultural Revolution. Bloomington, Indiana: The Indiana University Press.
Chen, S. K.
		1978 Modern Medicine in China. Taipei, Taiwan: Medicine Today Press. (In Chinese).
Cheng, T. A. et al.
		1979 A clinical experience of the transferred psychiatric patients under governmental
		social welfare funds. *In* 10 Years' Report. Taipei, Taiwan: Taipei City Psychiatric
		Center; pp. 187–199.
Chiang, P. E.
		1958 Comments on some conclusions of the 'Comparison of the Effects of Continuous
		Sleep Therapy and Prolonged Physiological Sleep Therapy on Neurasthenia.'
		Chinese Journal of Neurology and Psychiatry 4(3):256–257.
Chin, R. and Chin, A. L. S.
		1969 Psychological Research in Communist China: 1949–1966. Cambridge, Massachu-
		setts and London, England: The M.I.T. Press.
Chou, S. S., Pien, H. L., and Liu, C. Y.
		1957 Comparison of effects of continuous sleep therapy and prolonged physiological
		sleep therapy on neurasthenia. Chinese Journal of Neurology and Psychiatry 3(1):
		13–18.
Chu, G.
		1972 Drinking patterns and attitudes of rooming house Chinese in San Francisco.
		Quarterly Journal of Studies on Alcohol 33(1–2).
Chu, H. M.
		1972 Migration and mental disorder in Taiwan. *In* Transcultural Research in Mental
		Health. W. Lebra, ed. Honolulu, Hawaii: East-West Center Press.

Chu, L. W. and Lin, M. C.
1960 Mental diseases in Peking between 1933 and 1943. Journal of Mental Science 106:274.

Chung, Y. P.
1957 Observations on the therapeutic effects of the pharmacological sleep therapy on the exciting-exchausting type neurasthenia patients. Chinese Journal of Neurology and Psychiatry 3(1):19–24.

Claus, P. J.
1978 Spirit possession and spirit mediumship from the perspective of the Tulu oral traditions. Culture, Medicine and Psychiatry 2(4): 29–52.

Cooper, A. B. and Morgan, H.
1973 Epidemiological Psychiatry. Springfield, Illinois: Charles C. Thomas.

Cooper, J. and Sartorius, N.
1977 Culture and temporal variations in schizophrenia: A speculation on the importance of industrialization. British Journal of Psychiatry 130:50–55.

Crapanzano, V. and Garrison, V.
1977 Case Studies in Spirit Possession. New York: John Wiley and Sons.

Department of Health
1959 Guideline for the prevention and treatment of psychiatric illness. In Compendium of Laws and Regulations, July-December 1958, PRC. Edited by State Department. Peking: Legal Publishing Co.

Ewing, J. A., Rouse, B., and Pellizziri, E. D.
1974 Alcohol sensitivity and ethnic background. American Journal of Psychiatry 131:206–207.

Gallin, B.
1966 Hsin-Hsing, Taiwan, a Chinese Village in Change. Berkeley: University of California Press.

Gaw, A.
n.d. Report of a case of koro in a Chinese-American. Unpublished manuscript.

Gruenberg, E. M.
1974 The epidemiology of schizophrenia. In American Handbook of Psychiatry, Vol. II. S. Arieti, ed. New York: Basic Books; pp. 448–463.

Gurin, G. J., Veroff, J., and Feld, S.
1960 Americans View their Mental Health: A Nationwide Interview Study. New York: Basic Books.

Hollender, M. H. and Hirsch, S. J.
1964 Hysterical psychosis. American Journal of Psychiatry 120:1066–1074.

Hollingshead, A. B. and Redlich, F. C.
1958 Social Class and Mental Illness. New York: John Wiley and Sons.

Hsia, C. I. et al.
1958 Clinical analysis and follow-up interview of 2000 cases of schizophrenia. Chinese Journal of Neurology and Psychiatry 4(2):89–94.

Hsu, F. L. K.
1955 Americans and Chinese. London: Cresset Press.

Hsu, F. L. K.
1971 Eros, affect and pao. In Kinship and Culture. F. L. K. Hsu, ed. Chicago: Aldine; pp. 439–475.

Hsu, F. L. K.
1971b Psychosocial homeostasis and jen: Conceptual tools for advancing psychological anthropology. American Anthropologist 73:23–44.

Hughes, C. C., Tremblay, M., Rapoport, R. N., and Leighton, A. H.
1960 People of Cove and Woodlot. The Stirling Country Study, Vol. 2. New York: Basic Books.

Jew, C. C. and Brody, S. A.
   1967 Mental illness among the Chinese: Hospitalization rates over the past century.
         Comprehensive Psychiatry 8(2):129–134.
Kasamatu, A.
   1944 Über die vergleichend psychiatrische untersuchung in einem dorfs bei Cantong.
         Psychiatria et Neurologia Japonica 46:188–194.
Kenny, M. C.
   1978 *Latah* – The symbolism of a putative medical disorder. Culture, Medicine and
         Psychiatry 2(3):209–232.
Khoo, O. T. and Fernandez, P.
   1971 The problem of alcoholism in Singapore. Singapore Medical Journal 12:154–
         160.
Kleinman, A. K. et al. (eds.)
   1976 Medicine in Chinese Cultures. Washington, D.C.: U.S. Government Printing Office
         for Fogarty International Center, N.I.H.
Kleinman, A. M. and Mechanic, D.
   1979 Some observations of mental illness and its treatment in the People's Republic
         of China. The Journal of Nervous and Mental Disease 167:267–274.
Kleinman, A. M.
   1977 Depression, somatization and the "new cross-cultural psychiatry." Social Science
         and Medicine 11:3–10.
Kleinman, A. M.
   1978 The three faces of culture-bound disorders: An editorial. Culture, Medicine and
         Psychiatry 2(3):207–208.
Kleinman, A. M.
   1979 Patients and Healers in the Context of Culture: An Exploration of the Borderland
         Between Anthropology, Medicine and Psychiatry. Berkeley: University of
         California Press.
Koran, L.
   1972 Psychiatry in mainland China: History and recent status. American Journal of
         Psychiatry 128:970–977.
Koro Study Team
   1969 The *koro* epidemic in Singapore. Singapore Medical Journal 10: 234–242.
LaBarre, W.
   1946 Some observations on character structure in the Orient: The Chinese. Part I and
         II. Psychiatry 9:215–237, 375–395.
Langner, T. S. and Michael, S. T.
   1963 Life stress and mental health. *In* Rennie Series in Social Psychiatry, Vol. 2. A. L.
         Thomas, ed. New York: Free Press of Glencoe.
Leff, J.
   1977 Cross-cultural studies of emotions. Culture, Medicine and Psychiatry 1(4):317–
         350.
Leighton, A. H.
   1974 Social disintegration and mental disorder. *In* American Handbook of Psychiatry,
         Vol. II. S. Arieti, ed. New York: Basic Books; pp. 411–423.
Leighton, A. H.
   1959 My Name is Legion. The Stirling County Study, Vol. 1. New York: Basic Books.
Leighton, A. H., Lambo, T. A., Hughes, C. C., Leighton, D. C., Murphy, J. M., and Macklin,
D. B.
   1963 Psychiatric Disorders among the Yoruba. Ithaca, New York: Cornell University
         Press.
Leighton, D. C., Harding, J. S., Maclin, D. B., MacMillan, A. M., and Leighton, A. H.
   1963 The Character of Danger. The Stirling Country Study, Vol. 3. New York: Basic
         Books.

Lemkau, P. V.
  1964 Methodological problems in evaluating follow-up services to psychiatric patients. Mental Hygiene 48:161–171.
Leong, J. H. K.
  1974 Cross-cultural influences on ideas about drugs. Bulletin on Narcotics 26 (4): 1–7.
Li, C. H.
  1958 The therapeutic Effect of "Chiann-Naw pills" on 146 cases of neurasthenia. Chinese Journal of Neurology and Psychiatry 4(6):429–430.
Li, C. P., Li, T. S., et al.
  1958 Accelerated treatment of neurasthenia. Chinese Journal of Neurology and Psychiatry 4(5):351–356.
Lin, P. T. K.
  1973 APA lecturer says neuroses non-existant in mainland China. Psychiatric News 8:1, 13, June 20.
Lin, T. Y.
  1953 A study of the incidence of mental disorder in Chinese and other cultures. Psychiatry 16:313–336.
Lin, T. Y.
  1959 Effects of urbanization on mental health. International Social Science Journal 11(1):24–33.
Lin, T. Y.
  1963 Historical survey of psychiatric epidemiology in Asia. Mental Hygiene 47:351–359.
Lin, T. Y., Rin, H., Yeh, E. K., Hsu, C. C., and Chu, H. M.
  1969 Mental disorders in Taiwan, fifteen years later. In Mental Helath Research in Asia and the Pacific. W. Caudill and T. Y. Lin, eds. Honolulu, Hawaii: East-West Center Press.
Lin, T. Y. and Lin, M. C.
  1978 Service delivery issues in Asian-North American communities. American Journal of Psychiatry 135(4):454–456.
Lin, T. Y., Tardiff, K., Donetz, G., and Goresky, W.
  1978 Ethnicity and patterns of help-seeking. Culture, Medicine and Psychiatry 2(1): 3–14.
Liu, C. T.
  1957 Electroencephalographic (EEG) studies on neurasthenia. Chinese Journal of Neurology and Psychiatry 3(1):8–12.
Lo, W. H. and Lo, T.
  1977 A ten-year follow-up study of Chinese schizophrenics in Hong Kong. British Journal of Psychiatry 131:63–66.
Lyman, S., Maeka, V., Liang, P., eds.
  1939 Social and Psychological Studies in Neuropsychiatry in China. Peking: Peking Union Medical College.
Manschreck, T.
  1978 The atypical psychoses. Culture, Medicine and Psychiatry 2(3):233–268.
Martin, P. A.
  1971 Dynamic considerations of the hysterical psychosis. American Journal of Psychiatry 126:745–748.
Marsella, A. J., Kinzie, D., and Gordon, P.
  1973 Ethnic variations in the expression of depression. Journal of Cross-Cultural Psychology 4:435–458.
Marsella, A. J.
  1977 Depressive experience and disorders across cultures. In Handbook of Cross-Cultural Psychiatry. Culture and Psychopathology, Vol. 5. H. Triandis and J. Draguns, eds. Boston: Allyn and Bacon; pp. 30–72.

Marsella, A. J.
   1978 Towards a Conceptual Framework for Understanding Cross-Cultural Variations in
         Depressive Affect and Disorder. Paper delivered to the "Psychocultural Aspects of
         Ethnicity" Seminar. School of International Studies, University of Washington,
         April 18.
Marsella, A. J.
   1979 Cross-cultural studies of mental disorders. In Perspectives on Cross-Cultural
         Psychology. A. J. Marsella, R. Tharp, and T. Ciborowski, eds. New York: Aca-
         demic Press.
Merry, J.
   1975 A social history of heroin addiction. British Journal of Addiction 70:307–310.
Miller, M. H., Yeh, E. K., Alexander, A. A., Klein, M. H., Tseng, K. H., Workneh, F., and
Chu, H. M.
   1971 The cross-cultural student. Bulletin of the Menninger Clinic. 35:128–131.
Mitchell, R. E.
   1972 Levels of emotional strain in Southeast Asian cities. Project of the Urban Family
         Life Survey, Vols. I, II. The Chinese University of Hong Kong, Hong Kong. Taipei,
         Formosa: The Orient Cultural Service.
Mo, K. M. and Lian, J. K.
   1958 Treatment of neurasthenia with 1-glutamic acid. Chinese Journal of Neurology
         and Psychiatry 4(2):101–105.
Murphy, H. B. M.
   1954 The mental health of Singapore: Part I – suicide. Medical Journal of Malaya
         9:1–45.
Murphy, H. B. M.
   1959 Culture and mental disorder in Singapore. In Culture and Mental Health; pp.
         291–316. M. K. Opler, ed.
Neurasthenia Study Unit, Neurology Department, Peking Shie-Ho Hospital, Chinese Medical
Science Institute.
   1958 Observation on the treatment effect of meprobamate on neurasthenia. Chinese
         Journal of Neurology and Psychiatry 4(5):359–361.
Neutra, R., Levy, J. E., and Parker, D.
   1977 Cultural expectations versus reality in Navajo seizure patterns and sick roles.
         Culture, Medicine and Psychiatry 1:255–275.
Ngui, R. W.
   1969 The koro epidemic in Singapore. Australian and New Zealand Journal of Psy-
         chiatry 3:263–266.
Obeyesekere, G.
   1977 The theory and practice of psychological medicine in the Ayurvedic tradition.
         Culture, Medicine and Psychiatry 1:155–181.
Rao, V.
   1978 Some aspects of psychiatry in India. Transcultural Psychiatric Research Review
         15:7–38.
Rin, H.
   1959 Psychotherapy with six cases of obsessive-compulsive neurosis. Journal of
         Formosan Medical Association 59:189–200.
Rin, H., Wu, K. C., and Lin, C. L.
   1962 A study of the content of delusions and hallucinations manifested by Chinese
         paranoid psychotics. Journal of the Formosa Medical Association 61:46–57.
Rin, H. and Lin, T. Y.
   1962 Mental illness among Formosan Aborigines as compared with the Chinese in
         Taiwan. Journal of Mental Science 108:133–146.

Rin, H.
1965 A study of the etiology of *koro* in respect to the Chinese concept of illness. The International Journal of Social Psychiatry 11:7–13.
Rin, H., Chu, H. M., and Lin, T. Y.
1966 Psychophysiological reactions of a rural and suburban population in Taiwan. Acta Psychiatrica Scandinavica 42:410–473.
Rin, H.
1970 Twenty years' development of psychiatric epidemiology researches in Taiwan. Journal of the Formosa Medical Association 69:123–141.
Rin, H., Schooler, C., and Caudill, W. A.
1973 Symptomatology and hospitalization: Culture, social structure and psychopathology in Taiwan and Japan. Journal of Nervous and Mental Disease 157:296–312.
Rin, H., Chen, C. C., Lin, S. N., Wu, A. C. C., Huang, M. G., Chen, T., and Yeh, E. K.
1977 Attitude of members of welfare families towards mental illness. Bulletin of Chinese Society of Neurology and Psychiatry 3(2):31–39.
Rin, H.
1978 Psychiatry and Society. Taipei, Taiwan: Medicine Today Press. (In Chinese).
Robin, L. N.
1978 Psychiatric epidemiology. Archives of General Psychiatry 35:697–702.
Sartorius, N., Jablensky, A., and Shapiro, R.
1978 Cross-cultural differences in the short-term prognosis of schizophrenic psychoses. Schizophrenia Bulletin 4(1):102–113.
Singer, K.
1972 Drinking patterns and alcoholism in the Chinese. British Journal of Addiction 67:3–14.
Singer, K.
1974 The choice of intoxicant among the Chinese. British Journal of Addiction 69:257–268.
Singer, K.
1975 Depressive disorders from a transcultural perspective. Social Science and Medicine 5:289–301.
Srole, L., Langner, T. S., Michael, S. T., Opler, M. K., and Rennie, T. A. L.
1962 Mental health in the metropolis. *In* Rennie Series in Social Psychiatry, Vol. 1. A. C. Thomas, ed. New York: McGraw-Hill.
Sue, S. and McKinney, H.
1975 Asian-Americans in the community mental health care system. American Journal of Orthopsychiatry 45(1):111–118.
Taipale, V. and Taipale, J.
1973 Chinese psychiatry: A visit to a Chinese mental hospital. Archives of General Psychiatry 29:313–316.
Tan, E. S. and Carr, J. E.
1977 Psychiatric sequelae of *amok*. Culture, Medicine and Psychiatry 1:59–67.
Tan, E. S.
1969 The symptomatology of anxiety in West Malaysia. Australian and New Zealand Journal of Psychiatry 3:271–276.
T'ao, K. T. et al.
1957 Analysis of 1600 cases of schizophrenia. Chinese Journal of Neurology and Psychiatry 3(2):134–164.
Tao, K., Lin, J., and Zheng, Y.
n.d. Follow-up Study Related to Prognosis of 100 Cases of Childhood and Adolescent Schizophrenia. Nanking Neuropsychiatric Institute. Mimeographed report.

Teaching and Research Group of Psychiatry
  n.d.   Observation on 26 Cases of Graft Schizophrenia. Hunan Medical College, Chang-
          sha, China. Mimeographed report.
Teoh, J. I.
  1972   Transvestism treatment by aversive therapy. Medical Journal of Malaya 26:179–
          185.
Teoh, J. I.
  1974   Psychological problems among university students in an area of rapid socio-
          cultural change. Australian and New Zealand Journal of Psychiatry 8:109–120.
Teoh, J. I. and Dass, D.
  n.d.   Alcoholism and Culture: A Study of Chronic Alcoholism at the University
          Medical Center, Kuala Lumpur, Malaysia. Unpublished manuscript.
True, R. H.
  1975   Mental health services in a Chinese-American Community. *In* Service Delivery in
          Pan-Asian Communities. W. H. Ishikawa and N. H. Archer, eds. San Diego: Pacific
          Asian Coalition.
Tseng, W. S. and Hsu, J.
  1969   Chinese culture, personality formation and mental illness. International Journal of
          Social Psychiatry 16:5–14.
Tseng, W. S.
  1973   Psychopathological study of obsessive compulsive neurosis in Taiwan. Compre-
          hensive Psychiatry 14:139–150.
Tseng, W. S.
  1975   The nature of somatic complaints among psychiatric patients: The Chinese case.
          Comprehensive Psychiatry 16:237–245.
Tsuang, M. T.
  1972   Psychiatric genetics in Taiwan. International Journal of Mental Health 1:221–
          230.
Walls, C. Y., Walls, L. H., and Langsley, D. G.
  1975   Psychiatric training and practice in the People's Republic of China. American
          Journal of Psychiatry 132:121–128.
Wang, C. Y. and Tuan, S. C.
  1957   Clinical statistic analysis of the hospitalized patients of the Psychiatric Hospital
          of Peking Medical School in four year period. Chinese Journal of Neurology and
          Psychiatry 3(2):162–170.
Wang, R. P.
  1968   A study of alcoholism in Chinatown. International Journal of Social Psychiatry
          14:260–267.
Wen, J. K.
  1973   Social Attitudes towards Homosexuality. Thesis, College of Medicine, National
          Taiwan University, Taipei, Taiwan.
Wen, J. K.
  1978   Sexual attitudes of college students. Green Apricot 46:106–107. (In Chinese).
Westermeyer, J.
  1974   "The drunken Indian," Myths and realities. Psychiatric Annals 4(11):29–36.
Wolf, M.
  1972   Women and the Family in Rural Taiwan. Stanford, California: Stanford Univer-
          sity Press.
Wolff, P. H.
  1972   Ethnic difference in alcoholic sensitivity. Science 175:449–450.
Wolff, P. H.
  1973   Vasomotor sensitivity to alcohol in diverse Mongoloid populations. American
          Journal of Human Genetics 25:193–199.

Wong, K. C.
1950 A short history of psychiatry and mental hygiene in China. Chinese Medical Journal 68:44–48.

World Health Organization
1973 Report of the International Pilot Study of Schizophrenia, Vol. I. Geneva, Switzerland: World Health Organization.

Xia, Z., Yan, H., and Wang, C.
n.d. Mental Health Work in Shanghai. Shanghai Psychiatric Hospital. Mimeographed report.

Yap, P. M.
1958 Suicide in Hong Kong, with Special Reference to Attempted Suicide. Hong Kong: Hong Kong University Press.

Yap, P. M.
1960 The possession syndrome: A comparison of Hong Kong and French findings. Journal of Mental Science 106:114–137.

Yap, P. M.
1965 Phenomenology of affective disorder in Chinese and other cultures. *In* Transcultural Psychiatry. A. V. S. DeReuck and R. Porter, eds. Boston: Little and Brown; pp. 86–114.

Yap, P. M.
1965 *Koro*: A culture-bound depersonalization syndrome. British Journal of Psychiatry 3:43–50.

Yap, P. M.
1969 The culture-bound reactive syndrome. *In* Mental Health Research in Asia and the Pacific. W. Caudill and T. Y. Lin, eds. Honolulu, Hawaii: East-West Center Press; pp. 33–53.

Yap, P. M.
1974 Comparative Psychiatry. Toronto: University of Toronto Press.

Yeh, E. (ed.) and Tseng, W. S.
1971 Modern Life and Mental Health. Taipei, Taiwan: Buffalo Book Company. (In Chinese).

Yeh, E. K.
1972 Paranoid manifestations among Chinese students studying abroad: Some preliminary findings. *In* Transcultural Research in Mental Health, Vol. II. V. P. Lebra, ed. Honolulu, Hawaii: East-West Center Press; pp. 326–340.

Yeh, E. K., Chu, H. M., Ko, Y. H., and Lee, S. P.
1972 Student mental health: An epidemiological study in Taiwan. Acta Psychologica Taiwanica 14:1–26.

Yeh, E. K., Fan, B. Y., and Tien, S. J.
1979 A statistical study of the discharged patients from the Taipei City Psychiatric Center during 1969–1978. *In* 10 Years' Report, Taipei City Psychiatric Center. Taipei, Taiwan: Taipei City Psychiatric Center; pp. 209–248.

Yü, C. H., and Li, S. L.
1958 Statistical observations of the manic-depressive illness in Si-an area. Chinese Journal of Neurology and Psychiatry 4:288–291.

Young, D.
1979 Personal communication.

Young, D. and Li, H.
1979 Sporadic Virus Encephalitis with Mental Symptoms. Psychiatric Division, Hunan Medical College Hospital, Changsha, China.

APPENDIX

In the 5 March 1980 issue of the *Chinese Journal of Neurology and Psychiatry* (Volume 13, Number 1) and in a WHO Seminar on Psychiatric Epidemiology held in Paking in June 1980, psychiatrists from the People's Republic of China presented findings from more recent epidemiological investigations that significantly add to and extend the findings reviewed in this Chapter. While this new information (which appeared after this volume was in press) does change some of the particular details we have discussed, by and large it does not appear to significantly alter the general configuration we have drawn of mental illness in China. Nonetheless readers interested in this subject should be prepared for a substantial increase in the availability of relevant data owing to a more open policy of publication, new research, and collaboration with foreign researchers.

RANCE P. L. LEE

14. SEX ROLES, SOCIAL STATUS, AND PSYCHIATRIC SYMPTOMS IN URBAN HONG KONG

Mental health researchers have identified a number of social factors that may be associated with the prevalence of functional psychiatric illness. Some of the empirical findings are contradictory among studies using different methodologies or conducted in different times and places (Mishler and Scotch 1965; Turner 1972; and Dohrenwend 1975). It is recognized, however, that two of the highly consistent findings are the relationships of psychiatric illness to sex roles and social class. In general, the overall rates of psychiatric illness are higher among women than men (e.g., Davis 1962; Langner and Michael 1963; Phillips 1966; Phillips and Segal 1969; Gove and Tudor 1973; and Clancy and Gove 1974), and higher among members of lower socioeconomic groups (Faris and Dunham 1939; Hollingshead and Redlich 1958; Langner and Michael 1963; Leighton, et al. 1963; Kohn 1968; Dunham 1970; and Hodge 1970).

Sex and class differences in psychiatric illness were found not only in advanced industrial societies, but also in developing countries. In his study of psychophysiological symptoms in two Mexican cities, for instance, Langner (1965) observed that the high-income group reports fewer symptoms on the average than the low-income group, and that in general women report more symptoms than men, especially in a community where women's status is low.

The best known studies of mental health in Chinese society are the ones conducted by Lin and his associates (Lin 1953; and Lin, et al. 1969). In their successive studies of the prevalence rates of various types of mental disorders among all the inhabitants of three communities — a village, a small town, and a section of a city — in Taiwan in 1946–48 and in 1961–63, they discovered similar findings about the relationships of the overall rates of psychiatric disorders to sex and social class.[1] More specifically, Chinese females showed a significantly higher rate of psychoneurosis, while lower class individuals were most likely to suffer from schizophrenia, mental deficiency and psychopathic personality. It was noted that there was a significant increase in the prevalence of all mental disorders over the 15 years, and that the increase was mainly due to the marked increase of females with psychoneurosis. Immediately after the completion of the follow-up survey in 1963, the research team carried out an epidemiological study of psychophysiological reactions in a rural and suburban population — one of the above investigated communities — in Taiwan. An age-stratified random sample of 488 from 3,748 inhabitants over the age 15 were selected for the study. From the report by Rin, et al. (1966), we observe that the prevalence rate of psychophysiological symptoms was slightly higher among females than males, and that the prevalence rate tended to be higher among lower class individuals.

273

A. Kleinman and T.-Y. Lin (eds.), Normal and Abnormal Behavior in Chinese Culture, 273–289.
Copyright © 1980 *by D. Reidel Publishing Company.*

Another study of note is the sample survey conducted by Mitchell (1969) in the urban areas of Singapore, Hong Kong, Malaysia, Bangkok and Taipei in 1967–68. He found that among the Chinese population in these various areas, women were consistently more likely than men to be disturbed by emotional illness.[2]

Hong Kong is situated on the southeast coast of the China mainland. It is basically a Chinese society; a recent census indicates that about 98.3 per cent of the total population are Chinese. It is also noteworthy that Hong Kong has achieved a higher level of social and economic development than many other Chinese societies in the Asian region (Hopkins 1971; Cheng 1977). The major objective of the present study is to find out whether or not the above-mentioned findings about sex and social class differences in mental disturbance would hold in the highly modernized society of Hong Kong. Our findings may have implications for the future of other Chinese societies moving toward modernity.

In a clinical investigation of mental illness in Hong Kong, Yap (1965) found that there were more female than male in-patients with affective illness who had been admitted to hospital for the first time. Mitchell's (1969) sample survey of the Chinese adults in the urban sector of Hong Kong discerned a higher level of emotional illness not only among women, but also among economically deprived individuals. Yap's study included only individuals who were hospital in-patients. Mitchell collected data from a random sample of the community population and in this sense supplemented Yap's research. Mitchell, however, merely reported the bivariate distributions without making attempts to control for "third" variables such as age and education. Moreover, since Mitchell did not report on the validity of his measure of emotional illness, we are uncertain about the extent to which his 11 questions are indicative of mental morbidity.

The objective of this study is to examine and elaborate the relationships of sex roles and social class to the "true" prevalence of psychiatric symptoms among the urban residents of Hong Kong. The major questions raised here are: How is the distribution of psychiatric symptoms in a community population associated with sex roles and social class? Are the effects of sex roles and social class on psychiatric symptoms independent of each other, and also of other factors such as age and education? Why is or is not the prevalence of psychiatric symptoms related to sex roles and social class?

METHOD

Data were drawn from the Biosocial Survey conducted jointly by the Social Research Centre of The Chinese University of Hong Kong and the Human Ecology Group of Australian National University. A proportionate stratified random sample of 3,983 household heads between the ages of 20 to 59 were selected from the urban areas of Hong Kong in 1974. It is noteworthy that over 80 per cent of the four million people in Hong Kong resided in urban areas. In this study, census district and housing type were used as criteria for stratifying the urban households, and the tables devised by Kish (1965:388–401) were employed to insure randomness of the sample. The sampling fraction was 0.62 per cent for each stratum. An interview schedule was devised and used for collecting the information from respondents. The response rate was about 71 per cent. Unsuccessful interviews were replaced by cases randomly selected from a supplementary list. It is noted that the present research was in effect a study of the *non-institutionalized* adult population in the urban sector of Hong Kong.

The prevalence of psychiatric symptoms was measured by the 22 closed-end questions developed by Langner (1962) in the Midtown Manhattan Study. The items were translated into Chinese. Responses to each question were dichotomized into "pathognomonic" and "non-pathognomonic" categories. Scores on the 22 items were summed for each respondent, producing a scale with a range potentially from 0 to 22. A higher score in the scale was indicative of more psychiatric symptoms.

Langner's scale is one of the most common and best evaluated instruments to estimate the "true" prevalence of psychiatric symptoms in non-institutionalized populations through the use of field survey techniques (Langner and Michael 1963; Langner 1965; Manis, et al. 1963; Abramson 1966; Dohrenwend 1966; Phillips 1966; Haese and Meile 1967; Meile and Haese 1969; Phillips and Segal 1969; Dohrenwend and Crandell 1970; Phillips and Clancy 1970; Schader, et al. 1971; Gaitz and Scott 1972; and Gove and Tudor 1973).[3] The 22 items in the scale mainly deal with relatively mild forms of self-reported psychoneurotic and physiological symptoms, or possibly stress reactions. As Langner (1962:269) has pointed out,

(The scale) does not screen persons with organic brain damage, the mentally retarded, and the sociopaths. It does, however, provide a rough indication of where people lie on a continuum of impairment in life functioning due to very common types of psychiatric symptoms.

Examining the data in the present study, we found that the Alpha coefficient (Cronbach 1951) for the Chinese version of the total scale is .775, indicating a high degree of internal consistency among the 22 items. In an effort to determine the validity of the translated scale, Porritt and Miller (1976) found that every item of the scale could discriminate between the neurotic out-patients and a random sample of the "normal" population in Hong Kong at a statistically significant level, and that the correlations of Langner's scale to Bradburn's (1969) Positive Affect, Negative Affect, and Affect Balance scales are -.216, .497, and -.467, respectively. In view of these tests, the Chinese version of Langner's scale appears to have acceptable reliability and validity.[4]

Following Langner (1962), the point of discrimination between "well" and "sick" in the scale was made between the scores of 3 and 4 symptoms.[5] In other words, a score of 4 or more was arbitrarily used as the indicator of significant impairment.

Socioeconomic status (SES) of a family was indicated by housing status, family income, and material standard of the household. Housing status was dichotomized into low and high categories with scores of 0 and 1, respectively. Low housing status referred to those residing in Government's resettlement estates, simple stone structures, wooden sheds or roof-top cottages, while high housing status consisted of the remaining types of accommodation. Family income status was divided into four levels, scored from 0 to 3, indicating the gross monthly income of the household under HK$1000, $1000–$1499, $1500–$2499, and $2500 or above, respectively. The material standard of a household was assessed by the interviewer, and was divided into low, medium, high categories with scores 0, 1, and 2, respectively.

The relationships of the above three socioeconomic indicators to the prevalence of psychiatric symptoms were analyzed separately. In an effort to examine the overall relationship between socioeconomic status and psychiatric symptoms, the three indicators of socioeconomic status were dichotomized. Households with monthly income of HK$1499 or less were scored 0; otherwise, scored 1. Households with low material standard were scored 0; otherwise, scored 1. As the interelations among the three indicators were statistically significant ($p < .001$), their scores were summed for each respondent to form a SES scale. The total scores on the scale ranged from 0 to 3, with a higher score indicative of a higher level of family socioeconomic status.

Age and educational status of the individuals were introduced for control analysis. The four age-categories were 20–29, 30–39, 40–49, and 50–59 with scores from 0 to 3, respectively. Educational status was also divided into four categories which were no schooling, primary school or private tutoring, secondary school, and post-secondary school with scores from 0 to 3, respectively.

Gamma was employed to measure the strength of relationship, whereas chi-square was employed to test the statistical significance. In the control analyses the partial gamma was estimated (Davis 1971), which is a weighted average of the zero-order gammas in various subgroups.

RESULTS

The total scores on Langner's scale actually ranged from 0 to 19, with 31.6 per cent of the respondents having four or more symptoms. This percentage is rather close to the percentages typically found in American samples (with the same cut off point in Langner's scale). For instance, it is 31.2 per cent in Langner's (1962) sample of 1,660 adults in Midtown Mannhattan, and 33.6 per cent in Gaitz and Scott's (1972) sample of 1,441 adult residents in Houston.

From Table 1, it can be seen that psychiatric symptoms were more prevalent among women than men. The hypothesized relationship between sex and psychiatric symptoms was therefore confirmed.

It was found consistently that the lower the scores on the three indicators of socioeconomic status, the greater was the prevalence of psychiatric symptoms. All relationships were statistically significant at the .001 level. The gamma coefficients for the relationships of symptoms to housing status, income level, and material standard were -.20, -.17, and -.14, respectively. Table 1 shows that the overall relationship between socioeconomic status and psychiatric symptoms was also inverse and linear. The hypothesis about social class differences in symptoms was thus confirmed.

TABLE 1

Percent with 4 or more symptoms by sex roles and SES (Total N = 3983)

	Symptoms	N
Sex Roles*		
Male	24.8	1702
Female	36.7	2281
SES Scale**		
0 (Low)	39.5	598
1	34.6	963
2	31.7	1140
3 (High)	24.8	1107

* Chisquare = 63.74, p < .001; Gamma = .28
** Chisquare = 45.08, p < .001; Gamma = -.17

Since both sex roles and socioeconomic status have significant effects on psychiatric symptoms,[6] to what extent are their effects independent of one another? Table 2 shows the relationship between sex and symptoms after controlling for SES. In all SES groups, rates of psychiatric symptoms were consistently higher among women than men. Furthermore, the partial gamma was .28, which was equal to the original zero-order value. Evidently, the sex-symptoms relationship was independent of socioeconomic status.

TABLE 2

Percent with 4 or more symptoms among various sex and SES groups

Sex Roles	SES			
	0 (Low) [a]	1 [b]	2 [c]	3 (High) [d]
Male [e]	29.6	27.5	24.9	19.3
Female [f]	47.0	39.6	36.6	29.1

Sex differences in each SES group:
    (a) Chisquare = 17.96, p < .001; Gamma = .36
    (b) Chisquare = 14.64, p < .001; Gamma = .27
    (c) Chisquare = 17.15, p < .001; Gamma = .27
    (d) Chisquare = 13.60, p < .001; Gamma = .26
SES differences in each sex group:
    (e) Chisquare = 12.92, p < .01; Gamma = -.15
    (f) Chisquare = 33.03, p < .001; Gamma = -.19

Table 2 also indicates that the control on sex did not alter the inverse relationship between SES and psychiatric symptoms. In both sex groups, the lower the SES the greater was the proportion of respondents with four or more symptoms. The partial gamma was -.17, which was the same as the original gamma. Thus, it was found that the inverse relationship between family socioeconomic status and the prevalence of psychiatric symptoms was independent of sex.

Are the relationships of psychiatric symptoms to sex roles and socioeconomic status independent of age and education? It was noted that age-differences in mental disorder were small, although the relationship was more or less linear.[7] In general, older respondents tended to express more symptoms. The gamma coefficient, .05, also revealed the positive but slight relationship between age and psychiatric symptoms. Nevertheless, the relationship was significant at the .01 level. Education and psychiatric symptoms were also inversely related. The relationship was clearly linear and was statistically significant at the .001 level. The gamma was -.13.

Since age and education were significantly related to psychiatric symptoms, they must be controlled in the examination of the relationship between sex roles and symptoms and between SES and symptoms. It was found that there were more women than men with psychiatric impairment among various age and educational groups. The partial gamma for the relationship between sex roles and symptoms was .28 after controlling for age and was also .28 after controlling for education. These values were the same as the original zero-order gamma. The relationship between sex and symptoms was therefore independent of age and education.

Controlling for age and education separately did not alter the inverse relationship between SES and psychiatric symptoms. The partial gamma for the control of age was .17, and that for the control of education was .15. Since the original gamma was .17, it thus can be concluded that the inverse relationship between family socioeconomic status and psychiatric symptoms was independent of age and of education.

In short, controlling for age virtually had no effect on the relationships of psychiatric symptoms to sex and SES, while controlling for education had a minor effect on the SES-symptoms relationship but no effect on the sex-symptoms relationship.

In an effort to examine the joint effects and the possible interactions among variables, we introduced the stepwise multiple correlation analysis. The variable of sex roles was transformed into a "dummy" variable (Suits 1954), in which femaleness was scored 1 and maleness was scored 0. We learned from Table 3 that in addition to the variance explained by SES, age and education, sex roles could account for 1.57 (2.89—1.32) per cent of the variance in psychiatric symptoms, and that SES could explain 1.12 (2.89—1.77) per cent of the variance over and above that explained by sex, age and education. The zero-order correlations indicate that originally sex roles and SES accounted for 1.61 and 1.15 per cent of the variance, respectively, which were approximately equal

TABLE 3

Stepwise multiple correlations of sex roles, SES, age, education
and life satisfaction with psychiatric symptoms

Independent Variable(s)	Variance explained (%)
Sex Roles (female)	1.61
SES	1.15
Life Satisfaction	2.47
Sex, SES	2.86
Age, Education	0.58
Sex, Age, Education	1.77
SES, Age, Education	1.32
Sex, SES, Age, Education	2.89
Sex, SES, Age, Education, Life Satisfaction	5.10

All correlations, $p < .001$ (F-test)

to the additional variance contributed by them in the above stepwise correlation analyses. We thus observe that both sex roles and SES could make independent contributions to the explained variance in psychiatric symptoms.

INTERPRETATION

Why is the prevalence of psychiatric symptoms associated with sex and with family socioeconomic status? Under the influence of Merton's work on the concept of anomie, a number of researchers have argued, and have verified in one way or another, that the relationships between certain social factors and mental disorder may be a product of the stress resulting from the discrepancies between aspiration and achievement (Merton 1959; Dunham 1964). For instance, both the investigations by Hollingshead, Ellis and Kirby (1954) and by Rinehart (1968) have empirically demonstrated that educational and occupational discrepancies were more prevalent, and also greater in magnitude, among patients than non-patients. After a comprehensive review of the research literature, Kleiner and Parker (1963) concluded that this mobility orientation is a significant factor in the genesis of mental illness, and that larger discrepancies between achievement and aspiration may be more prevalent among individuals in lower socioeconomic groups. In other words, individuals with lower socioeconomic status are less able to achieve their aspirations and are consequently more likely to be mentally impaired.

The theoretical postulate of achievement-aspiration discrepancies has been employed to explain not only the relationship between mental disorder and socioeconomic status, but also the sex-differences in mental disturbance. In an elaborate discussion of the relationship between sex roles and mental illness, Gove and Tudor (1973) have strongly argued that in modern industrial societies more women than men become mentally ill because women find their position in society to be more frustrating and less rewarding.

Hong Kong has become a modern industrial society. Concomitant with its rapid modernization and industrialization is the rising level of aspirations. From a sample survey of 1,065 adults in a larger-scale (about 600,000 residents) middle and lower class community of Hong Kong, Shively (1972) reported that achievement was considered important by 50.7 per cent of the respondents and not important by only 18.7 per cent. Lau (1977) studied a random sample of 550 adults from the entire urban populations of Hong Kong and found that even if the respondents were already well-fed and well-clothed, most of them (58.9 per cent) still expressed yearnings for more money, and only a minority (29.6 per cent) did not cherish such an aspiration.

In view of the previous studies in the West and the relatively high level of aspirations in Hong Kong, it is worth asking: Is the relationships of psychiatric symptoms to sex and SES in the present study a result of discrepancies between aspiration and actual achievement? We did not find any information in the Bio-social Survey which could be used as a direct measure of discrepancies between achievement and aspiration. We found, however, one item in the questionnaire which in a way reflects the level of discrepancies. The item asks: Generally speaking, are you satisfied with your daily life (your status, the things you do, and the situation around, etc.)? This item is, in effect, a general measure of life satisfaction. It was assumed in the present study that a lower level of life satisfaction was indicative of larger discrepancies between achievement and aspiration. It should be recognized that this is a rather indirect indicator and hence the findings to be reported may be more suggestive than affirmative.

The variable of life satisfaction was trichotomized into low (strongly or fairly dissatisfied), medium (so-so), and high (strongly or fairly satisfied), which were then scored from 0 to 2, respectively. It was found that life satisfaction was inversely (gamma = -.28) and significantly ($p < .001$) related to the prevalence of psychiatric symptoms. 51.7 per cent of the respondents with low satisfaction reported four or more symptoms as compared with 33.1 per cent of those with medium satisfaction and 27.4 per cent of those with high satisfaction.

The stepwise multiple correlations in Table 3 show that in addition to the variance explained by sex roles, SES, age and education, life satisfaction could account for 2.21 (5.10–2.89) per cent of the variance in psychiatric symptoms. The additional variance was almost equal to the proportion of variance (2.47 per cent) that was originally explained by life satisfaction alone. This demonstrates the usefulness of life satisfaction as an explanatory variable. Its added contribution to the explanation of psychiatric symptoms was not only substantial, but was also independent of other variables under study.

Life satisfaction was also significantly ($p < .001$) related to sex roles and SES. As expected, there was a positive relationship between life satisfaction and SES (gamma = .34). It was, however, unexpected to find that more women than men were generally satisfied with their daily life (gamma = .14).

The introduction of life satisfaction greatly affected the relationship between SES and psychiatric symptoms. The partial gamma was -.12, which was smaller than the original zero-order value of -.17. Hence, life satisfaction could partially, but not entirely, explain the SES-symptoms relationship. Table 4 provides more detailed information about the partial relationships. It was noted that the inverse relationship became statistically insignificant and very weak among the respondents with low (gamma = -.01) and with medium (gamma = -.06) satisfaction. Dissatisfaction with life, therefore, had played an important role in the genesis of psychiatric symptoms among individuals of various socioeconomic groups. It was observed, however, that the inverse relationship between SES and symptoms was still strong and statistically significant among those with high satisfaction (gamma = -.19). Further studies are needed to find out why in the conditions of high satisfaction, lower SES individuals are still more likely to have psychiatric symptoms. It is noted that life satisfaction is a subjective feeling. It could be that among those with high satisfaction some objective factors in the low class environment, which are not perceived by the individuals as important bases for life satisfaction, are in fact harmful to their psychophysiological states. These factors may include, for instance, overcrowding, air and noise pollution, and the relative inaccessibility to qualified medical care.

Table 4 indicates that control of life satisfaction did not affect the original relationship between sex roles and symptoms. In each level of satisfaction, more women than men expressed symptoms. The gamma coefficients among respondents with low, medium and high satisfaction were .37, .30 and .33, respectively. All these were somewhat greater than the original zero-order gamma of .28.

TABLE 4

Percent with 4 or more symptoms by sex roles and SES among various levels of life satisfaction

	Life-Satisfaction		
	L	M	H
Sex Roles			
Male	43.5 [a]	25.3 [b]	19.6 [c]
Female	62.4	38.6	32.7
SES			
0 (Low)	53.3 [d]	34.5 [e]	37.6 [f]
1	51.6	33.9	30.8
2	48.8	34.4	28.0
3 (High)	53.7	27.6	21.5

(a) Chisquare = 14.92, p < .001; Gamma = .37
(b) Chisquare = 17.46, p < .001; Gamma = .30
(c) Chisquare = 49.41, p < .001; Gamma = .33
(d) Chisquare = 0.68, N. S.;   Gamma = -.01
(e) Chisquare = 2.61, N. S.;   Gamma = -.06
(f) Chisquare = 32.31; p < .001; Gamma = -.19

Furthermore, the partial gamma was .33 which also exceeded the original gamma. Life satisfaction was therefore unable to explain the relationship between sex roles and psychiatric symptoms. On the contrary, it may behave as a "suppressor" variable (Rosenberg 1968). In other words, the sex-differences in psychiatric symptoms would have been greater were it not that women had a higher level of life satisfaction than men. The factor of life satisfaction has, in effect, obscured the sex-symptoms relationship.

The concept of achievement-aspiration discrepancies has often been used for the interpretation of the associations of mental disorder with sex roles and socio-economic status. In the present study, we have used the general satisfaction with daily life as an indicator of discrepancies. We found that it could partially account for the relationship between SES and psychiatric symptoms, but could not explain the relationship between sex and symptoms. Its failure to account for the sex-differences in psychiatric symptoms may, of course, be due to the kind of indicator being used. It is possible that the use of more refined and relevant indicators, such as those used by Rinehart (1968), may produce different results. Nevertheless, the validity of life satisfaction as an indicator of achievement-aspiration discrepancies appears to be acceptable, since we found in this study that it was significantly associated with SES and with psychiatric symptoms in the expected directions.[8] We therefore tend to believe that sex-differences in psychiatric symptoms are due to factors other than the achievement-aspiration discrepancies.

One of the most often discussed factors in relation to sex-differences in psychiatric symptoms is the response bias in field studies. Both Dohrenwend (1966) and Phillips and Clancy (1970) have empirically demonstrated that there are group differences in modes of responding to mental health items such as those developed by Langner (1962). In particular, Phillips and Segal (1969) have suggested that sex differences in psychiatric symptomatology, as measured by Langner's 22 items, are not real but are only a reflection of the differences between women and men in admitting certain unpleasant feelings. They argued that in modern Western cultures, it is more appropriate and acceptable for women than men to be expressive about their personal difficulties (also see Cooperstock 1971; and Nathanson 1975).

As our data do not lend support to the "real differences" explanation, the "women are more expressive" hypothesis probably works in the Hong Kong society. For many centuries, the Chinese society has been dominated by males. To maintain the dominant role, men are expected to be strong and tough and are not supposed to make complaints to others. There are old Chinese sayings (Chen 1973), for instance, "as a man one should rather die than bend" (大丈夫寧死不屈) and "he should rather bleed than weep" (流血不流淚). As a man has to show to others that he is indeed a "man", he must suppress his feelings and should not make complaints about his physical or psychological weakness.

On the other hand, women have played a submissive role in Chinese society. They are expected to be weak and gentle, rather than strong and tough. It appears to be generally accepted not only by men but also by women themselves that females are weaklings (女人是弱者). Both the case study by Fanny Cheung (forthcoming) in Hong Kong and the questionnaire survey by Aline Wong (1975) in Singapore confirmed that Chinese women tend to have a negative self-image. Most of them feel inferior and rather useless, and are neither proud nor confident of their contributions to the family and the society. As a result, it is widely believed that a gracious lady usually has an unfortunate life (紅顔多薄命). As women tend to accept the inferior status and the unfortunate experience as a way of life, it is not a shame to express and admit their own personal difficulties. After all, it is considered normal, rather than abnormal, for a woman to be psychologically or physically weak.

In view of the aforementioned contrasting beliefs and expectations about men and women in Chinese society, it seems likely that women are more expressive than men about their personal problems. When we conducted the survey in Hong Kong, therefore, the female interviewees might be more willing than the male interviewees to tell our interviewers about their psychiatric symptomatology. The differential modes of expressing distress among male and female respondents produced a response bias, which may account for our findings about the sex-differences in self-reported psychiatric symptoms.

The above observation on the contrasting expectations for women and men in Chinese society is indirectly supported by some empirical findings. In a sample survey of urban residents, Shively and Shively (1972) found that in Hong Kong lower class individuals were more likely to stick to traditional Chinese social norms. This finding suggests that the aforementioned contrasting social expectations would have greater influence upon lower SES males and females. In other words, there should be greater difference between men and women in expressing their personal difficulties in the low SES group as compared with the higher SES groups. Consequently, the sex-differences in psychiatric symptoms would be relatively greater in the low SES group. Our data in Table 2 suggests that this was in fact the case. The percentage difference between men and women in the low SES group was 17.4, whereas differences in higher SES groups were around 10 to 11 per cent. The gamma value in the low SES group was also clearly greater than those in other groups. It seems, therefore, that the "women are more expressive" hypothesis is plausible in the context of Hong Kong.[9]

Does the response bias in field studies affect the inverse relationship between socioeconomic status and self-reported symptoms? Investigations by Dohrenwend (1966) and Phillips and Clancy (1970) tend to suggest that differential expressiveness may produce certain effects on the class-symptoms relationship. Their findings, however, are not clear-cut. As Phillips and Clancy (1970) have found, the relationship between socioeconomic position and mental health is affected by people's evaluations of the desirability of mental health inventory items, but the existence of the relationship is not *just* an artifact of the distortions arising from a response bias. In the present study, we found that the control of life satisfaction affected the class-symptoms relationship. More specifically, the inverse relationship almost disappeared among respondents with low or medium satisfaction, but remained strong and significant among those with high satisfaction. These findings are not consistent with the "differential expressiveness" explanation, which predicts that the inverse relationship between SES and symptoms will hold across the three categories of life satisfaction. We have not found any reasons to believe that the expressiveness explanation works for respondents with high satisfaction but not for the other two groups of respondents. It should be noted here that in the present study the distributions of men and women among the four socioeconomic groups were approximately the same. Therefore, even if expressiveness might affect the sex-differences in mental disturbance, it would not affect the class-symptoms relationship. In sum, our findings tend to support the position that the inverse relationship between socioeconomic status and psychiatric symptoms is real and is not a result of differential modes of expressing distress. Mental health inventory items, like those devised by Langner, may be useful for the study of class-symptoms relationship, but may not be a valid instrument for the study of sex-differences in mental illness.

CONCLUSION

The major objective of this paper was to conduct a cross-cultural examination of two well-known propositions which were developed in the West, i.e., the relationships of psychiatric symptoms to sex roles and social class. The data were collected from a probability sample of 3,983 adults, aged 20 to 59, in the urban areas of Hong Kong. The prevalence of psychiatric symptoms was measured by Langner's 22 items. The Chinese version of the scale was found to have acceptable reliability and validity.

We found that there were higher rates of psychiatric symptoms among women than men, and among members of lower socioeconomic groups. The effects of sex roles and socioeconomic status on psychiatric symptoms were independent not only of each other but also of age and education.

The concept of achievement-aspiration discrepancies was introduced to interpret the findings. Using the general satisfaction with daily life as an indicator of discrepancies, we found that it partially accounted for the relationship between socioeconomic status and psychiatric symptoms. Hence, the "discrepancies" explanation is probably valid. Individuals in lower socioeconomic position were more likely to be mentally impaired, partly because of their greater discrepancies between achievement and aspiration.

The control of life satisfaction, however, led to an increase rather than a reduction of the relationship between sex roles and psychiatric symptoms. This resulted from a higher level of life satisfaction among women than men. We proposed that explanations other than achievement-aspiration discrepancies should be considered; and we suggested that, in Chinese society, the relationship between sex roles and symptoms might be an artifact of the response bias in field studies using mental health inventory items. Chinese social norms tend to permit women rather than men to be expressive of their distress.

ACKNOWLEDGEMENT

This paper used part of the data in the Hong Kong Biosocial Survey which was funded by the Nuffield Foundation. The survey was mainly designed and conducted by Stephen Boyden and Sheelagh Millar of the Australian National University and Y. K. Chan of The Chinese University of Hong Kong. The analysis of the data for this paper was supported by the Social Research Centre of The Chinese University of Hong Kong. The author wishes to express his appreciation to Fanny Cheung, John Jones and Sheelagh Millar for their suggestions and comments, and Yuet-wah Cheung for his research assistance.

NOTES

1. Both surveys were conducted by the same research team, using an identical research technique and similar diagnostic criteria (Lin, et al. 1969: 67–68).
2. In Mitchell's study, emotional illness was indicated by 11 questions on symptoms, including shortness of breath, heart beating hard, spells of dizziness, nightmares, losing weight, hands sweat, can't get going, trouble getting to sleep, headaches, nervous, and loss of appetite. Those with four or more of these symptoms were labelled emotionally ill.
3. It should be recognized that the use of Langner's scale has recently been criticized on both conceptual and methodological ground. See, for instance, Seiler (1973) and Dohrenwend and Dohrenwend (1976).
4. It needs to be underscored that the present study measures psychiatric morbidity as defined by Langner's 22 items. In effect, we look for "universals" for the purpose of making a comparison between Hong Kong and the West. A study of this kind has its own significance, as it provides a cross-cultural validation of professional psychiatric constructs. However, as Kleinman (1977) has argued, the study may have committed a "category fallacy". That is, we may have superimposed the Western psychiatric categories on the mental states of the Chinese population in Hong Kong. Since somatization exists to a greater extent in Chinese culture than in the West (Wong 1976; Kleinman 1977), the use of Langner's scale in this study may have missed some stress symptoms which are important to the Chinese people, such as the feeling of having insufficient blood and "ch'i" (vital essence), of excessive heat and "fire" inside the body, and of over-accumulation of "gas" in the chest. Furthermore, some of the items (e.g., fainting, loss of appetite, heart beating, and acid stomach) in Langner's scale may be defined by the local population as indications of physical instead of mental sickness, thus creating a gap between the Western professional judgement and the indigenous definition of psychiatric morbidity. We agree with Kleinman (1977) that there is a need for detailed phenomenological descriptions in Hong Kong, and believe that such accounts of cultural specifics would supplement studies (like the present one) which emphasize cultural universals.
5. However, it should be pointed out that the cut off point is essentially arbitary. In their validity studies of the scale, for instance, Mannis (1963) argued that the scale is valid only for scores of 10 or higher, whereas Haese and Meile (1967) concluded that the best cut off point is between 6 and 7 symptoms.

6. It should be made explicit here that this paper adopts the social causation approach, which assumes that the formation of psychiatric symptoms is a consequence of socially-induced stress on the individual (for discussions see, for instance, Dunham 1964; Dohrenwend 1966; and Lee 1976). With the present data, we were unable to provide an adequate test of this assumption. Readers should bear in mind that there are alternative hypotheses. It may be, for instance, that the sex-differences in symptoms are due to physiological factors rather than social roles, and that instead of social causation the social class differences are due to the social selection of individuals with symptoms into lower class status. Further studies are needed to examine these alternative propositions (for some suggestions, see Dohrenwend 1975; and Lee 1976).

7. Gaitz and Scott (1972) also found very little relationship between age and symptoms. Their measurement of psychiatric symptoms is identical to ours, although the age-categories are not the same.

8. An issue of concern is that since life dissatisfaction could be a result, or a component, of psychiatric morbidity, the life satisfaction finding in this study may be an artifact. We would like, however, to remind the readers of an important assumption underlying this study, i.e., the questionnaire item on life satisfaction is used as an indicator of achievement-aspiration discrepancies. Analytically, therefore, life satisfaction (as an indicator of the concept of discrepancies) is distinct from the concept of psychiatric symptoms, and it can be conceived as a determinant of psychiatric symptoms.

9. As an alternative proposition, it may be argued that relative to their male counterparts, the low SES females tend to suffer from greater deprivation than the higher SES females. Consequently, the sex-differences in psychiatric symptoms were greater in the low than the higher SES groups. This argument, however, does not seem to be in line with our data. In a further analysis, we found that females were significantly more satisfied with life than males in all SES groups, and that the magnitudes of sex-differences in life satisfaction were also about the same in these various SES groups.

REFERENCES

Abramson, J. H.
1966 Emotional disorder, status inconsistency and migration. Milbank Fund Quarterly 44 (January): 23–48.
Bradburn, N. M.
1969 The Structure of Psychological Well-Being. Chicago: Aldine.
Chen, John T. S.
1973 1001 Chinese Sayings. Hong Kong: Chung Chi College Press.
Cheng, T. Y.
1977 The Economy of Hong Kong. Hong Kong: Far East.
Cheung, Fanny
Forthcoming Self perception, cultural norm and development: Case studies of 36 Chinese women. To be published in the Journal of The Chinese University of Hong Kong.
Clancy, K., and Walter Gove
1974 Sex differences in mental illness: An analysis of response bias in self-reports. American Journal of Sociology 80 (July): 205–16.
Cooperstock, Ruth
1971 Sex differences in the use of mood-modifying drugs: An explanatory model. Journal of Health and Social Behavior 12 (September): 238–44.
Cronbach, Lee J.
1951 Coefficient alpha and the internal structure of tests. Psychometrika 16 (September): 297–334.

Davis, James A.
  1962 Stipends and Spouses. Chicago: University of Chicago Press.
  1971 Elementary Survey Analysis. N. J.: Prentice-Hall.
Dohrenwend, Bruce P.
  1966 Social status and psychiatric disorder: An issue of substance and an issue of method. American Sociological Review 31 (February): 14–34.
  1975 Sociocultural and social-psychological factors in the genesis of mental disorders. Journal of Health & Social Behavior 16 (December): 365–92.
Dohrenwend, Bruce P., and Dewitt L. Crandell
  1970 Psychiatric symptoms in community, clinic, and mental hospital groups. American Journal of Psychiatry 126 (May): 1611–21.
Dohrenwend, Bruce P., and Barbara S. Dohrenwend
  1976 Sex differences and psychiatric disorders. American Journal of Sociology 81 (May): 1447–54.
Dunham, H. W.
  1964 Anomie and mental disorder. In Anomie and Deviant Behavior. B. Clinard, ed. N.Y.: Free Press; pp. 128–157.
  1970 Social class & mental disorder. British Journal of Social Psychiatry and Community Health 4:76–83.
Faris, R. E., and H. W. Dunham
  1939 Mental Disorders in Urban Areas. Chicago: University of Chicago Press.
Gaitz, C. M. and J. Scott
  1972 Age and the measurement of mental health. Journal of Health & Social Behavior 13 (March): 55–67.
Gove, W. R., and K. Clancy
  1976 Response bias, sex differences, and mental illness: A reply. American Journal of Sociology 81 (May): 1463–70.
Gove, W. R., and J. F. Tudor
  1973 Adult sex roles and mental illness. American Journal of Sociology 76 (January): 812–35.
Haese, Philip, and Richard Meile
  1967 The Relative effectiveness of two models for scoring the mid-town psychological disorder index. Community Mental Health Journal 3 (Winter): 335–42.
Hodge, Robert W.
  1970 Social integration, psychological well-being, and their socioeconomic correlates. In Social Stratification, Edward O. Laumann, ed. N.Y.: The Bobbs-Merrill; pp. 182–206.
Hollingshead, A. B., and F. C. Redlich
  1958 Social Class and Mental Illness. N.Y.: John Willey & Sons.
Hollingshead, A. B., R. A. Ellis, and E. L. Kirby
  1954 Social mobility and mental illness. American Sociological Review 19 (October): 511–20.
Hopkins, K., ed.
  1971 Hong Kong: The Industrial Colony. London: Oxford University Press.
Kish, Leslie
  1965 Survey Sampling. London: John Wiley & Sons.
Kleiner, Robert J., and Seymour Parker
  1963 Goal-striving, social status, and mental disorder: A research review. American Sociological Review 28 (April): 162–203.
Kleinman, Arthur M.
  1977 Depression, somatization and the new cross-cultural psychiatry. Social Science & Medicine 11: 3–10.

Kohn, M. L.
    1968 Social class & schizophrenia: A critical review. *In* The Transmission of Schizo-
         phrenia, David Rosenthal and Seymour S. Kety, eds. London: Pergamon; pp.
         155–173.
Langner, Thomas S.
    1962 A twenty-two item screening score of psychiatric symptoms indicating impair-
         ment. Journal of Health & Social Behavior 3 (Winter): 269–76.
    1965 Psycho-physiological symptoms and status of women in two Mexican com-
         munities. *In* Approaches to Cross-Cultural Psychiatry, J. M. Murphy and A. H.
         Leighton, eds. Ithaca, N.Y.: Cornell University Press.
Langner, T., and S. T. Michael
    1963 Life Stress and Mental Health. N.Y.: The Free Press.
Lau, S. K.
    1977 Utilitarianistic Familism: An Inquiry into the Basis of Political Stability in Hong
         Kong. Research Report of the Social Research Centre, The Chinese University of
         Hong Kong.
Lee, Rance P. L.
    1976 The causal priority between socioeconomic status and psychiatric disorder: A
         prospective study. The International Journal of Social Psychiatry 22 (Spring):
         1–8.
Leighton D. C., J. S. Harding, D. B. Macklin, A. M. Macmillan, and A. H. Leighton
    1963 The Charter of Danger. N.Y.: Basic Books.
Lin, T. Y.
    1953 A study of incidence of mental disorders in Chinese and other cultures. Psychiatry
         16: 313–36.
Lin, T. Y., H. Rin, E. K. Yeh, C. C. Hsu, and H. M. Chu
    1969 Mental disorders in Taiwan, fifteen years later: A preliminary report." *In* Mental
         Health Research in Asia and the Pacific, W. Caudill and T. Y. Lin, eds. Honolulu:
         East-West Center; pp. 67–91.
Manis, J., M. Brawer, C. Hunt, and L. Kercher
    1963 Validating a mental health scale. American Sociological Review 28 (February):
         108–16.
Meile, Richard, and Philip N. Haese
    1969 Social status, status incongruence, and symptoms of stress. Journal of Health
         & Social Behavior 10 (September): 237–44.
Merton, Robert
    1959 Social Theory and Social Structure, Revised and Enlarged Edition. Glencoe: Free
         Press.
Mishler, Elliot G., and Norman A. Scotch
    1965 Sociocultural factors in the epidemiology of schizophrenia: A review. Inter-
         national Journal of Psychiatry 1 (April): 258–305.
Mitchell, R. E.
    1969 Levels of Emotional Strain in Southeast Asian Cities, Vols. I & II. A Project of the
         Urban Family Life Survey, The Chinese University of Hong Kong, Hong Kong.
Nathanson, C. A.
    1975 Illness and the feminine role: A theoretical review. Social Science & Medicine
         9: 57–62.
Phillips, D. L.
    1966 The "true" prevalence of mental illness in a New England state. Community
         Mental Health Journal 2 (Spring): 35–40.
Phillips, Derek, and Kevin Clancy
    1970 "Response biases in field studies of mental illness." American Sociological Review
         35 (June): 503–15.

Phillips, D. L., and B. F. Segal
1969 Sexual status and psychiatric symptoms. American Sociological Review 34 (February): 58–72.
Porritt, D., and S. Millar
1976 Psychometrics of the dependent variables. Unpublished manuscript, Australian National University.
Rin, H., et al.
1966 Psychophysiological reactions of a rural and suburban population in Taiwan. Acta Psychiatrica Scandinavica 42:410–473.
Rinehart, James W.
1968 Mobility aspiration-achievement discrepancies and mental illness. Social Problems 15 (Spring): 478–88.
Rosenberg, Morris
1968 The Logic of Survey Analysis. N.Y.: Basic Books.
Schader R., M. Ebert, and J. Harmatz
1971 Langner's psychiatric impairment scale: A short screening device. American Journal of Psychiatry 128 (November): 569–601.
Seiler, Lauren H.
1973 The 22-item scale used in field studies of mental illness: A question of method, a question of substance, and a question of theory. Journal of Health & Social Behavior 14 (September): 252–64.
Shively, A. M.
1972 Kwun Tong Life Quality Study: Data Book. Unpublished document of the Social Research Centre, The Chinese University of Hong Kong.
Shively, A. M., and Stanley Shively
1972 Value changes during a period of modernization: The case of Hong Kong. Occasional paper of the Social Research Centre, The Chinese University of Hong Kong.
Suits, D. B.
1954 Use of dummy variables in regression equations. Journal of American Statistical Association 52: 548–51.
Turner, R. Jay
1972 The epidemiological study of schizophrenia: A current appraisal. Journal of Health & Social Behavior 13 (December): 360–69.
Wong, Aline
1975 Women in Modern Singapore. Singapore: University Education Press.
Wong, C. L.
1976 An appraisal of psychiatric symptoms, with special reference to psychiatric private Practice in Hong Kong. Hong Kong Journal of Mental Health 5 (December): 5–7.
Yap, P. M.
1965 Phenomenology of affective disorder in Chinese and other cultures. In Transcultural Psychiatry, A. V. S. DeReuck and R. Porter, eds. Boston: Little, Brown; pp. 84–114.

MAVIS TSAI, L. NEAL TENG, STANLEY SUE

15. MENTAL HEALTH STATUS OF
CHINESE IN THE UNITED STATES

Among the more intriguing issues regarding Chinese in the United States is the mental health status of this population. Owing to the increased influx of Chinese immigration, emerging public images of Chinese-American socio-economic success, and expanded interest in ethnic cultures in the United States, social scientists have made greater attempts to understand the psychological well-being of this group.

The purpose of this chapter is to analyze the mental health status of Chinese in the United States, a minority group conservatively estimated to number about 800,000 individuals by 1980 (Owan 1975). First, rates of mental disorders and personality are discussed. Second, social stressors that influence psychological well-being are outlined. Third, special Chinese populations at risk for mental disorders as well as special problems such as juvenile delinquency and suicide are given particular attention. Finally, implications for mental health are drawn. It should be noted that in discussing Chinese-Americans, one is inevitably confronted with the diverse within-group differences in terms of degree of acculturation, generational status in the United States, area of residence, primary language facility (Cantonese, Mandarin, or English), etc. Although the heterogeneity of Chinese-Americans limits the applicability of generalizations, for heuristic purposes we shall try to indicate the interaction between Chinese culture and living in the United States.

RATES OF MENTAL DISORDERS

There have been two major methods used to determine the incidence or prevalence of mental disorders in the population: (1) the use of untreated cases and (2) the use of treated cases. The former method involves survey techniques (interviews or psychological tests) to assess the mental health status of a representative sample of a population of interest. To our knowledge, there are no studies of this kind on the Chinese population in the United States. The latter method — use of treated cases — estimates the rates of mental disorders on the basis of the number of individuals in a population who receive treatment for mental disorders in mental health facilities (e.g., hospitals, clinics, and community mental health centers) or by private practitioners. The use of treated cases essentially assumes that demand for mental health services is a reflection of a population's mental health needs.

Research on the utilization of mental health facilities by Chinese-Americans consistently demonstrated three findings. First, relatively few Chinese are admitted as psychiatric patients. Jew and Brody (1967) investigated the hospital-

A. Kleinman and T.-Y. Lin (eds.), Normal and Abnormal Behavior in Chinese Culture, 291–310.

ization rate (first admissions) between 1854–1961 in California. They found that although the Chinese hospitalization rate has gradually increased during the last century, Chinese still have significantly lower rates of first admissions to mental hospitals than non-Chinese. Similar findings have been reported by Berk and Hirata (1973), Brown, Stein, Huang, and Harris (1973), and True (1975) in California. Sue and McKinney (1975) found that in 17 community mental health facilities only 0.1% of the patients were Chinese when the population areas served by these facilities included 0.6% Chinese. Second, the small proportion of Chinese who utilize psychiatric facilities tended to be more severely disturbed than Caucasian patients. This observation appears to be true regardless of the type of patient, type of facility, and type of assessment procedure. For example, Brown et al. (1973) reported that Chinese inpatients in a psychiatric hospital were more disturbed than their Caucasian counterparts on the basis of behavioral ratings on Lorr's Twelve Psychotic Syndromes scale. On the basis of MMPI performances, Chinese-American students exhibited greater psychopathology than Caucasians at a university psychiatric service (Sue and Sue 1974). Finally, Sue and McKinney (1975) found that Chinese and other Asian-American patients at community mental health centers were more likely to be given a psychotic diagnosis than were Caucasian patients. Third, there is evidence that Chinese have a greater tendency than Caucasians to express emotional disorders through somatic complaints (Kleinman 1975; Marsella, Kinzie, and Gordon 1973; Sue and Sue 1974; Tseng 1975; Tseng & Char 1974). The mind-body distinction is, perhaps, less pronounced in Chinese than in Western industrialized cultures. In summary, research on Chinese-Americans suggests that they underutilize mental health facilities, they are more disturbed when seen as patients, and they express psychological disturbance through bodily symptoms.

It would be tempting but unwarranted to conclude that because of the low utilization rates of mental health facilities, Chinese-Americans have low rates of mental disturbance. Utilization reflects "illness behavior," that is, what one does when experiencing emotional problems. There are many additional factors besides emotional problems that determine utilization. The following have been proposed as factors inhibiting self-referral for professional mental health services:

(1) *Stigma and shame over mental disturbance and illness behavior.* Although all families, not just Chinese, become upset over the mental disturbance exhibited by a family member, the stigma of mental illness seems much greater among Chinese than among the general U.S. population. The Chinese are particularly affected because kinship relationships are considered extremely important. The integrity or "goodness" of the family is threatened when one member shows deviant behavior. A related reason for the stigma attached to mental illness among Chinese is the belief that mental illness may be inherited — its presence in a family can lead to the labeling of that family's offspring unfit for marriage (Kleinman 1977). The family's feelings of shame and desires to keep the disturbed member's behaviors from public attention may inhibit utilization of professional mental health resources.

(2) *Availability of alternative resources.* The stigma of mental illness, combined with kinship loyalty and a sense of obligation to care for the mentally ill family member, frequently result in efforts by emotionally disturbed individuals to seek help from their families, friends, respected intermediaries, etc., rather than mental health professionals. In a study of ethnicity and patterns of help-seeking in Vancouver, Canada, Lin, Tardiff, Donetz, and Goresky (1978) found that the help-seeking pattern of Chinese patients was characterized by early, prolonged efforts by the family to intervene with problems. Remarkably advanced psychotic symptoms were tolerated as long as there was no excessively disruptive behavior. When external assistance was sought, patients' somatization of their psychological problems led them to general practitioners and medical clinics rather than mental health clinics. For Chinese and other ethnic groups, cultural resources such as herbal medicine or acupuncture may also be used.

(3) *Cost of mental health services.* Mental health services can be financially costly and many Chinese may not be able to afford such services. Although financial considerations are important, offering free mental health services does not necessarily increase utilization. For example, Brown et al. (1973) reported a program whereby mental health services were offered free of charge at a facility in Chinatown, Los Angeles. There was no significant increase of admissions to the facility.

(4) *Location and knowledge of facilities.* The location of mental health services (i.e., the accessibility) and knowledge about these services are important in influencing utilization. If facilities are located far away and are inconvenient to use and if there is inadequate knowledge of the availability of services, these resources will not be employed. For example, Kim (1975) found that about one-third of Chinese who participated in a survey reported that they often failed to seek help for problems because they did not know where to go. Insufficient knowledge was particularly a strong factor for immigrant and women respondents. Note that convenient location and adequate knowledge do not ensure utilization for emotional problems. Rather, these two factors are necessary but not sufficient conditions for seeking professional mental health services.

(5) *Hours of operation.* Many Chinese, particularly those who work in Chinatowns, have unusual or long working hours. If mental health facilities provide most of their services during normal business hours, many Chinese are simply unable to use services.

(6) *Belief systems about mental health.* Belief systems, expectations, and causal attributions for mental disturbance influence help seeking behaviors. Traditional modes of treatment in mental health facilities such as psychotherapy, behavior therapy, group therapy, etc., may be perceived as being ineffective to those persons who have non-Western beliefs about behaviors and emotions. For example, Chinese and other Asians are more likely than Caucasians to believe that mental health is due to the avoidance of morbid thoughts and that mental illness is due to organic factors (Sue, Wagner, Ja, Margullis, and Lew 1976). If

this is the case, then Chinese-American patients who are asked by therapists to talk about personal and emotional problems (i.e, to discuss "morbid" thoughts) may feel uncomfortable and may believe that psychotherapy is of little benefit. It also follows that if many Chinese perceive mental illness as an organic disorder, somatic forms of treatment may be more readily accepted and expected. Brown et al. (1973) indicate that medication and problem solving approaches appear to be more effective than insight-oriented therapy for many Chinese patients. The main point is that an emotionally disturbed person is not likely to seek help from mental health agencies if the person believes that mental health agencies do not address the right issues and problems in treatment.

(7) *Responsiveness of services.* In the previous discussion regarding belief systems, it is obvious that Chinese may find treatment procedures strange or inappropriate. A larger issue is whether current psychotherapeutic practices are effective with this patient group. The lack of bilingual therapists is a major problem encountered by Chinese patients who mainly speak Chinese. In Kim's (1975) survey, Chinese considered a bilingual staff as the most important characteristic of a service agency. Helpfulness of staff was the next most important characteristic. Helpfulness presumably refers to concerned and dedicated staff who show respect for clients and who are effective and understand the cultural values and experiences of clients. Interestingly, convenient access to agencies, confidentiality of services, and cost of services, while important to some respondents, were clearly of secondary importance.

DISCUSSION

Our ability to estimate the rate of mental disorders in the Chinese-American population is extremely limited. Surveys of mental disturbance in untreated cases do not exist. Utilization patterns of mental health facilities (i.e., treated cases) suggest that few Chinese seek help from these facilities. The important issue concerns the reasons for the low utilization patterns. The argument that low demand for services is due to low needs for mental health services appears to be weak. While Chinese are underrepresented as psychiatric patients, there is evidence that those who seek help are severely disturbed. A reasonable hypothesis is that the most severely disturbed individuals become psychiatric patients because they have no other resources with which to deal with their problems. Chinese with milder problems may simply avoid using services for a variety of reasons. The unresponsiveness of treatment programs, the stigma of mental illness, financial cost, availability of alternative resources, location and knowledge of services, hours of available services, and beliefs about mental health are factors that influence illness behavior and utilization of professional services. Rates of mental disturbance have probably been severely underestimated for Chinese-Americans. This will become more apparent as we examine research on personality and social stressors encountered by this ethnic group.

PERSONALITY

There is now growing recognition that psychological well-being is not simply the absence of mental disorders. One can be free of mental disorders and yet show poor mental health — low feelings of self-esteem, of environmental mastery, of autonomy, and of self-actualization. Therefore, in order to understand the psychological well-being of Chinese-Americans, mental health and personality must also be examined.

Studies that have used various personality measures to assess the psychological characteristics of Chinese-Americans have consistently shown that they differ from Caucasian-Americans on a number of personality attributes. For example, Sue and Kirk (1972; 1973) systematically compared Chinese-American students with the general population of students at the University of California, Berkeley. The following assessment measures were used: Omnibus Personality Inventory, Strong Vocational Interest Blank, and the School and College Ability Test. Chinese, compared to the general student body (mainly Caucasians), were (a) higher on quantitative and lower on verbal performances on the Ability Test, (b) more interested in physical sciences and applied-technical fields and less interested in social sciences, aesthetic-cultural fields, and verbal-linguistic vocations, and (c) more conforming and less socially extroverted, preferring concrete-tangible approaches to life and reporting greater emotional distress. Subsequent analysis of the data (Sue and Frank 1973) suggests that there is considerable heterogeneity within the Chinese-American group but that ethnic differences are distinguishable. Similar findings have been shown in other studies. Abbott (1976) compared the responses of Chinese in Taipei versus Chinese in San Francisco on the California Personality Inventory. Mean profiles for the two groups were strikingly similar when age and sex were controlled. The overall Chinese profile included high scores on self-control, good impression, and femininity in both sexes; however, lower scores were found on poise, ascendancy, self-assurance, tolerance, intellectual efficiency, well-being, and flexibility. Scofield and Sun (1960) found a group of Chinese immigrant students to be more withdrawn, shy, emotionally insecure, sensitive, suspicious, and aloof than Caucasian-American college students. The overall findings from these studies suggest that Chinese in the United States differ from Caucasian-Americans and that the differences favor greater emotional disturbance (i.e., less mental health) for Chinese.

The issue of whether Chinese-Americans actually do exhibit less mental health has plagued researchers. Certainly, personality studies appear to show more emotional problems among Chinese than Caucasians. Before the issue can be resolved, three questions must be answered. First, since most studies have examined college students, what is the generality of research findings with respect to the entire population of Chinese in the United States? Second, how valid are assessment procedures? This question deals with the culture fairness of assessment measures that are standardized in the United States and used with culturally different groups. A related problem is that response sets may differ between Chinese and Caucasian-Americans. For example, Chinese may self-report more psychological distress simply because they are more honest, less defensive, or more serious in their test-taking task. Third, how should personality differences between Chinese and Caucasians be interpreted? That is, even if ethnic differences exist, what is the relevance of these differences for evaluating mental health? The fact that Chinese-Americans are more conforming, less extroverted, less flexible, etc., can be seen as positive rather than negative attributes. Since Americans generally value independence, individualism, extroversion, assertiveness, and flexibility, there is a tendency to define differences exhibited by other ethnic groups as deficits. It is clear that mental health cannot be solely defined by one cultural group's standards and then applied to different groups.

Our belief is that Chinese-Americans do experience conditions that lower mental health. It is not that characteristics such as conformity, introversion, etc., are intrinsically maladaptive. Rather, when behavioral patterns learned through one's family or subculture are negatively valued by the larger or dominant culture, then serious conflicts may arise for that individual. Let us now examine the conditions that create stress and conflict for Chinese-Americans.

SOCIAL STRESSORS

In a previous paper, Sue and Chin (in press) argued that Chinese-Americans encounter stress because of culture conflict, rapid social change, and prejudice and discrimination. Since mental health is influenced by stressors, it is important to examine these phenomena.

1. Culture Conflict

Culture conflict presumably exists whenever members of one culture come into contact with another culture in which norms, values, and behavioral patterns are significantly different; and whenever conformity to each culture is either rewarded and socialized or is punished by the other culture.

As the family is the fundamental unit of Chinese culture, and the primary socializing agent for offspring, a description of traditional Chinese families will provide a better understanding of cultural values. A social hierarchy exists in the family system assigning a prescribed status to each individual on the basis of generation, age, and sex. The members of a senior generation are considered superior to those of a junior generation, while within each generation older members take precedence over younger members. In addition, males occupy a superior position relative to females; sons are valued over daughters (Fong 1973). The primary allegiance of a son is to the family; obligations as a father and husband are secondary. Daughters are expected to do domestic work, to marry, to help their mothers-in-law, and to bear children. Whenever economically feasible, the extended family system encourages the habitation of several generations of blood relatives under one roof.

In the traditional family, elders are viewed with great reverence. Unquestioning obedience and loyal devotion to parents are encouraged. Parent-child relationships are characterized by a formal, respectful expression of role expectations. Independent behavior which might deviate from traditional norms is suppressed to keep the family intact. Children are taught to sacrifice self-expression and to restrain emotional displays in the interest of maintaining family solidarity. The inculcation of guilt and shame are the principal techniques used in controlling the behavior of family members. Deviant behavior of one individual is considered to reflect negatively on the entire family. High value is placed on the attainment of a good education and the building of a respectable reputation in the community.

Although the traditional family structure and its subcultural values are in transition, many values from the past are still retained by Chinese parents in the United States (Young 1972). In a study of the child-rearing attitudes of various subcultures in America, Krigler and Kroes (1973) reported that Chinese mothers are stricter with their children than are their Jewish and Protestant counterparts. Interview data by Sollenberger (1968) showed that Chinese parents are much stricter in controlling their children's aggression than are American parents. The Rorschach performances of Chinese adolescents in Hawaii differed qualitatively from those of a Chicago sample of American youth (Hsu, Watrous, and Lord 1961). When faced with a novel situation, they were seen to be typically cautious, constricted, and conventional. Chinese-American responses showed more conformity to parental wishes and tended to suggest a submissive acceptance of the environment.

In the process of growing up in the United States, one's commitment to Chinese cultural norms can be eroded by the influences of the peer group, the school system, and the mass media. When Chinese children enter the American school system, they learn new social values which conflict with those of their parental culture (Fong 1968). The American way of life emphasizes "individual-centeredness" (Hsu 1970) — autonomy, assertiveness, and independence — within a youth-oriented perspective (Barnett 1958). These values are in direct contrast to the Chinese values of generational continuity, family solidarity, respect for elders, and situation-centeredness whereby individual impulses are subordinated to the will of the family or group.

The detrimental effects of exposure to different cultural demands are well-documented. A study by Kurokawa (1969) suggests that acculturation conflict may be related to accident or injury-proneness in Chinese-and Japanese-American children. It was found that acculturated children with unacculturated parents are more likely to have accidents than are unacculturated children. The former are caught between contradictions: traditionally oriented parents teach their children to be cautious, to control their impulses, and not to show initiative; while their schoolmates stress daring and athletic prowess. Kurokawa speculates that the child in this situation was likely to receive injuries for two reasons: (1) due to conflicts at home, he/she is more apt to be tense, to lack alertness, and to be less capable of coping with hazardous situations, and (2) he/she may be more anxious for recognition by the white peer group and will court danger in order to prove his/her courage.

The conflcit over parental authority seems to heighten during adolescence (Fong 1968; Chun-Hoon 1971; R. H. Lee 1960; Sung 1971). Such conflicts have been vividly depicted in two autobiographies by Chinese-Americans – *Fifth Chinese Daughter* by Jade Snow Wong (1950) and *Father and Glorious Descendant* by Pardee Lowe (1943). In reviewing the case study of a Chinese-American client, Sommers (1960) notes that the incompatibility of Oriental-Occidental values may lead to severe difficulties in developing a stable identity. Similarly, Bourne (1975) argues that acculturation cannot be achieved without exacting a toll in terms of psychic and emotional turmoil. He found that Chinese-American clients from a large West Coast university mental health clinic exhibited intense anxiety over inability to reconcile parental wishes regarding filial piety and academic achievement. Male problems clustered around social isolation, passivity, and academic achievement needs; whereas females experienced guilt developed from liaisons with Caucasian men. These findings are comparable to those of Weiss (1970), who investigated the dating attitudes of Chinese-Americans in a field study, postulating that the acculturation process can create intense conflicts. He suggests that Chinese-American females are more acculturated and have received more complimentary stereotypes than males. Therefore, they come to expect the males they date will behave boldly and aggressively in the Western manner; and they can be quite vehement in their denunciation of Asian male traits. Chinese-American males, on the other hand, are under strong pressures to achieve academically and have fewer opportunities to learn adaptive social skills.

The above studies have shown that exposure to cultural diversity with concomitant demands for allegiance to opposing forces is a stressor which can be detrimental to mental health. Three different reactions to this stress have been described (Sue and Sue 1971). A person may: 1) remain allied to the values of his/her own culture; 2) attempt to become over-Westernized and reject Chinese ways; or 3) attempt to integrate aspects of both cultures which he/she believes are functional to his/her own self-esteem and identity.

2. Social Change

In a transitional world, conflict is generated as old roles are undone and new ones emerge (Fong 1973). Social change can be quite stressful to the extent that it occurs faster than one's ability to find adjustive techniques and resources.

A growing body of evidence suggests that major life changes can diminish physical and mental health. Holmes and Masuda (1974) have found that life events (e.g., death of spouse, change in residence, a new job, child leaving home) can be assigned numerical values that indicate the magnitude of social readjustment required. Furthermore, the accumulation of many life changes over a short period of time has been found to negatively correlate with well-being (Dohrenwend and Dohrenwend 1974). This is particularly true if the life events are undesirable (e.g., death of spouse) rather than desirable (e.g., marriage). Hinkle (1974) investigated a sample of China-born persons in the United States who had undergone considerable cultural and social changes. Results of medical examinations and psychological tests revealed that as a group these Chinese experienced greater medical problems than a comparable age group of Americans. It seems that many intense life changes over short time spans create stress which strains the adaptive capacity of individuals. Such findings have been confirmed cross-culturally (Holmes and Masuda 1974). Although social change is experienced by everyone, we shall focus on the issues confronting three groups at risk for extensive life changes – immigrants, the elderly, and women.

Approximately 20,000 Chinese immigrate to the United States each year. The Chinese population in this country is increasingly becoming an immigrant group. In fact, the Chinese-American population has increased by 89% since 1960, two-thirds of these being immigrants (Bridge 1975). Immigrants undoubtedly experience severe life changes. Being in a foreign country, experiencing disruption of previous social relationships, trying to find a job, and encountering prejudice and discrimination are major life events that require substantial social readjustment. Persons who do not have resources to facilitate transition from one culture to another are likely to be at risk for physical and psychological disturbances. Many post-1955 immigrants have come to the United States without adequate financial resources or knowledge of English. Consequently they are forced to accept menial jobs. Given jobs with low wages and long hours, they are unable to improve their position because of the lack of time to learn English or new skills (Chen 1970).

In order to have more familiar surroundings, many Chinese immigrants live in Chinatown although living conditions for its residents are deplorable. They are afflicted with complex social problems such as inadequate health care, overcrowding, unemployment, poverty, and crime. A case in point is San Francisco's Chinatown, the largest in this country. It spans 42 square blocks and contains 885 persons per acre, ten times the national average. One-third of the families have incomes which fall below the federal poverty level (Yee 1970). This level of indigence is related to the fact that the lack of English language facility compelled many immigrants to seek employment in garment factory sweatshops, notorious for compensation well below minimum wage and for deplorable working conditions (Allard 1975). Certain sections of Chinatown's economic-political establishment appear to perpetuate poverty by threatening employees with deportation if they complain about the long hours, low pay, and unsanitary working conditions (Chen 1970). The 67% rate of substandard housing contributes to abnormally high rates of tuberculosis. Two-thirds of the residents have received less than a seventh grade education. Moreover, high rates of delinquency have become acknowledged by the community (Yee 1970). Similar problems have been documented for Chinatowns in New York (Yuan 1966), Philadelphia (Jung 1976), and Boston (Murphy 1971).

Roughly 90% of the elderly Chinese in San Francisco are immigrants; very few are fluent in English (Kalish and Yuen 1971). For many of them the material comfort, esteem, and prestige traditionally accorded the aged in Asia have assumed dimensions of poverty, misunderstanding, and social and physical alienation from the dominant culture in America (Kalish and Moriwaki 1973; Yuen 1972).

Compounding cultural and language barriers has been the erosion of traditional generational continuity and filial piety among younger Chinese-Americans (Fujii 1976). Today two-thirds of the immigrant aged live independently of their families, and their American-born grandchildren do not speak Chinese. Discrepancies between the elderly's expectations and the actual practices of their middle-aged progeny are reflected in areas of loyalty, respect, devotion, living arrangements, and financial support (Wu 1975).

The consequences of social change and of culture conflict can also be seen in sex roles. In the United States sex roles are moving in the direction of greater equality. The impact of such changes is unclear although both Chinese-American women and men must reconcile contemporary sex roles with past sex roles in traditional Chinese culture. For example, the educational ambitions of contemporary Chinese females have broadened, but their emerging role is not fully accepted by all segments of Chinese society (Fong 1973). The tension between the need to develop a greater capacity for self-assertion and achievements on the one hand, and the pressure to maintain "sex appropriate" traditional roles (as daughter, wife, or mother) on the other, must be resolved (Fujitomi and Wong 1973). Fong and Peskin (1969) hypothesized that Chinese female students would experience greater conflict with, and rebellion against, Chinese culture than Chinese males. That is, since the role of student has been encouraged more strongly for Chinese males than for the females, those females who attended college would exhibit more alienation with their traditional Chinese sex roles. Results on the California Psychological Inventory supported this hypothesis. Sue and Kirk (1975) also believe that a domestic versus a feminist role conflict may be quite intense for Chinese-American female students. They found that Chinese-American females extensively used the counseling services at a major West Coast university for vocational and personal problems. In summary, rapid social change especially for immigrants, the elderly, and females may place individuals under a great deal of stress and strain.

3. Prejudice and Discrimination

Racial prejudice and discrimination against Chinese in the United States is an ill-concealed fact. It has been abundantly documented in areas of Congressional anti-Chinese legislation (Lyman 1974), multiple aspects of health, education, and welfare (Owan 1975), and distorted stereotypes (Chin 1972). Whether racial discrimination by the white majority is an antecedent, a concomitant, or a direct causative factor in the mental health of Chinese-Americans has not been conclusively determined. What the bulk of evidence does suggest is that exposure to either covert or overt racial discrimination is an additional stressor which, like any other major stressor, places the mental health of a population at higher risk. Racism appears to complicate successful coping with life tasks in several distinct psychological areas, particularly in the achievement of an adequate self-concept, interpersonal intimacy, and feelings of control over one's fate.

While many individuals readily admit that Chinese in the United States have suffered racial prejudice and discrimination in past years, some feel that Chinese are no longer victims of racism. This view, supplemented by statistics regarding high median family incomes, high educational attainments, and upward occupational mobility, maintains that discrimination is a thing of the past. We do not want to belabor the point, except to indicate that Chinese still encounter prejudice and discrimination. An ethnic minority can show upward mobility as a group and still experience discrimination (Sue 1977). It is also true that within such a group, variability in achievement patterns may be quite high.

Negative or inaccurate stereotypes in the mass media, lack of responsiveness to the needs of Chinese-Americans, differential treatment on the basis of race, etc., all have effects on psychological well-being. For example, racial self-hatred, poor self-esteem, and conflicts in self-identity may emerge in Chinese-American children (Fox and Jordan 1973). Sue (1977) believes that prejudice and discrimination against a group can result in perceptions of noncontrol whereby outcomes are not dependent upon individual behaviors but are related to race. That is, the outcome of personal initiative may be affected more by racial prejudice than individual merit. In such a situation, one learns to be helpless and feels unable to control fate (Seligman 1975), which in turn influences mental health. Kuo, Gary, and Lin (1975) found that (1) many Chinese-Americans reported that they felt unable to control their fates or destinies (i.e., an external locus of control) and (2) degree of externality was positively related to psychological distress.

In summary, mental health is influenced by the nature and extent of stress. Because of culture conflict, rapid social change, and discrimination, Chinese-Americans are under a substantial amount of stress. We have assumed from the available research that rates of mental disturbance have been underestimated for Chinese-Americans and that in view of the many stressors experienced by them, their positive mental health is being affected.

OTHER FORMS OF DEVIANT BEHAVIOR

As mentioned previously, research on deviant behaviors among Chinese-Americans has been lacking. We would now like to briefly discuss the available knowledge on specific problems such as juvenile delinquency, suicide, drug abuse, and alcoholism, realizing that studies have been conducted on selected Chinese samples and the research methodology used is often limited.

1. Juvenile Delinquency

One of the most salient aspects of the growing Chinese population in America is the surge in youthfulness, made possible by the balancing of the sex ratio and the formation of nuclear families with children. For many years, the Chinese population was heavily overrepresented by older males who came to this country as laborers. With the signing of a new immigration act by President Johnson in 1965, females and youths could more freely enter the United States. This meant that the number of youths could increase through immigration and through the formation of families which was not as likely to occur when the population of Chinese females was small.

Until the late 1960's it was believed that juvenile delinquency among Chinese was very rare. Abbott and Abbott (1968) found that the rate of juvenile delinquency among Chinese-Americans in San Francisco was extremely low. A number of explanations have been brought forth to account for this low rate. First, the low rate may be more apparent than real. Methods of sampling and collecting data may simply undercount Chinese delinquency. Second, past studies showing low rates of Chinese juvenile delinquency may actually be reflecting the small proportion of juveniles (youths). As noted before, the Chinese population for many decades was overrepresented with older males. Third, many persons feel that Chinese cultural values, family patterns, strict control over aggressive and antisocial behaviors, etc., have inhibited juvenile delinquency. All three factors have probably been responsible for the low official rates of juvenile delinquency among Chinese.

One fact is certain, however. Within the past 10 years, there has been a tremendous increase in gang violence in some of the larger American China-towns. In San Francisco, at least 17 persons were slain between 1971 and 1973, and this figure doubled to at least 35 between 1973 and 1975 (Allard 1975). Youth gangs or youth gang members have been involved with murder, other forms of violence, extortion, and robbery. There seems to be no single factor that can fully explain why these problems have occurred. Many of the gang members are immigrants, school dropouts, and poor. Unaccepted by the traditional Chinese organizations and social groups, they have a difficult time functioning outside of the Chinese community. Most feel angry, frustrated, and alienated. Gangs seem to have several functions such as providing members with status possibilities, belongingness, protection, and economic gains (through extortion). Territorial disputes and other conflicts have arisen between rival gangs.

2. Suicide

Intense emotional and psychological stress and isolation may lead to loneliness and hopelessness. The suicide rate for Chinese throughout the United States in unknown. Bourne (1973) conducted a study of the suicide rate among Chinese in San Francisco for the period of 1952–1968. He noted that over the 16 year period, the rate of suicide for Chinese equalled that of the general San Francisco population. (Incidentally, the San Francisco rate is among the highest in the nation.) While suicide was once four to five times more prevalent among Chinese males than females, the ratio has steadily changed in recent years with a growing incidence of Chinese women committing suicide. For both sexes, suicides are most likely to occur between 55 and 65 years of age, although the mean age of male suicides has been progressively decreasing. Some other interesting patterns were also noted. Consistent with city-wide trends, barbiturate overdose has become the most frequent mode of suicide although among Chinese women hanging is more common. Firearms have not been used by Chinese men in a single case since 1965. Suicide in the Chinese male is most often imputed to despondency over poor physical health, as contrasted with the Chinese female who typically has suffered interpersonal conflicts and sometimes a past history of identified psychiatric disorder. Increasing assimilation may cause Chinese suicide patterns to approximate those of the general population.

3. Drug Abuse

Studies of drug usage in various parts of the country suggest that there is an overrepresentation of drug abuse in the Asian (including Chinese)-American population. In California, a state with one of the highest concentrations of Asians, they comprise 3% of the population. The percentage of Asians in the penal system is 4%, and of these 95% are incarcerated for drug-related offenses (Namkung 1972). In a study of the records of Chinese narcotic addicts at the U.S. Public Health Service Hospital in Lexington, Kentucky from 1957 to 1962, Ball and Lau (1966) found Chinese constituted almost 3% of the 32,209 male addicts treated at the hospital. The Chinese, however, comprised less than one-fifth of one percent of the U.S. male population. Nakagawa and Watanabe (1973) surveyed the Asian junior and senior high school population in Seattle, Washington, to determine the incidence of drug usage. Of the 65% of students who returned the questionnaires on personal usage of hard drugs (excluding marijuana and alcohol), 12% of the males and 17% of the females were classified as "users." They concluded that a drug problem exists within the Seattle Asian-American community.

Although two of these studies included Chinese with other Asian ethnic groups and although use of treated cases to estimate prevalence of drug abuse may be a poor procedure, the findings do suggest that drug abuse is a serious problem among Chinese-Americans. It is interesting to note that Hsu (1970) has indicated that Chinese have traditionally used drugs as medication, and some as a result become addicted. Most addicts have also been among older rather than younger persons. Drugs apparently serve to enhance their harmony with the environment by reducing conflict. Caucasian-American addicts tend to be younger, to seek "highs," and to act out personal predilections. Hsu points to the cultural differences between Chinese and Americans in drug use. It follows from Hsu's analysis that Chinese-American patterns of drug use may become increasingly similar to those of Caucasian-Americans as increased assimilation occurs. What is interesting but unclear at this point is whether Chinese-Americans who are bicultural Americans will develop behavioral patterns unique to a bicultural heritage – neither "Chinese" nor "American."

4. Alcoholism

As in the case of the other disorders discussed, solid empirical data on the incidence of alcoholism are lacking. Available evidence suggests that the rate of Chinese-American alcoholism is low, according to anthropological studies of Chinatowns, hospital admission rates, and small sample surveys (Sue, Zane, and Ito 1979). Two explanations have been proposed to account for this low rate of alcoholism: (1) genetic racial differences in alcohol sensitivity; and (2) cultural differences in attitudes and values toward the use of alcohol. As indicated by Sue et al. (1979), some studies have shown that Chinese are far more likely than Caucasians to show facial flushing after the ingestion of alcohol. This differential flushing was demonstrated even after testing Chinese who were raised on American diets, after drinking less alcohol per person than Caucasians, and after testing Chinese versus Caucasian infants. The hypothesis is that Chinese have greater autonomic nervous system reactivity to alcohol or that they have aversive reactions to alcohol. The alternative explanation is that excessive drinking behavior is discouraged by family and community attitudes, values, and sanctions. However, Chinese often freely consume alcohol at meals or social functions in moderation.

It is difficult to compare the adequacy of the genetic and cultural explanations for several reasons. First, genetic differences may exist between the races and cultural values may have evolved because of these differences. Second, genetic racial differences such as flushing may exist but may not directly influence drinking behaviors. Third, cultural proscriptions against excessive alcohol consumption may be the underlying basis for observed or self-reported physiological reactions. Finally, both genetic and cultural factors may be important in drinking patterns.

To test the importance of cultural factors, Sue et al. (1979) surveyed reported drinking behaviors, demographic characteristics, and values of Chinese, Japanese, and Caucasian-Americans. Findings indicated that Chinese reported much less alcohol consumption than Caucasians. Degree of assimilation to Western values was directly related to self-reports of drinking among Chinese. Chinese were also more likely than Caucasians to report negative attitudes (their own and those of their parents) toward drinking alcohol. The results supported the importance of cultural factors in drinking patterns.

In this section, we have tried to briefly indicate specific problems such as juvenile delinquency, suicide, drug abuse, and alcoholism. The paucity of research on the rates of these disorders and on hypotheses regarding their nature and causes severely limits our ability to characterize Chinese-Americans. Another confounding factor is that with the arrival of new immigrants, changes in the nature of Chinese communities, and other rapid changes, results from studies are quickly dated. Thus, caution must be exercised in analyzing available research.

CHINESE-AMERICAN RESOURCES

Thus far, we have indicated that (1) rates of mental disorders have been under-estimated for Chinese-Americans; (2) personality and mental health are affected by stressors such as culture conflict, rapid social change, and prejudice and discrimination, paricularly in the case of immigrants, the elderly, and women; and (3) little is known about juvenile delinquency, suicide, drug abuse, and alcoholism at this point. Our discussion has mainly focused upon deviant behavior and stress. It should also be mentioned that resources and strengths also exist within the Chinese-American population. These strengths include community, familial, and individual resources (Sue and Chin in press).

Chinese communities throughout the United States have become increasingly organized to provide mental health and human services. In areas where there are relatively large numbers of Chinese and other Asians, community mental health facilities, bilingual schools, social services, and other educational, legal, and welfare programs have developed. Community leaders still point to the unmet needs of Chinese and the problems created by years of neglect by local and federal governments. Nevertheless, bilingual and bicultural services are con-tinuing to evolve. An increasing number of Chinese are utilizing these programs in San Francisco, New York, Seattle, Boston, Honolulu, and Chicago.

Many Chinese-Americans also have networks of resources that, at times, serve to alleviate emotional disturbance. For example, third parties or intermediaries (shopkeepers, friends, respected leaders, acupuncturists, herbalists, benevolent association members) may be called upon to help a distressed person.

While we have indicated that Chinese family values may conflict with Western values, the family is often a major source of mental health strengths. The kinship system of the Chinese encourages a mutual dependence which forms the basis of a psychological security for both the old and the young. Hsu (1970) believes that Chinese children are socialized to see the world in terms of a network of relationships. From the beginning, children are conditioned to the multiple authority of not only their parents but also grandparents, aunts, uncles, and in-laws. The feelings toward parents and other adult authority figures being divided and diluted, the child generally does not develop a paralyzing attachment to, or strong repulsion against, the elders. Even less reason exists for the emergence of the Oedipal triangle in which the child is allied to one parent or the other. Chinese parents, on the other hand, have little reason for anxiety as their children mature. First, the Chinese parent-child relationship is considered to be immutable, and not subject to individual acceptance or rejection. Second, Chinese social structure is such that age, far from being a handicap, is a blessing. Chinese parents have no reason to regret their children's maturity, for it assures not a lesser role but a more respected place for themselves. Thus, the family and kinship system of the Chinese encourages a sense of belongingness, inter-relationship, and security that allows one to minimize emotional lability and feelings of isolation.

Finally, despite the stressors such as culture conflict and prejudice, many Chinese have developed a strong and healthy bicultural or multicultural identity. This identity allows one to successfully function in a more "Chinese" or "American" setting and to integrate aspects of both cultures. For example, young married couples who are Chinese may consider their own nuclear family as being the most important relationship (which is more of a Western pattern) and yet show strong affectionate bonds to their parents or to elder relatives (which is more of a Chinese pattern). In other words, many Chinese-Americans have developed coping strategies to deal with the problems in society.

SUMMARY

In this article, we have tried to indicate the mental health status of Chinese in the United States. On the one hand, we have argued that despite popular beliefs, Chinese-Americans are not particularly immune to mental disorders. In fact, we believe that their rates of mental disorder have been underestimated. On the other hand, despite stressors such as culture conflict, rapid life changes, and prejudice, Chinese-Americans do have strengths, resources, and effective coping strategies. We have only limited knowledge of problems involving juvenile delinquency, suicide, drug abuse, and alcoholism. It is apparent that much more research using appropriate and sensitive methodology should be conducted in order to determine the frequency and nature of mental disturbances as well as the means to foster mental health.

REFERENCES CITED

Abbott, K. A.
  1976 Culture change and the persistence of the Chinese personality. In G. DeVos (ed.), Responses to Change: Society, Culture, and Personality. New York: Van Nostrand.
Abbott, K. A. & Abbott, E. L.
  1968 Juvenile delinquency in San Francisco's Chinese American community: 1961–1966. Journal of Sociology, 4: 45–56.
Allard, W. A.
  1975 Chinatown The Guilded ghetto. National Geographic 148(5): 627–643.
Ball, J. C. & Lau, M. P.
  1966 The Chinese narcotic addict in the United States. Social Forces 45(1): 68–72.
Barnett, M. L.
  1958 Some Cantonese-American problems of status adjustment. Phylon 1: 420–427.

Berk, B. B. & Hirata, L. C.
1973 Mental illness among the Chinese: myth or reality? *In* S. Sue & H. Kitano (eds.), Asian Americans: A Success Story? Journal of Social Issues, 29(2): 149–166.
Bourne, P. G.
1973 Suicide among Chinese in San Francisco. American Journal of Public Health 68(8): 744–750.
Bourne, P. G.
1975 The Chinese student – Acculturation and mental illness. Psychiatry, 38(3): 269–277.
Bridge
1975 An Asian American perspective. Facts and Figures – a Closer Look at the 1970 Census 3(4): 34–38.
Brown, T. R., Stein, K. M., Huang, K., & Harris, D. E.
1973 Mental illness and the role of mental health facilities in Chinatown. *In* S. Sue & N. Wagner (eds.), Asian-Americans: Psychological Perspectives. Palo Alto: Science and Behavior Books, Inc.
Chen, P. N.
1970 The Chinese community in Los Angeles. Social Casework 51(10): 591–598.
Chin, F.
1972 Confessions of the Chinatown cowboy. Bulletin of Concerned Asian Scholars 4(3): 58–70.
Chun-Hoon, L.
1971 Jade Snow Wong and the fate of Chinese-American identity. Amerasia Journal 1: 36–49.
Dohrenwend, B. S. & Dohrenwend, B. P. (eds.)
1974 Stressful Life Events: Their Nature and Effects. New York: Wiley.
Fong, S. L. M.
1968 Identity conflicts of Chinese adolescents in San Francisco and the United States. *In* E. B. Brody (ed.), Minority Group Adolescents in the United States. Williams and Wilkins.
Fong, S. L. M.
1973 Assimilation and changing social roles of Chinese Americans. Journal of Social Issues 29(2): 115–127.
Fong, S. L. M. & Peskin, H.
1969 Sex-role strain and personality adjustment of China-born students in America: A pilot study. Journal of Abnormal Psychology 74: 563–567.
Fox, D. J. & Jordan, V. B.
1973 Racial preference and identification of Black, American Chinese, and White Children. Genetic Psychology monographs 88(2): 229–286.
Fujii, S. M.
1976 Elderly Asian Americans and use of public services. Social Casework 57(3): 202–207.
Fujitomi, I. & Wong, D.
1973 The new Asian-American woman. *In* S. Sue & N. Wagner (eds.), Asian-Americans: Psychological Perspectives. Science and Behavior Books, Inc.
Hessler, R. M., Molan, M. G., Ogbru, B. and New, P. K. M.
1975 Intraethnic diversity: Heath care of the Chinese Americans. Human Organization 34: 253–262.
Hinkle, L.
1974 The effect of exposure to culture change, social change, and changes in inter-personal relationships on health. *In* B. S. Dohrenwend & B. P. Dohrenwend (eds.), Stressful Life Events: Their Nature and Effects. New York: Wiley.

Holmes, T. & Masuda, M.
    1974 Life change and illness susceptibility. *In* B. S. Dohrenwend & B. P. Dohrenwend
          (eds.), Stressful Life Events: Their Nature and Effects. New York: Wiley.
Hsu, F.
    1970 Americans and Chinese. Garden City, N.Y.: Doubleday.
Hsu, F., Watreus, B. G. & Lord, E. M.
    1961 Culture pattern and adolescent behavior. International Journal of Social Psychiatry
          7: 33–53.
Jew, C. C. & Brody, S. A.
    1967 Mental illness among the Chinese: Hospitalization rates over the past century.
          Comprehensive Psychiatry 2(8): 129–134.
Jung, M.
    1976 Characteristics of contrasting Chinatowns: 1. Philadelphia, Pennsylvania. Social
          Casework 57(3), 149–154.
Kalish, R. & Mariwaki, S.
    1973 The world of the elderly Asian American. Journal of Social Issues 21(2): 187–
          208.
Kalish, R. & Yuen, S.
    1971 Americans of East Asian ancestry: Aging and the aged. The Gerontologist 2:
          36–47.
Kim, B. L.
    1975 A study of Asian Americans in Chicago: Their socio-economic characteristics,
          problems, and service needs. Unpublished Monograph.
Kleinman, A.
    1975 Explanatory models in health care relationships. *In* National Council for Inter-
          national Health: Health of the Family: 159–172. Washington, D.C.,; National
          Council for International Health.
Kleinman, A.
    1977 Depression, somatization and the "new cross-cultural psychiatry." Social Science
          and Medicine 11: 3–10.
Krigler, S. F. & Kroes, W. H.
    1972 Childrearing attitudes of Chinese, Jewish, and Protestant mothers. Journal of
          Social Psychology 86: 250–210.
Kuo, W. H., Gary, R., & Lin, N.
    Locus of Control and Symptoms of Psychological Distress Among Chinese Americans.
          Paper presented at the Meeting of the Society for the Study of Social Problems.
          San Francisco, California.
Kurokawa, M.
    1969 Beyond community integration and stability: A comparative study of Oriental
          and Mennonite children. Journal of Social Issues 25(1): 195–213.
Lee, R. H.
    1960 The Chinese in the United States of America. Hong Kong: Hong Kong University
          Press.
Lin, T. Y., Tardiff, K., Donetz, G. & Goresky, W.
    1978 Ethnicity and patterns of help-seeking. Culture, Medicine and Psychiatry 2(1):
          3–13.
Lowe, P.
    1943 Father and Glorious Descendant. Boston: Little & Brown.
Lyman, S.
    1974 Chinese Americans. New York: Random House.
Marsella, A. J., Kinzie. D. & Gordon, P.
    1973 Ethnic variations in the expression of depression. Journal of Cross-Cultural
          Psychology 4(4);435-458.

Murphy, B.
   1971 Boston's Chinese: They have problems, too! Opportunity 1(3): 18–24.
Nakagawa, B. & Watanabe, R.
   1973 A Study of the Use of Drugs Among the Asian-American Youth of Seattle. Seattle: Demonstration Project for Asian-Americans.
Namkung, P. S.
   1972 Asian American Drug Addiction – The Quiet Problem. Paper presented at the National Conference on Drug Abuse.
Owan, T.
   1975 Asian-Americans: A Case of Benighted Neglect. Paper presented at the National Conference of Social Welfare, San Francisco.
Scofield, R. W. & Sun, C.
   1960 A comparative study of the differential effect upon personality of Chinese and American child training practices. Journal of Social Psychology 52: 221–224.
Seligman, M. E.
   1975 Helplessness. San Francisco: Freeman and Company.
Sollenberger, R. T.
   1968 Chinese-American child-rearing practices and juvenile delinquency. Journal of Social Psychology 74: 13–23.
Sommers, V. S.
   1960 Identity conflict and acculturation problems in Oriental Americans. American Journal of Orthopsychiatry 30(3): 637–644.
Sue, D. W. & Frank, A. C.
   1973 A typological approach to the psychological study of Chinese and Japanese American college males. Journal of Social Issues 29(2): 129–148.
Sue, D. W. & Kirk, B. A.
   1972 Psychological characteristics of Chinese-American students. Journal of Counseling Psychology 19(6): 471–478.
Sue, D. W. & Kirk, B. A.
   1973 Differential characteristics of Japanese-American and Chinese-American college students. Journal of Counseling Psychology 20: 142–148.
Sue, D. W. & Kirk, B. A.
   1975 Asian Americans: Use of counseling and psychiatric services on a college campus. Journal of Counseling Psychology 22(1): 84–86.
Sue, S.
   1977 Psychological theory and implications for Asian Americans. Personnel and Guidance Journal 55: 381–389.
Sue, S. & Chin, R.
   In press Chinese-American children: Psychosocial development and mental health. In G. Powell, A. Morales, & J. Yamamoto (eds.). The Psychosocial Development of Minority Group Children. New York: Brunner/Mazel.
Sue, S. & McKinney, H.
   1975 Asian Americans in the community health care system. American Journal of Orthopsychiatry 45(1): 111–118.
Sue, S. & Sue, D. W.
   1971 Chinese American personality and mental health. Amerasia Journal 1(2): 36–49.
Sue, S. & Sue, D. W.
   1974 MMPI comparisons between Asian American and non-Asian students utilizing a student health psychiatric clinic. Journal of Counseling Psychology 21(5): 423–427.
Sue, S., Wagner, N., Ja, D., Margullis, C., & Lew, L.
   1976 Conceptions of mental illness among Asian and Caucasian American students. Psychological Reports 38: 703–708.

Sue, S., Zane, N. & Ito, J.
   1979 Reported alcohol drinking patterns among Asian and Caucasian Americans. Journal of Cross-Cultural Psychology 10(1): 41–56.
Sung, B. L.
   1971 The Story of the Chinese in America. New York: Collier.
True, R. H.
   1975 Mental health services in a Chinese American community. In W. H. Ishikawa & N. H. Archer (eds.) Service Delivery in Pan Asian Communities. San Diego: Pacific Asian Coalition.
Tseng, W. S.
   1975 The nature of somatic complaints among psychiatric patients: The Chinese case. Comprehensive Psychiatry 16: 237–246.
Tseng, W. S., & Char, W. F.
   1974 The Chinese of Hawaii. In W. Tseng, J. McDermott, & T. Maretzki (eds.), People and Cultures in Hawaii. 24–23. Honolulu: University of Hawaii School of Medicine.
Weiss, M. S.
   1970 Selective acculturation and the dating process: The pattern of Chinese-Caucasian inter-racial dating. Journal of Marriage and the Family 32: 273–278.
Wong, J. S.
   1950 Fifth Chinese Daughter. New York: Harper.
Wu, F. Y.
   1975 Mandarin-speaking aged Chinese in the Los Angeles area. Gerontologist 15(3): 271–275.
Yee, M.
   1970 Chinatown in crisis. Newsweek Feb. 23: 57–58.
Young, N. F.
   1972 Independence training from a cross-cultural perspective. American Anthropologist 74(3): 629–638.
Yuan, D. Y.
   1966 Chinatown and beyond: The Chinese population in metropolitan New York. Phylon 27: 321–332.
Yuen, S.
   1972 The Chinese elderly poor in San Francisco. In Chinese Americans: School and Community Problems. Chicago: Integrated Education Associates.

MARJORIE H. KLEIN, MILTON H. MILLER, AND A. A. ALEXANDER

16. THE AMERICAN EXPERIENCE
OF THE CHINESE STUDENT:
ON BEING NORMAL IN AN ABNORMAL WORLD

The young person who leaves home to study or work in a foreign land is in an ironic position. Ordinarily a quite well-adapted person, with achievements great enough to be eligible for study abroad, he/she moves deliberately into a position of stress and personal vulnerability. In the new environment, he/she must learn new and strange ways of doing things in order to continue to function at the accustomed high degree of excellence. Thus by taking on the role and the experience of the stranger in a strange land, the foreign student enters into a kind of voluntary or forced deviance.

There are various ways that this abnormality is experienced and dealt with by the sojourner, but the common denominator of any pattern is conflict — role conflict and its psychological risks: identity conflict, identity change, or identity diffusion. The conflict always involves forces in the home and host culture, and tension between an individual's public and private self. Needs for security and stability work against needs for growth, curiosity, and change. In addition to a new sensitivity to the clear-cut value differences between cultures, what one finds in the natural situation of cross-cultural contact is a shift of perspective. The accommodation of the individual to the socio-cultural environment, an adaptation which we generally take so for granted that we are unaware of it, becomes a more salient and compelling part of the conflict. This altered consciousness, particularly a heightened sense of self and concern about the other, is the core of the experience of being a stranger. Thus in 'culture shock' the problem goes beyond the experience of competing values, manners, or goals to the core question: Who am I?

This chapter is based on research spanning one decade and two continents, with a particular focus on the adaptation processes of Chinese students. The studies reported here cover the whole of their cross-cultural experience: The first study of background, goals, and concerns in the predeparture phase was done in Taiwan with the most valuable collaboration of Eng-Kung Yeh and Hung-Ming Chu. Our own research at Wisconsin considered the social and emotional experiences during the first critical years abroad, as well as the determinants of physical and psychological health during longer periods of study lasting 6 years or more. Here the collaboration of K. H. Tseng and Fikre Workneh provided an essential and invaluable perspective.

Each of the studies in this chapter considers patterns of motives and personal resources as important determinants of the quality of an individual's sojourn experience. Each touches upon the theme of role conflict and personal identity. Thus we have focused on the lived life experience of deviance and the ways that the Chinese students learned to cope with it over their time in the United States.

311

A. Kleinman and T.-Y. Lin (eds.), Normal and Abnormal Behavior in Chinese Culture, 311–330.
Copyright © 1980 by D. Reidel Publishing Company.

More specifically we have considered questions such as: Are those Chinese who choose to go abroad deliberately inviting role or identity conflict? That is, are they seeking to be different at the start? Are they psychologically more flexible and adaptive than those who stay at home? Is their anchorage to the home culture as strong as for those who remain at home? And once the Chinese student goes abroad, what happens then? To what extent has the individual's 'set', the pattern of motives, attitudes, resources and concerns shaped the over-seas experience? What is the nature of their contact with the host culture and their involvement with the co-national subculture fashioned by each sojourner within the host culture? And finally, how do these patterns and social experi-ences contribute to the rate and nature of maladaptation in Chinese students?

In approaching all of these issues we have thought in terms of a range of experiences and adaptations, each offering different solutions to the underlying role and identity conflicts that are inherent in cross-cultural travel. Our own work with foreign students (e.g., Klein et al. 1971) as well as the results of a number of studies carried out in the 1950's and 1960's by others (e.g., Kelman et al. 1962; Bennett et al. 1958; Lambert et al. 1956; Morris 1960; Coelho 1958) seemed to indicate that the following patterns of adaptation are characteristic for visiting students from a number of different cultures:

Instrumental Adaptation

Characteristic of those with clear professional-academic goals; major interaction and involvement organized around specific tasks; extra-curricular social life continuous with home, i.e., contact maintained with fellow nationals; major tensions and adjustments in task performance; social adjustment and contact with host minimal and limited to professional role; changes primarily to satisfy academic needs and interests; minimal readjustment on return home unless professional roles are very different (e.g., adjusters).

Identification

Primary interest in involvement with host culture; academic or professional goals secondary to cross-cultural contact; major adjustments made to facilitate con-tacts and interaction with new culture, exploration of the community; interest in learning local customs. Interpersonal problems are the greatest source of stress for this group, with the level of tension high. Satisfying interactions are likely to lead to positive and/or differentiated attitudes toward the host country and to shifts in identification and interpersonal style. There is danger of alienation and readjustment tensions.

Withdrawal

Initial interest in involvement with host and academic or task purposes secondary to goal of new experience and cross-cultural contacts; efforts made to contact host and to explore the community; tensions arise in the interpersonal context and impede adjustment; there is a shift from disappointing relations with the host culture to primary contact with fellow nationals; efforts are directed at restoration-maintenance of national identity. This pattern represents an attempt on the part of the sojourner to cope with unsatisfying social experiences. It is likely that cultural tendencies for sensitivity and withdrawal will predispose this pattern. It is also noted that negative attitudes toward and selective perception of the faults of the host culture will prevail and that strong identification with home reference groups will be maintained where possible.

Resistance

The role of cultural ambassador is most salient; primary social contacts are maintained with own national group or other foreigners; interaction with host is organized around exchange of information about culture and the attitudes are largely dependent on the status accorded to the home country. Attitude change is minor with no significant shift in national identification.

The consequences of these general adaptational styles are varied. Each pattern has its unique mix of costs and benefits. Instrumental adaptation and identification both facilitate positive sojourn experiences, but alienation from home is a clear risk for identification. Identification, on the other hand, leads to more profound and enduring changes in outlook, including greater flexibility, tolerance and 'internationalism.' Withdrawal and resistance are costly because the aims of international exchange are not met, and because the individuals suffer. Withdrawal is the more stressful and frustrating of the two, and more likely to lead to enduring negative attitudes that reinforce negative stereotypes of the host culture.

These patterns suggest the major questions for the studies summarized in this chapter. The predeparture study compared background, motives, concerns and resources of those who are planning to go out with those who stay at home. Studies of social adaptation reported next questioned the influence of these motives, etc., on the quality of the social experience in the host culture. The final set of studies considered the relationship of these patterns to indices of maladaptation, specifically rates of emotional and physical illness.

PREDEPARTURE: ARE THOSE WHO STUDY ABROAD DIFFERENT AT THE START?

In order to get at the question, "Who goes out?", we undertook in 1967 a collaborative study with our colleagues, Drs. Eng-Kung Yeh and Hung-Ming Chu, at the National Taiwan University (Chu et al. 1971; Yeh and Chu 1974). We gave a questionnaire to 132 Chinese students who were preparing to go to the United States for graduate study (*Go* group) and to a sample of 108 students who were staying in Taiwan for their graduate study (*Stay* group) who were matched as carefully as possible to the *Go* subjects. The questionnaire (with questions in

TABLE 1

Comparison of Chinese Going to U.S. for Study (*Go* n = 132) and Staying at Home (*Stay*, n = 108): Demographic and Background

Variable (% of all R's)				*Chi Square* [a] (Stay vs. Go)
Birthplace				
	Father	R*		
Taiwan	60	57		
Mainland	39	38		Not Significant
Other	1	5		
Religion				
	Father	Mother	R	
None	35	28	48	
Buddhist or Taoist	33	35	9	Not Significant
Protestant or Catholic	12	17	21	
Parent's Education				
	Father	Mother		
College	27	13		
Secondary or Vocational	41	33		
Elementary or less	33	57		Not Significant
Father's Occupation				
Business	23			
Government	17			
Agriculture	14			
Professional	10			
Education	7			Not Significant
Other	13			
Sibling's Education		*Stay %*	*Go %*	
No Sibling in College	41	50	34	
Some or All in College	59	50	16	
		$X^2=5.97$,	df	1, $p < .05$
Position in Family				
Oldest or Only	37			
Middle	49			Not Significant
Youngest	15			
Age				
21–25 years	63			
Over 25 Years	37			Not Significant
Martial Status				
Single	82			
Engaged or Married	17			Not Significant

a Chi Squares are for frequences

Percentages do not always total 100 because nonresponses, etc., are not tabled.

Chinese and English), covered: 1) life experiences and family background, including previous travel, assessments of school performance and current health; 2) reasons and goals for overseas study (asked hypothetically for the *Stay* group); 3) anticipated adjustment problems or difficulties for overseas study; and 4) images of self, Chinese peers, and Americans.

Table 1 lists demographic and background variables in the two groups. The groups were essentially similar: most (57%) were Taiwan born of parents also born in Taiwan. Religious backgrounds varied (although Mainlanders are most often Christian). Most fathers were educated at the secondary level or beyond, with a range of middle and upper level occupations represented. The only significant difference in background between the *Go* and *Stay* groups was that more of the *Go* group had siblings in college, possibly reflecting greater family financial resources. Beyond this, there were no differences in respondents' age, position in family, or marital status at the time of the sojourn: most (92%) were single, and two-thirds were below the age of twenty-five.

Recent educational-occupational experiences were also similar (see Table 2). The only differences found were for field of study and field of previous job, with more of the *Go* group in science, engineering, or medicine; more of the

TABLE 2

Comparison of Go and Stay Groups:
Educational-Occupational Background and Future Plans

Variable (% of all R's)		*Chi Square* (Stay vs. Go)	
Years of Education			
9 – 15	5		
16 – 17	70	Not Significant	
18 or more	26		
Major Field		*Stay %*	*Go %*
Agriculture	22	15	27
Science or Med.	36	42	33
Engineering	17	10	22
Humanities, Soc. Sci. or Education	26	34 $X^2 = 15.99$, df 3, p $<$.01	18
Satisfaction with Major Dept. in Taiwan			
Very Satisfied	24		
Satisfied	59	Not Significant	
Less Satisfied	17		
Rank of Major Dept. in Taiwan			
First	48		
2 – 5	37	Not Significant	
6 or less	14		
Previous Job in Future Field			
Yes	23		
No	65	Not Significant	

Table 2 (continued)

Field of Job		*Stay %*	*Go %*
Engineering, Science, Med.	12	9	15
Business, Agriculture	5	8	6
Education, Humanities, Social Sciences	7	8	1
		$X^2=13.57$, df	2, p $<$.01
Length of Job			
One Year or Less	17	Not Significant	
More Than One Year	18		
Does R Have Job Awaiting Return?			
Yes	26	Not Significant	
No	74		
Level of Extracurricular Activities		*Stay %*	*Go %*
Above Average	21	13	30
Average	44	39	48
Below Average	35	48	23
		$X^2=19.69$, df	2, p $<$.001
Degree Expected		*Stay %*	*Go %*
None	4	0	6
MA or MS	17	4	24
Ph.D.	80	96	71
		$X^2=17.94$, df	2, p $<$.001
Certainty of Return Home			
Very Certain	30		
Probably	50	Not Significant	
Uncertain	19		
Definitely Not	0		

Stay group in humanities, social science, or education. It is paradoxical that those in fields at the 'growing edge' of the mainstream of the Taiwanese economy were more readily able to go abroad to develop their skills, where they could become vulnerable to cultural isolation or to the 'brain drain'. The only other educational history variable that distinguished the two groups was their reported level of extra-curricular activity, with the *Go* respondents reporting themselves to be slightly more active than the *Stay* respondents. This hint of greater outgoingness in the *Go* group was also reflected in their responses to a question about ease of making friends: the *Go* group rated themselves as significantly more able to make friends than did the *Stay* group.

Responses to questions about future plans in Table 2 also suggested that respondents may be part of a new wave of immigration. Only 25% reported definite job plans after their studies. Most were seeking the Ph.D., and expected this to take three or more years (our experience indicates four to six years would be more realistic). Although there was a greater proportion of M.A.'s expected in the *Go* group, this was probably more related to immediate support programs than to the students' ultimate intentions. Thus, only 30% of both groups were "certain" they would be living in Taiwan after their studies. As we know foreign students to be very circumspect about their plans for leaving home, we suspect that a sizable proportion of the 50% who said they "probably" would return or remain home changed their minds later.

What of the previous international experiences of the sojourners, or experiences in independent living which may foster breadth of experience and flexible adaptive skills? Table 3 shows that very few respondents in either group reported previous travel, and the few trips reported were within Asia. Most in both groups, however, had had some experience in independent living. The *Go* group was significantly more likely to report previous living away, however.

TABLE 3

Comparison of Go and Stay Groups: Overseas Experience

Variable (% of all R's)		*Chi Square* (Stay vs. Go)	
Previous Travel From Taiwan			
Yes	5	Not Significant	
No	95		
Lived Away From Family		*Stay %*	*Go %*
Never	17	16	17
Away at One Time	31	16	43
Away at Time of Sojourn	45	59	33
		$X^2 = 23.50$, df 2, p $<$ .001	

If travel abroad is a substantial potential stress, then the traveler's coping skills, specifically social resources, prior experience with members of the host culture, and sense of health and resilience should be important, both as indicators of normality and as predictors of adjustment during the sojourn. Table 4 shows that those who were going out reported significantly more

TABLE 4

Comparison of Go and Stay Groups: Overseas Experience

Variable (% of all R's)		*Chi Square* (Stay vs. Go)	
Contact With Americans in Taiwan		*Stay %*	*Go %*
Yes	43	27	57
No	54	73	43
		$X^2 = 19.47$, df 1. p $<$ .001	
Who was Contact		*Stay %*	*Go %*
Friend or Classmate	25	13	37
Teacher	12	9	15
Co-worker	3	2	5
		$X^2 = 1.02$, df 2. p $<$ .75	
R Knows Someone Who Has Studied Overseas		*Stay %*	*Go %*
Yes	88	82	92
No	12	18	8
		$X^2 = 3.99$, df 1, p $<$ .05	

previous contact with American peers and also more acquaintance with fellow nationals already overseas. Turning to data concerning health, reported in Table 5, we see that while reports of actual health problems were similar in the two groups, the *Go* group rated themselves significantly more healthy, both physically and psychologically.

TABLE 5

Comparison of Go and Stay Groups: Health Status

Variable (% of all R's)			*Chi Square* (Stay vs. Go)	
Illness				
	Family	R		
None	82	95	Not Significant	
Yes	18	5		
R's Rating of Physical Health			*Stay %*	*Go %*
Above Average		53	47	58
Average		45	48	42
Below Average		2	5	0
			$X^2=7.83$, df 2, p $<$.02	
R's Rating of Mental Health			*Stay %*	*Go %*
Above Average		66	53	77
Average		30	40	21
Below Average		1	3	0
			$X^2=15.67$, df 2, p $<$.001	

These differences were reflected even more clearly in responses to questions concerning goals for the sojourn, problems anticipated, and expectations for interactions with Americans. Ratings of 15 goals for importance were first factor-analyzed, and scores on the four resulting factors were compared for the *Go* and *Stay* groups (Table 6). The groups differed for three of the four factors: the *Go* group scored significantly higher on three factors – "cross-cultural curiosity" (p $<$ .01), "desire for self-improvement combined with a desire to please parents" (p $<$ .01), "desire for training in specific field" (p $<$ .01). The groups did not differ on the fourth factor, "desire for new experiences". Considering the greater importance placed on the training and self-improvement factors relative to cross-cultural curiosity, one might conclude that the *Go* group stood out more with respect to their desire for professional mobility or achievement than their motive to loosen or shed cultural ties.

Comparison of factors derived from responses to 20 potential problem areas also indicated that the *Go* group was less concerned with problems in general, significantly less so for two of the five factors: "academic adjustment" (p $<$ .05) and "distance from family" (p $<$ .05). Considering the relative rank of all factors, the respondents were again more concerned with academic adjustment and acceptance by Americans than with distance from family, home-sickness, and least of all with making social contacts with Americans.

This relatively modest expectation of the *Go* group for contact with

TABLE 6

Comparison of Go and Stay Groups: Goal and Problem Factor Scores

Factor	Average Rating[a]		p value[b]
	Stay	Go	
Goals			
1. Cross-cultural Curiosity[c]: Live Away From Home, Know U.S. Life, Meet Different People, Know U.S. Culture	1.84	2.29	$<.01$
2. Personal Change: Have Different Experiences, Find Self, See U.S.	2.94	3.04	NS
3. Family Advancement: Improve Family Finances, Please Parents, Get Degree	2.38	2.63	$<.01$
4. Home Oriented Achievement: Training in Field (positive)	3.32	3.62	
See U.S., Live Away From Home (negative)	1.90	1.96	$<.01$
Problems Anticipated			
1. Academic Adjustment: School Work, Study Time, Money	2.13	1.97	$<.05$
2. Contact With U.S.: Chance to Meet Americans, Make American Friends, Opposite Sex Contact	1.77	1.70	NS
3. Cultural Adaptation: Speaking English, Understanding English, Place to Live	2.02	1.92	NS
4. Lifestyle Change: Strange Food, Homesickness, Climate	1.86	1.75	NS
5. Distance From Family: Worry About Family, Contact With Home, Racial Discrimination	1.93	1.75	$<.05$

[a] Average of ratings on items loading above 30.
[b] p value for Analysis of Variance of factor scores.
[c] The three items with the highest loadings are listed.

Americans was further clarified in a series of questions (not asked of the *Stay* group) regarding the importance of various activities with Americans. As Table 7 shows, respondents valued contacts related to academic goals (talk about courses and studies) much more than other more purely social contacts.

In sum, the differences that had emerged so far suggested that while the *Go* and *Stay* groups were alike in many respects, the *Go* group saw themselves as

TABLE 7

Importance of Activities With Americans for Go Group

Activity	Importance Rating %		
	Not At All	Somewhat	Very
Talk About Courses or Studies	1	25	74
Talk About Art, Literature, etc.	14	62	23
Visit in Homes	7	64	30
Talk About Family or Life at Home	13	64	23
Talk About Intimate or Personal Matters	9	60	30

more ambitious, more gregarious, less concerned with adaptational problems, and more healthy psychologically and physically. They also had more experience with independence and more contact with Americans. With regard to their forth-coming trip to the United States, they placed greater value on academic goals than on cross-cultural contacts, although they valued contacts more highly than the *Stay* group. In terms of the patterns of adaptation described earlier, they seemed like those who make 'instrumental' adaptations.

Evidence of loosened cultural ties in the *Go* group was more apparent in their

TABLE 8

Adjectives Rated Significantly More True of Chinese Than of Americans

	% True of Chinese	% True of Americans
Calm	92	42
Respectful	92	63
Cautious	90	58
Gentle	89	71
Obedient	86	22
Serious	86	25
Reserved	86	10
Spiritual	85	49
Stable	84	50
Intellectual	83	74
Considerate	81	66
Shy	79	7
Formal	73	13
Tolerant of Differences	73	45
Treats People as Equals	72	55
Emotional	62	50
Distant	46	21
Suspicious	31	22
Aloof	30	12

From Yeh and Chu 1974

self images, especially as contrasted with images of fellow nationals and Americans. (See Yeh and Chu 1974; Chu et al. 1971 for a fuller description of these data analyses). Respondents were given a list of adjectives and asked to indicate the extent to which each was true or false of themselves, people their own age in their home country, and Americans. All respondents clearly differentiated between Chinese and American character traits. Table 8 lists the 19 adjectives that were rated by all to be significantly more true of Chinese peers than Americans; Table 9 lists the 23 adjectives rated to be more true of

TABLE 9

Adjectives Rated Significantly More True of Americans Than of Chinese

	% True of Americans	% True of Chinese
Active	100	30
Optimistic	98	58
Frank	98	46
Self-Confident	98	66
Practical	97	69
Cheerful	97	56
Responsible	97	75
Materialistic	95	34
Cooperative	94	73
Spontaneous	94	46
Forceful	91	40
Helpful	86	78
Outgoing	83	60
Eager for Change	83	21
Bold	80	14
Aggressive	79	19
Boastful	77	25
Changeable	55	23
Noisy	48	12
Irritable	30	16
Rebellious	26	10
Demanding	23	13
Bitter	18	7

From Yeh and Chu 1974

Americans. If these can be thought of as the respondents' perceptions of differences in Chinese and American character, then it is of interest to compare their self concepts. In general the self-descriptions in both the *Go* and *Stay* groups fell in between these two extremes; that is, the students saw themselves as more active, optimistic, frank, cheerful, aggressive, etc., than their Chinese peers, and rated other "Chinese" traits to be less true of themselves (e.g., shy, formal, emotional, distant, aloof, obedient, and reserved). Yeh and Chu interpreted this difference to indicate that the Chinese graduate students as a whole saw themselves as more self-confident than their Chinese peers. Since most of these characteristics were 'American' character traits in the respondents' eyes, it can also be concluded that both the *Go* and *Stay* groups had somewhat more Americanized or Westernized self concepts. Further, the greater self-confidence and the greater Westernization was more striking in the *Go* group than in the *Stay* group. In all cases where there were significant differences in self-ratings of the two groups, the *Go* group saw themselves as having less of the Chinese characteristics (specifically, less considerate, shy, and aloof) and more of the American characteristics (specifically, more active, optimistic, spontaneous, forceful, and aggressive). When this finding is coupled with the fact that all of the differences between the *Go* and *Stay* group's ratings of Americans were in the direction of more favorable perceptions on the part of the *Go* group (Americans were seen as more tolerant, equalitarian, eager for change, stable, and agreeable; less suspicious, changeable, noisy, selfish, and hypocritical), it can be interpreted to suggest that even before their departure, respondents in the *Go* group were more favorably disposed toward and more identified with American norms.

In general, we have concluded from this predeparture study that the going out students were more socially mobile, had more experience with independence and, most importantly, saw themselves as healthier, more confident, more sociable, and more resourceful than their counterparts who remained at home. It was also true that the Chinese students who left home to study abroad perceived themselves as less similar to reference groups in the home culture, even before departing. In some sense then, these sojourners were deviant with respect to traditional home country norms, but deviant in a way that would enable easier integration or adaptation to Western ways. Still, their goals for overseas study were dominantly task-oriented, and the students were openly devoted to living out family aspirations. Few were motivated by the desire to change or to sever ties with home. Thus these young people going out from Taiwan in the late 60's were more representative of the internationally-oriented growing edge of the mainstream of their culture than of an alienated minority who were bound to leave that culture behind.

SOCIAL ADAPTATION AND EXPERIENCES OF CHINESE STUDENTS IN THE UNITED STATES

While we have seen that Chinese students on the eve of their departure for the United States placed more weight on academic and personal achievement than on cross-cultural social contacts, we also found that these sojourners were at the same time ready to enter into relationships with the host people in the sense that they were more favorably disposed toward them and saw themselves as already sharing aspects of the American character.

One series of studies we have carried out in Wisconsin concerned with the social experiences of Chinese students showed us, however, that the actual course of social contact was limited even beyond the sojourners' very modest expectations. Indeed, two repeated trends emerged from these studies that bear on the theme of this paper: 1) the visiting student experienced him/herself to be a stranger; that is, there was a sense of separateness and strangeness initially that made the sojourner vulnerable or sensitive to negative experiences with the host people. 2) This sense of strangeness was at the same time softened and sharpened by the pull of the co-national subculture which functioned both as a buffer against the pain of the contacts with the host people, and as a salient force for the maintenance of home values in a foreign land.

The course of social contact between Chinese students and American hosts that has emerged from the several studies can be summarized as follows. Chinese students initially had a guarded optimism about their ability to fit into American social life. At least one-half desired contact; that is, they placed a high premium on intimacy with the host people initially, but at the same time they expected these contacts to be somewhat difficult. This was reflected in their image of Americans as friendly, outgoing people, but at the same time, as lacking qualities usually associated with deep friendship in Chinese society: consideration for others, patience, sensitivity, seriousness, attention to formality and conduct. The origins of this expectation could be traced to contacts with Americans abroad — particularly from experiences of seeing Americans form co-national sub-groups in Taiwan, as well as to reports of returning students and media images of Americans. Thus, the arriving Chinese both feared and at the same time knew that "real" intimacy with the American people might be a struggle — that the American "big hello", the warm but superficial invitation to join in time-limited, pleasant, and mutually uncommitted social activities would predominate.

What actually happened? In one follow-up study of 59 Chinese students (Klein et al. 1971; Klein et al. 1974) questionnaires from the Fall (upon entry to the University) and from the Spring revealed the students' disillusionment with the host nationals. Despite ample opportunity to get to know host nationals, despite efforts of organizations, advisors, and some American friends, we found social contacts in a "typical week" to be limited. Thirty-nine percent of the respondents reported no social contact or sense of friendship with Americans, one-third reported one or two contacts, and one-third reported *none* over the entire six months covered by the study. In response to other questions, about 40% of the respondents expressed their sense of disillusionment more strikingly: 36% reported Americans to have been difficult to get to know (although reports of outright indifference on the part of Americans were rare) and only 11% reported finding Americans easy to befriend. Interviews with some of these students brought the details to light: one theme that ran through the interviews was what seemed to the respondents a puzzling lack of the Americans' willingness to follow through on initial social contacts. Time and again we heard of the Chinese students meeting Americans at work or at social gatherings where promises to meet again were exchanged, but never honored. Sometimes the students would meet a casual American acquaintance on the street and suffer the humiliation of not being recognized. Few of the host people were inclined to take the time to establish intimacy in the Chinese style. Part of the difficulty, of course, stemmed from cultural differences in the meaning and expectations associated with friendship. The Chinese we talked to consistently had found that what they thought to be a close friendship in their culture was different from the way Americans defined close friendship. When pressed for details, responses involved both specific expectations (e.g., open-ended standing invitations; importance of etiquette and politeness) but also the disturbing intrusion in the encounter of the sense of being a stranger. When Americans were questioned about their contacts with Chinese, we saw the reciprocal: confusion about expectations, concern about what is misperceived as dependency, and awkwardness about how to deal with "alien" formality and politeness. Thus any opportunity for miscommunication seemed to heighten vulnerability on both sides, especially when either party to the contact was feeling a stranger. It was our sense that the more self-conscious either the guest or the host became, the more likely there was to be a cycle of vulnerability and sensitivity that was very difficult to break. Thus it was not surprising that a combination of opportunity and self-image variables was predictive of rates of social contact and levels of satisfaction with these contacts in the Chinese sample. Those who had more American friends in the Spring had anticipated, in the Fall, few problems communicating with or befriending Americans. They also had, in their first six months, more opportunity to meet Americans (in their living arrangement), and found their optimistic predictions confirmed. The result was, by the time of the Spring questionnaire, a greater sense of satisfaction and well-being, both socially and academically. If we start with the premise that cross-cultural contacts generate vulnerability, and assume that a kind of "role playing" is needed to overcome vulnerability, to bridge the gap of different values and social customs, and to create new ways of communicating, it is not surprising that the more socially confident and extroverted do better.

A second study that we carried out among members of a local Formosa Association showed that these problems and concerns are not just problems of newcomers. In this sample, unlike the first, most respondents were married, had lived in Madison more than one year (with 11% more than four years) and had before that lived other places in the United States. Overall, this group reported satisfaction with the quality of their academic experiences and their personal achievement. When questioned in detail, however, about contacts with Americans and fellow nationals, they reported consistently less contact with Americans than with co-nationals, and this became more striking for the more intimate contacts. Thus, while the frequency of contacts between Americans and co-nationals was quite similar for activities such as talking about courses and studies or talking about daily events, the gap widened significantly with talk about politics, about family life or personal matters. Thus it was not surprising that we found that for 40% of the respondents in this group, a visit to an American family was a very rare event (7% never, 34% only once).

If there was indeed a push away from Americans (whether realistic or imagined) the pull of the co-national subgroup was equally powerful. Time and again in our interviews we were touched by the degree to which intimacy with the co-national group in the United States replaced ties with friends and family. We also learned of the degree to which this subgroup either subtly or openly reinforced home social divisions (e.g., Taiwanese vs. Mainlander) and home values; members of the co-national group who moved too close, especially in sexual relationships with Americans, came to know very readily of the group's disapproval. This in conjunction with the real help and support offered by the group, and their ability to serve as family surrogates in many matters (even to the extent of subtly arranging marriages), served as a powerful reinforcer and source of stability and security. This force for security, however, was also a powerful force against the achievement of truly international contact. Viewed from the context of the theme of this chapter the co-national group at the same time perpetuates and exacerbates the role conflict for the visiting student. And in the case of those who attempt to cross beyond the limits posed by the sub-culture, they may further heighten it. Related to this is our observation over ten years clinical contact that the most psychiatrically-troubled foreign students are usually those who have managed to become estranged, not only from Americans, but also from fellow nationals.

It is difficult to know exactly in what perspective to view this situation. From the point of view of those who value adaptation and international contact, the experience of the Chinese student and the role of the co-national subculture in maintaining isolation must be quite disappointing. From the perspective of the students and the sub-group, the reverse may be true: that is, the American world, or at least those elements of the American world with discrepant values and ways, provided the deviant background against which the co-national sub-group offered an island of stability and normality, a focus for identity, and the cultural continuity necessary for a smooth transition and return to the home culture. In any case, for the sojourner, a sense of separateness and alienation (whether from Americans or from co-nationals) may be a permanent and ines-capable aspect of the overseas experience, a sort of psychological baggage that is difficult to unpack or leave behind. While the internationally minded may regret this deviance and this experience, the culturally faithful may see it as the only way to survive a difficult situation.

PHYSICAL AND PSYCHOLOGICAL HEALTH DURING THE SOJOURN

Our clinical experience with culture shock has led us to view both physical and psychological problems as indicators of maladaptation. We have observed that the student in emotional or physical trouble experiences him/herself as deviant in both worlds: ties with the home world are lost and at the same time there is a sensed failure to function in the new world. The co-national subculture, or the individual's image of home are not strong enough to soften the impact. We have also observed that while different individuals have different motives and needs for the sojourn (e.g., maintenance of home country identification vs. cross-cultural adaptation), it is the failure of these needs (whatever they are) to be met that leads to psychological or physical pain. Thus in this section our focus is on the relationship between motivational, background and personal resource patterns as predictors of a variety of health problems.

Culture shock can be mild or severe. Indeed, we view it as a continuum of stress reaction to experienced conflict, varying all the way from the mild and nagging dysphoria and heightened vulnerability that all experience when travel-ing abroad to extremes of depression, fear and suspicion that are treated clinical-ly. The basic experience seems to have universal and common elements. There is usually a feeling of depression or dysphoria, a sense of loss and threat, with anxiety reflected both in fears of others and in heightened sense of self-consciousness. With this, there is also usually a heightened somatic concern. It is this modality of the experience that is the major focus of the data analysis to follow.

As background, some theoretical comments are in order. First, with regard to the depressive component of culture shock, several current theories of depres-sion suggest a special risk for travelers. Views of depression-as-loss are consistent with the loss of social anchorage, loss of status, disruption of basic social skills and ties with loved ones that are almost inevitable in crossing international boundaries. It is rare indeed that one moves whole, taking all sources of self-esteem intact, recreating familiar support systems in a new social context. When it can be done, for example through the presence of home country subcultures as we have discussed earlier, culture shock and perhaps particularly the depres-sive aspect can be minimized. When this loss cannot be minimized, however, or when the sojourner wishes to leave the home culture behind and actively en-counter the new culture, the risk for depression may be greater. The recent applications of the learned helplessness model for depression are also germane (e.g., Seligman 1974). One way to describe what changes in intercultural travel is to speak of the breakdown of habitual contingent relationships between stimulus and response, between behavior and its consequences in the social context. At home the effective person knows, usually implicitly, the rules that guide social interactions, so that one can control reinforcements. Abroad, one must learn new rules and until this takes place, the visitor is plunged into a state of helplessness, perhaps not learned in the strict sense, but analogous to that of the ineffective person with no control over reinforcement. It takes skill, particu-larly social skills, to learn new rules and to get reinforcement from new settings.

The second key components of the culture shock experience are heightened self-consciousness on one hand and increased concern with others' reactions, and intentions, on the other; the feeling "everyone is looking at me and my mistakes" and the sense "they will use and exploit me" are common experiences. What is important is that they may readily lead to somatic concern and psycho-somatic vulnerability. Concern with the self, in the absence of involving relationships with others creates perhaps a heightened awareness of natural physiological arousal or stress reactions (e.g., heart pounding in new situations). Other concerns may stem from the depressive experience — feelings of retardation, insomnia, or fatigue. Fears of illness may be further reinforced as the inevitable digestive upsets are combined with concerns with adaptation to emerge as fears of illness and worries about contamination by strange food and germs.

Thus we would argue that the psychological experience of culture shock has a strong somatic component. The feelings involved have somatic effects, and this facet of the experience may become especially salient for individuals who are not psychologically-minded.

In a survey of all the student health service visits made in one week in December by all University of Wisconsin students, we found no difference in overall health service use for U.S. and foreign students. If anything, the foreign students tended to use the health services less. However, looking at visits by organ system and type of complaint involved, we did find significant differences in rate of visits for the following categories: foreign students had more gastrointestinal complaints (38% versus 17% for U.S. students), more complaints classified as generalized or undifferentiated (12% versus 6%), more visits for psychosomatic complaints (19% versus 7%), and more pain complaints (19% versus 5%). There was, however, no difference in the rate of psychiatric complaints.

We also know from speaking with and treating foreign students with psychological distress that the medical services rather then psychological and counseling services are the preferred sources of help. This stems not only from a tendency to somatize psychological problems but also from a fear of psychiatric labels. In our experience the foreign student who eventually gets psychiatric intervention invariably started by seeking medical help for physical or for mixed physical and psychological complaints. Perhaps for these reasons, we have found the rate of psychiatric help-seeking and treatment to be quite low in Chinese students: of a sample of 113 Chinese whom we followed for more than five years, only three ever sought psychiatric help for depression.

In contrast, there were many more health service visits: over more than five years, 87 of the 113 made a total of 854 visits, an average of 7.6 visits per person. Table 10 presents a breakdown of these visits by organ system and by type of complaint. Most visits were for ear, nose, and throat or respiratory problems (infections and allergies); second were skin problems (usually irritations), followed by gastrointestinal complaints (usually stomach pains or bowel upsets). The rate of psychosomatic and psychiatric complaints was lower still.

In order to see if any background or motivational variables measured at the start of the sojourn were predictive of this type of maladaptation, we did regression analyses considering seven background factors, nine factor scores for goals and concerns, and five aspects of the self image as predictors of student health visits for 1) "more somatic" and 2) more "psychological" types of complaints. Very few of the variables considered predicted visits of either type, and the

TABLE 10

Organ System and Type of Complaint for 854 Student Health Service Visits of
113 Chinese Students

Organ System	%	Complaint	%
Ear, Nose or Throat	25	Infection	30
Skin or Connective Tissue	20	Irritation	14
Respiratory	12	Allergy	14
Gastro-intestinal	11	Injury	13
Muscular-Skeletal	8	Pain	10
Genito-Urinary or OB	5	Psychosomatic	7
Eye	5	Preventive	4
Generalized or Undifferentiated	3	Psychiatric	2
Emotional	3		
Neurological	2		
Dental-Oral	2		
Cardio-vascular	1		

relationships for the variable of time away from family was inconsistent. Rates of injury and infection were negatively related to experience away from family; rates of more psychological complaints were positively associated with this variable, as well as with a higher level of academic concerns. Without extensive replication of these findings our interpretation is best restricted at this time to the comment that it was the students' subjective sense of being at risk in the area that is central to the sojourn (academic achievement) that is predictive of psychological maladaptation.

TREATMENT OF CHINESE

In an earlier article (Alexander et al. 1976) we attempted to summarize our experiences treating psychological problems of Chinese students. In effect, we have come to view the therapist as a mediator in the range of role conflicts that are part of the overseas experience. Perhaps the most common and pressing conflict is between the student's predeparture wishes, aspirations or fantasies about the sojourn and its reality. Many have relied on their proven capacity for hard work to overcome their own concerns and fears so that they would continue to distinguish themselves academically. Often, by the time they are seen professionally, they have been defeated — as much by the United States university system or their own worries and sensitivities as by the subject matter. A corollary conflict also lies in the difference between their having left home with the sense they must bring honor to themselves, their families, and their country; and their contemporary fear that by not performing as they had hoped they will disgrace, disappoint, and. dishonor the large subjective audience they carry around. We have seen the nature of their perceived failure to vary widely. For many it concerned issues of scholastic performance; for others it was about either having immersed themselves too much or not enough in the host culture;

for others still, it took a more idiosyncratic form such as failure to obtain the proper occupational position in either the home or host country, or having indulged in the differing sexuality of the host culture. For many, at the end of the sojourn, the conflict has centered about their intuitive sense of having changed in ways that elders and peers at home would not approve.

The proper role of a therapist is to alleviate these discrepancies between what is and what "should" be, and between what was and what now is. Sometimes a reappraisal in realistic terms of goals and expectations can be useful, and the patient's own experience examined from a non-judgmental perspective is the best data from which to work. At other times, attempts to bind the wounds to the foreign students' ego is a most useful role for the therapist — so long as a trusting and authoritative relationship has developed. Specific techniques are described more fully in our prior publication, but they can all be covered by saying that the therapeutic issue for foreign patients will be to reestablish a concept of themselves with which they can once again be comfortable. The ravages of trying to be normal in what is an "abnormal" world often coalesce around the notion that it is the foreigner who is either entirely sound and right, or entirely unsound and wrong. It is not surprising that paranoia and depression are the two most commonly seen categories of psychiatric disorders in foreign students, for each is merely the most extreme way of resolving the difference between what one is and the world in which one finds him/herself.

TABLE 11

Variables Related to Health Service Visits of Chinese Students

Type of Visit	Predictor Variable[a]	Multiple R
Infection – Injury	Lived away from family before (−)	.220*
Pain, Psychosomatic or Psychiatric	Lived away from family before (+) Academic concerns (+)	.296**

[a]Results of Stepwise Multiple Regression Analysis; variables significant at 10% level or below are listed.
**p .01
*p .05

ACKNOWLEDGEMENT

These studies were supported by Ford Foundation Grant 133–5653, by the Wisconsin Psychiatric Institute and the University of Wisconsin Medical School Research Committee. The authors wish to express their appreciation to Dean Henry Hill and to members of the International Committee of the University of Wisconsin for their support and interest in this project and to Dr. Gregory Barnes and Dean Anne Corry for their help and cooperation. Thanks are also due to Sandra Bass, Christine Carey and Elizabeth Huesemann for their assistance with data gathering and analysis.

REFERENCES

Alexander, A. A., F. Workneh, M. H. Klein, and M. H. Miller
  1976 Psychotherapy and the foreign student. *In* P. Pederson and R. Wintrob (eds.), Cross-Cultural Counseling. Honolulu: Cultural Learning Institute, University of Hawaii.
Bennett, J. W., H. Passin, and R. K. McKnight
  1958 In Search of Identity – The Japanese Overseas Scholar in America and Japan. Minneapolis: University of Minnesota Press.
Chu, H. M., E. K. Yeh, M. H. Klein, A. A. Alexander, and M. H. Miller
  1971 A study of Chinese students adjustment in the U.S.A. Acta Psychologica Taiwanica 13:206–218.
Coehlho, G. V.
  1958 Changing Images of America: A Study of Indian Students' Perceptions. Glencoe, Illinois: The Free Press.
Kelman, H. C., and L. Bailyn
  1962 Effects of cross-cultural experience on national images: A study of Scandinavian students in America. Journal of Conflict Resolution 6:319–334.
Klein, M. H., A. A. Alexander, K. H. Tseng, M. H. Miller, E. K. Yeh, and H. M. Chu
  1971 Far Eastern students in a big university – Subcultures within a subculture. Science and Public Affairs: Bulletin of the Atomic Scientists 27:10ff.
Klein, M. H., M. H. Miller, A. A. Alexander, K. H. Tseng, F. Workneh, E. K. Yeh, and H. M. Chu
  1974 When young people go out in the world. *In* Lebra, W. P. (ed.), Youth, Socialization, and Mental Health: Vol. III of Mental Health Research in Asia and the Pacific. Honolulu: University of Hawaii Press.
Lambert, R. D. and M. Bressler
  1956 Indian Students on an American Campus. Minneapolis: University of Minnesota Press.
Morris, R. T. and O. M. Davidsen
  1960 The Two-Way Mirror: National Status in Foreign Students' Adjustment. Minneapolis: University of Minnesota Press.
Seligman, M. E.
  1974 Depression and learned helplessness. *In* R. J. Friedman and M. M. Katz (eds.). The Psychology of Depression: Contemporary Theory and Research. Washington, D.C.: V. H. Winston.

17. MENTAL ILLNESS AND PSYCHOSOCIAL ASPECTS OF MEDICAL PROBLEMS IN CHINA

BACKGROUND

This chapter is based on observations made by the authors of psychiatric and medical facilities in China during June 1978.[1] As members of the Rural Health Care Systems Delegation of the Committee on Scholarly Communication with the People's Republic of China, we visited production brigade health stations, commune hospitals, county hospitals, municipal and provincial hospitals, university teaching centers, and psychiatric facilities in six provinces of north and south China.

Our view of mental illness in the People's Republic of China (PRC) derives from several sources: visits to two departments of psychiatry and one outpatient neurology clinic in teaching hospitals in three urban areas; reports on or observation of psychiatric patients in general hospitals and medical clinics in rural areas; and interviews with patients with psychosocial problems secondary to physical disease or somatization of psychological problems in rural clinics.

There is a long history of stigmatization of mental illness in China prior to 1949, and such stigma continues in present-day Taiwan, Hong Kong, and overseas Chinese communities (Chin and Chin 1969; Gaw 1975; Kleinman 1975, 1976; Lamson 1935; Tseng and Hsu 1969). We simply cannot gauge its magnitude in the PRC today based on our brief visit, but we were frequently told by cadres and health workers that they were improving this problem through popular education. However, the cultural reticence that Chinese display worldwide regarding mental illness and psychiatry can be inferred from the hesitancy, embarrassment, and limited extent to which public health and health care personnel in China are willing to inform visitors on this subject. This cultural reticence may receive further support from an overly simple reading of Marx and Mao that associates mental illness with the "evils" of capitalist society and assumes that it should not be present in a socialist state.

For these and perhaps other reasons, mental illness is not highlighted in the People's Republic. Most strikingly, during a meeting on June 9, 1978, with China's Vice Minister of Public Health, Tan Yun-ho, we were informed that " . . . in the countryside mental illness is not a major problem and its incidence is not high." The fact that mental illness is not regarded a major public health or health care problem was reiterated in discussions with Lu Chin-chun, Fu I-cheng, and Chao Chu-gen, respectively Vice President, Deputy Secretary-General, and Leading Member, Peking Branch of the Chinese Medical Association. These views were largely affirmed by officials and medical and public health personnel during our visits to county, commune, and production brigade health facilities.

331

A. Kleinman and T.-Y. Lin (eds.), Normal and Abnormal Behavior in Chinese Culture, 331–356.
Copyright © 1980 by D. Reidel Publishing Company.

Seymour Kety (1973), in ending his observations on psychiatry in China in 1973, posed a seemingly perplexing question. Why, he asked, are the Chinese so reticent to talk about psychiatry or to acknowledge mental illness when there are indications of progressive care and accomplishment? Kety, a prominent researcher, describes the difficulties he had in getting to meet colleagues and to visit psychiatric facilities. Most visitors seem to be directed to the same institutions — the #3 Hospital in Peking and the Shanghai Mental Hospital, the former we visited too. Visits to this hospital have also been noted by Sidel (1973) and Lowinger (1978). At this hospital we saw a planned performance by psychiatric inpatients, and we also noted a listing of psychiatric diagnoses in English mounted under glass plating on a desk, presumably to be responsive to English-speaking visitors. A report by Lowinger (1978) could serve as a partial transcript of our own visit. Any generalizations on the basis of these visits to specially selected institutions, thus, must be made with the greatest caution.

A point to remember is that the Chinese usually speak in normative rather than empirical terms. The descriptions they give are often ideal descriptions of the way they would like things to be. The use of models serves to educate their own people as to goals and means and is not intended to be representative of the average or usual. In the psychiatric area we experienced the largest difficulty of access and the greatest discordance between ideology and what we could see with our own eyes even in model institutions. It has been maintained and reported by Sidel (1973:291), for example, that after liberation "isolation and binding of patients were ... prohibited," but in one teaching institution there were a series of locked isolation rooms in which we saw three patients bound by their hands and legs. We were assured that psychiatric units we visited were not locked, yet we could see the physician holding a key in preparation as we approached certain units. Much of what we saw of inpatient care was based on principles of social influence; when we asked "sensitive questions" about social aspects of mental illness, however, we were told that psychiatry in China was a biological discipline, not "social psychiatry." Despite repeated requests to see nonteaching psychiatric units, and our knowledge that they were sometimes close by in areas we were visiting, we were repeatedly told that the institutions were too far away. Although we would be driven into rural areas for four or five hours to see model production brigades when there were brigades within walking distance of the compound where we stayed, it was impossible to see psychiatric units when they were ten minutes away.

It is exceedingly difficult to evaluate the claims made that there is little mental illness in China because only rarely were there data to support such claims, and the data that were available were highly inadequate. China is largely a rural nation dependent on simple agricultural methods and one in which there are strong family ties and cohesive social organizations at production team, brigade, and commune levels. Such contexts more easily shelter impaired persons and can provide sufficient social support and restraints that help contain the more bizarre manifestations of mental illness. Moreover, because mental illness is seen as equivalent to psychosis and apparently is still stigmatizing for families, it may be more readily ignored, normalized, or handled as physical illness or as issues of social control. It is possible that "adequate maternal and child care, economic security, and the solidarity of the people with a common purpose — national reconstruction — are all factors likely to reduce the rate of mental disorders" (Ho 1974), but the link between such factors and psychosis remains problematic. Given the absence of epidemiological data, we can say very little about the incidence of mental disorder in China. Our visits and discussions, however, provide some sense of pathways into treatment and contexts of care.

Findings from psychiatric epidemiological studies conducted in other Chinese communities disclose roughly the same amount of psychiatric morbidity with respect to the major psychoses as in Western societies (see article by Lin, Klein-man, and Lin above), though alcoholism and homosexuality have a decidedly low prevalence. Lacking epidemiological evidence from the PRC that disconfirms the findings from other Chinese populations, it is plausible that the prevalence rate for psychiatric disorders there is roughly similar to that of Chinese in Hong Kong (see the article by Lee above), Taiwan (Lin et al. 1969), Singapore (Murphy 1959), and the United States (see the article by Tsai, Teng and Sue above).

SOMATIZATION AND PSYCHOSOCIAL PROBLEMS IN MEDICAL CARE

Studies have determined that most mental illness among Chinese is somatized (i.e., manifested as somatic rather than psychological complaints) (see Kleinman 1977; and Chapters 13, 15, and 18 in this volume), and our own observations in the PRC are consistent with this view. Tseng (1975) discovered, for example, that 70 percent of patients who visited the psychiatric clinic at National Taiwan University Hospital and were later demonstrated to be suffering from psychiatric disorders complained of physical ailments as their chief problem. Because we encountered instances of somatization of depression at all levels of the health care system we visited in China, it is plausible to believe that a similar magnitude of psychiatric problems are somatized in the PRC and that, as a consequence, public health and health care personnel fail to appreciate the true prevalence of mental illness because of their concepts of illness and the absence of epidemio-logical data.

In Taiwan, minor mental illness (depression, anxiety neurosis, hysteria, hypochondriasis) is most frequently labeled as "neurasthenia" (*shen-ching shuai-jo*) or given culture-specific diagnoses ("wind disease," "kidney deficiency"). These labels connote for laymen — and often even for practitioners — physical rather than psychological distress, and sanction a medical rather than a psychiatric sick role (Kleinman 1979). Depression among Chinese, when labeled as "neurasthenia" or "kidney deficiency" (*shen-k'uei*), is not only categorized as a physical disorder, but appears to be experienced vegetatively, not intra-psychically (see Lin et al. above). Choice of health care services follows this somatic conceptualization of personal and interpersonal distress. Patients with mental disorders initially go to Chinese-style doctors, Western-style general practitioners, or shamans, and not to psychiatrists or psychologists. Only if their disorders worsen significantly and they perceive them as severe and untreatable by usual practitioners do they enter psychiatric treatment facilities (cf. Lin and Lin below and Lin et al. 1978 for data on Chinese in Vancouver).

Chin and Chin (1969) suggest that at least until the Cultural Revolution "neurasthenia" may have served the same function in China as in Taiwan and other Chinese communities. It was our general impression that "neurasthenia" represents the largest single illness category of psychiatric patients in outpatient practice in China and accordingly that most patients with psychiatric disorders are treated in general medical and neurological rather than in psychiatric settings.

In all medical care systems, illness serves as an important and legitimate means for reducing burdensome expectations that strain the person or for justifying personal failures. In Western medical care systems it has been estimated that a significant proportion of patients seek the physician's assistance because of symptoms associated with psychosocial problems. Depending on cultural patterns, such patients may openly acknowledge their psychological distress or express such distress through vague somatic complaints or physiological concomitants of anxiety and depression. Given the pervasiveness of such problems, it is appropriate to ask how the medical care system in rural China relates to psychosocial difficulties in the life of the peasant.

Life for the average peasant has improved a great deal, but it is still a hard life requiring good health, energy, and good fortune. There are undoubtedly many psychosocial problems that occur in families, teams, and brigades, and the household's income depends on the work points earned by its workers. In the rural areas there are few acceptable excuses for able-bodied workers not to perform their share of the work, and even in the case of illness there is no sick leave, sickness insurance, or disability payments, with the exception of work-related accidents. A household member who fails to meet work obligations reduces the earnings of the household and thus increases the burden on others. In all likelihood therefore, there must be great informal pressure to carry one's share of the effort.

Sickness, even without compensation, is an acceptable excuse, one more likely to bring sympathy and concern from family and neighbors than condemnation. The sick role, thus, is an important mechanism to relieve tension and to facilitate restoration of the social unit. The production brigade health station provides ready accessibility to those desiring assistance, and Chinese traditional medicine provides both the theoretical basis and the treatments necessary to encourage restoration in an acceptable and face-saving way. It was therefore not surprising that many patients we interviewed at all levels of care had vague and unspecified gastrointestinal complaints, and that patients who suffered from depression, anxiety, and a variety of psychophysiological complaints (typically diagnosed as neurasthenia) were more commonly seen in the traditional Chinese clinic.

Understanding how such complaints are expressed and managed requires understanding of Chinese cultural patterns. In Chinese culture the maintenance and restoration of interpersonal relationships are a central theme, and an introspective orientation, particularly in relation to negative affective states, is discouraged (Hsu 1971). Mental illness, furthermore, has traditionally been highly stigmatized (and this apparently has persisted). The Chinese thus do not have an elaborate psychological vocabulary to characterize the quality of distress, and negative emotion appears to be muted or suppressed (Kleinman 1979; Tseng and Hsu 1969). Instead distress seems to be expressed somatically with less obvious evidence of depressive affect or anxiety (Kleinman 1977; Tseng 1975). One finds, however, as we did in our interviews, frequent complaints of the vegetative symptoms usually associated with a diagnosis of depression in Western nations. It was clear from our interviews that such patients were commonly diagnosed as having neurasthenia, and that they were more frequently referred, or referred themselves, to the traditional Chinese medical clinic. Some examples of such syndromes, the way they were interpreted, and the way they were managed in nonpsychiatric settings are discussed below. Concepts of neurasthenia as they relate to American and Chinese conceptions of diagnosis are discussed in more detail in Lin et al. above.

Case Vignette: In the Luen-tsun Commune Hospital in Chang-an County, Shensi, we observed doctor-patient interactions in the Chinese medical clinic. The doctor staffing this clinic had received both Western and traditional training, but treated patients with only herbal medication. In this clinic we saw consultations with a 51-year-old mother and her 22-year-old unmarried daughter. The daughter had many presenting complaints including back pain, headaches, difficulty breathing, and poor appetite. The mother reported that the daughter does not want to do anything and feels out of sorts all of the time. She said that the daughter does not work in the house and does not have the energy to do outside work. She described the symptoms of her daughter as *huo-ch'i ta* (excessive internal hot energy). The girl looked obviously depressed, and when we questioned her she reported depressed affect and sleep disturbance with early morning wakening. The daughter, a middle-school graduate, began to feel this way at graduation, when she was 18 years old, but could not associate these feelings with any personal or social problem.

When we asked her what she thought the problem might be, she denied illness and indicated that she was brought to the clinic by her mother and the barefoot doctor. We asked her what might make her better, and she answered that if there was "peace in the family" she would be better. These possible social issues were not pursued in any way by the doctor, and he explained that she had a Chinese illness due to an imbalance of *yin* and *yang*. Although he acknowledged hysteria and depression, he indicated that the girl had a physical illness that must be treated with herbs, and he wrote an elaborate herbal prescription.

The mother was later treated by the same doctor, but quite independently of her daughter. She complained of trouble with eating, a burning sensation in her stomach, and a feeling of nausea. She also reported headaches, cough, and occasional stomach pains. She had no problem with her chest or heart. Further, she reported that when she goes to work she feels a lack of energy, a fogginess in her head, and a tiredness in her legs. In response to the doctor's question, she indicated that she was not sure whether she had a "hot" or a "cold" constitution. The doctor on "reading her pulse" reported it as "high, strong, and fast." In response to our follow-up questions, the mother reported feeling somewhat depressed but indicated her illness was not the same as her daughter's, although it was made worse by her daughter's illness. She reported that there were eleven people in her family living in four rooms, including five children, a mother, and an aunt. She said there was constant noise and turmoil, and she had the feeling that she "couldn't work with" the problems in her family.

It would be presumptuous of us, given so little information and the possibilities of misunderstandings, to analyze these cases or to attribute any general significance to the importance of the particular comments made.[2] There are some observations, however, consistent with so many of our other observations and interviews in Chinese and internal medicine clinics that we can suggest them with considerable confidence. Here we emphasize the response of personnel in the conventional medical context.

At no time did we observe doctors pursuing psychosocial problems of patients in assessment or management although they readily seemed to recognize "neurasthenia" and hysterical complaints. At no time either in assessing the patient or in treatment were psychosocial issues seen as relevant, and these complaints were always dealt with as evidence of a physical disease. Although doctors in the Chinese medical clinic used traditional concepts to explain the condition, and Western-trained doctors viewed the complaints as evidence of neurological disease, the treatment always involved some form of direct medication and never any exploration of possible nonphysical influences. We have no way of assessing the extent to which such issues are taken up in the context of the family or production team, or the way criticism or small group influence is used to mediate psychosocial stress. Nor can we assess the population of problem types that these referrals come from and the way they might relate to other psychosocial problems that are not referred. What seems clear is that the medical system, for whatever reason, chooses to ignore the psychosocial dimensions of these consultations, but there seems to be a dependence on the Chinese traditional clinic more than on internal medicine to deal with this type of condition. Given Chinese culture and the problems of managing psychosocial issues, we are not in a position to assess whether the dominant response is appropriate or inappropriate.

Case Vignettes: During the same clinic session we observed a consultation with a 34-year-old man who was a farmer, but who was formerly a teacher. He complained of feeling weak and tired, pain in the back, and a constant feeling of anxiety. He also reported some depression, a poor appetite, and sleep disturbance with early morning wakening. The patient reported that he had lots of troubles with people and that he thought he had neurasthenia. Similar patients were apparent at all levels of care. For example, in the Western county hospital in Tao Yuan County in Hunan Province we interviewed a 25-year-old woman who reported a variety of complaints for "long years." More recently she had a feeling of dizziness and developed palpitations when feeling tense. She denied any affective symptoms. She reported that she had three children and much work to do. Recently she felt her heart rate quicken in response to her feeling that there was too much work to do. She has been treated regularly by the barefoot doctor with both Western and traditional medicines and also acupuncture.

She has been told that her symptoms can be helped but not cured. A third patient, a 35-year-old man, was interviewed at the Chinese medical clinic at the Kweilin Central Hospital. He reported having had many symptoms for some time, including dizziness and a feeling of heaviness in the head. More recently he lacked energy, had a feeling of weakness and fatigue, and suffered from a poor appetite and sleep disturbance with early morning wakening. This man had seen his barefoot doctor and doctors at both the Kweilin Central Hospital and the Municipal Workers' Hospital, but has experienced no improvement in symptoms. The doctor at the workers' hospital told him that he had a Chinese disease and referred him to the Chinese medical clinic at the central hospital, which he was revisiting. The doctor indicated that the diagnosis was a *yin* disorder which had produced an excess of "cold" elements in the patient's constitution, for which he was prescribing traditional medicines.

We interviewed a 30-year-old female patient undergoing acupuncture treatment at the Institute of Acupuncture and Moxibustion. She had a history since adolescence of more that 30 discrete, multiple, recurrent physical complaints, involving at least 9 separate areas of the body. Some of these problems had never received a definitive diagnosis. This history is consistent with Briquet's syndrome (hysteria). Recently she had exhibited the vegetative complaints of depression with depressed affect and anhedonia as well as physical complaints. She reported problems at work and in her family. The Chinese-style doctors agreed with me the patient was depressed, but they stated that acupuncture would relieve her psychological symptoms along with her physical symptoms. According to them the psychological disorder was the result of an underlying organic problem that would respond to acupuncture.

Similarly the doctors in the Department of Chinese Medicine of the Mi-yun County Hospital outside of Peking, stressed herbal rather than acupuncture treatment, reporting that they frequently were referred patients from internal medicine with chronic illness or neurasthenia in which there were psychological problems. But they treated these problems solely with herbal and other traditional Chinese somatic therapies, which they believed were specific remedies for psychological as well as physical problems, not with "talk" therapy. Much the same was reported to us by a Chinese-style pharmacist preparing herbs to treat neurasthenia at the Tachai Commune Hospital. Of the seven cases we observed in the Chinese Medicine Clinic of Luen-tsun Commune Hospital, Chang-an County, outside of Sian, six seemed to us cases with primary psychological problems and secondary somatization, yet the doctor gave neither supportive care nor psychologically-minded treatment.

Case Vignette: One patient was a 41-year-old man with headaches, pains in joints, insomnia, "too many dreams," loss of appetite, weakness, and the belief that there was something wrong with his brain that caused his scalp to sweat excessively. It seemed to us this patient had a depressive syndrome associated with a fixed idea, which could have been a somatic delusion. In treating him, the doctor diagnosed a skin disease of the scalp which was making the man depressed. He prescribed herbal medicine that he claimed would improve the scalp problem and through it the patient's "brain function." That in turn would cure the depression. In the entire interchange doctor and patient discussed illness and treatment solely in somatic terms.

In interviews we conducted with 138 patients in general medical outpatient clinics in production brigade health stations and county and commune hospitals, 4% of all primary complaints and 8% of identified secondary complaints involved psychological problems. In almost all of the cases that appeared to us as probably somatization of depression or other psychiatric disorders (N = 17), physician and patient viewed the underlying disease as a physical one. When they recognized psychological problems, they were viewed as caused by the underlying physical disorder. Rarely was a diagnosis of mental illness entertained by the participants. Moreover, these problems were not managed with psychosocial interventions in the general medical care setting either at primary or more specialized levels of care. Even the Chinese medicine clinics in county and commune hospitals, which, as we have already noted, appear to manage such problems routinely (12% of our interviews were in traditional Chinese medicine clinics, but 24% of these patients reported what seemed to be primary psychological complaints and 35% secondary psychological complaints), did not provide psychosocial exploration or care. Vague and diffuse complaints were interpreted in a somato-psychic frame of reference and treated solely with somatic therapies. Neither the Chinese-style doctors nor the Western-style physicians we observed inquired into personal, family, or social network problems. In two situations in which we elicited information on such social tensions in our interviews, our hosts became upset, concerned that we might misinterpret what we heard.

Our observations of the practice of barefoot doctors were very few, but in no case we saw treated by barefoot doctors was specific attention given to experiential or interpersonal aspects of illness. These impressions fit with research findings from Taiwan that disclose that Chinese-style and Western-style physicians do not usually provide psychosocial interventions, whereas sacred folk practitioners do (Kleinman 1979). Because the latter have been prohibited from practicing in the PRC, one can only wonder where, outside the context of the family, psychological and social aspects of sickness are dealt with. Do the ubiquitous "small groups" play such a role? Are these problems recognized and responded to in informal social networks? These questions cannot be answered based on the limited information obtained in visits such as ours.

PSYCHIATRIC DISORDERS AND THEIR TREATMENT

The delivery of psychiatric care in China, especially in rural areas, is based on the restricted meaning given to the terms "mental illness" and "psychiatric disease." These terms are largely limited by the Chinese to denote psychotic disorders, mental retardation, and other severe forms of behavioral pathology. Although concepts of mental illness may differ from place to place and from one practitioner to another, we found that such terms as "mental illness," "schizophrenia," and "psychosis" were all used interchangeably. Most inpatients were diagnosed as schizophrenic, and a distinction was made between excited and passive schizophrenics, with the passive type predominating. In one teaching center we were told that excited schizophrenic patients respond to Lithium carbonate, supporting our hypothesis that many of these patients would probably be diagnosed as bipolar depression in Western countries. Manic-depressive disorder, we were told repeatedly, is infrequently diagnosed, and depression was also rarely seen. The fact that most depression is manifested as somatic complaints results in few cases identified or referred to psychiatrists by other health personnel. Other common inpatient disorders included primarily organic disorders such as senile psychosis and arteriosclerotic disease.

The psychiatric outpatient departments in the hospitals we visited were also primarily directed toward the management of schizophrenic patients. The psychiatrists in the #2 affiliated Hospital of the Hunan Medical College, however, told us that as many as half of the outpatients were neurotics, predominantly patients with neurasthenia, but also some were hysterics and obsessive neurotics. Such diagnoses as anxiety neurosis, phobia, hypochondriasis, and reactive depression were only rarely made. In the neurology outpatient service of the Chung Shan Medical College we were told that neurasthenia was very common.

In theory, the treatment of mental illness is organized in tiers, akin to the general organization of medical care. The lowest level is the barefoot doctor in the production brigade who may identify patients in need of care and who assists in administering medication for patients in the brigade. The second level is the commune hospital which may treat schizophrenic patients for as much as three months as inpatients if they are not so agitated that they disrupt the work of the hospital. Patients who do not improve sufficiently to return to their homes may be sent to a psychiatric hospital that may provide either short-term (up to six months) or long-term care (several years) depending on the geographic area and the other facilities available. Some chronic cases who cannot return to the community may spend long periods of time in large chronic disease institutions (referred to as sanitaria) associated with large factories and state industries which treat both the mentally ill and other chronic patients. We were told that sanitaria did not keep patients for decades, although several years of care might be provided. Many chronic patients were returned to their brigades and treated in "home beds" by families and barefoot doctors. In urban areas, there are also municipal and provincial mental hospitals, but we could not get a consistent picture of the types of patients treated or average lengths of stay. Details will be provided later for specific areas we visited.

It was difficult to arrive at a clear picture of the way schizophrenic patients were managed at the brigade level in the areas we visited. For the most part, the existence of mental illness is not recognized, and the concept plays only a small part in the total medical care picture in rural areas. Some schizophrenic patients are retained in the community in "home beds" which, as we understood the concept, meant that they received special attention from the barefoot doctor assisted by staff from commune hospitals and special psychiatric institutions if they existed in the area. The Chinese doctors frequently referred to prevention of mental illness. Close questioning revealed that "prevention" referred to (1) alerting the families to dangers of suicide; (2) instructing on necessary medications; (3) paying attention to food habits and feeding the patient; and (4) instructing the families as to what to observe and report to health personnel.

The simplicity of Chinese agriculture and industry, the strong family network, and the tight system of social organization provide considerable flexibility
in managing patients in the community. Family members and commune officials
are involved in patient "planning," and cooperate in arriving at work assignments
patients can manage. Patients may do more simple tasks and receive assistance
at the work place in managing daily activities. Mental illness in China is not a
confidential relationship between patient and doctor, but a social issue involving
the home, the work place and the production brigade. We were told repeatedly
that educational efforts were being made to reduce the stigma of mental illness,
and were also told that marriage was possible for schizophrenic patients.

Schizophrenia in rural areas is initially diagnosed in commune and county
hospitals. Such cases may be treated for periods up to three months or referred
immediately to provincial psychiatric hospitals. Psychiatric care in commune and
county hospitals is provided by Western-style physicians with general medical
training. These hospitals generally do not have psychiatrists. But at the county
and prefecture level, general hospitals may contain Western-style physicians who
have received special courses in the diagnosis and treatment of mental illness,
such as those provided by the department of psychiatry of the Hunan Medical
School. Psychiatric personnel from specialty hospitals also may visit general
hospitals in rural areas as part of special mobile health teams to provide consultation and instruction.

Provincial and municipal psychiatric hospitals form part of China's chronic
disease hospital system. This system includes tuberculosis and leprosy hospitals,
and this triad itself suggests that stigma and isolation from the mainstream of
general medical care may affect China's psychiatric services for chronic mental illness in the same way it affects psychiatric care throughout Asia. Because we did
not observe long-stay hospitals or "home bed" psychiatric care by barefoot doctors, we are limited in commenting on the management of chronic mental illness.

Our visits and interviews illustrate our general observations. At the Mi-yun
County Hospital in the far suburbs of Peking, we were told that when a psychotic patient was first seen in the outpatient clinic, he was evaluated and usually
sedated with a neuroleptic drug by the Western-style doctors in the Internal
Medicine Clinic. Then he was sent immediately to Stability Hospital in Peking.
Because this county hospital was relatively close to a large municipal psychiatric
hospital, it did not treat patients with mental illness but referred them directly
to this specialty hospital. At the Chen-ke chuan Production Brigade in the same
county, the barefoot doctor's medical kit contained injectable chlorpromazine,
which we were informed was occasionally used to treat chronic schizophrenic
patients who were maintained in their production teams and treated at the
brigade health station or in "home beds."

At the Tachai Commune Hospital (serving 11,600 people) we were told that
over the past year only two or three cases with psychosis were treated as inpatients at the hospital. None was referred to the provincial psychiatric hospital
located in this county. Here as elsewhere we were informed by local cadres that

the small number of cases of mental illness reflected the fact that mental illness was caused by bad social conditions especially affecting women in China prior to 1949, whereas the People's Republic, by vastly improving social conditions, removed the root cause of mental illness. Dr. Tu Hsieh-chih, director of the hospital, went on to say that depression (*yu-ping*), which they rarely saw, was a psychotic disorder and therefore a mental illness, whereas minor "psychological problems" (*hsin-li wen-t'i*), which were fairly common in their outpatient clinic, were caused by neurasthenia or "insomnia" and were not mental illness (*ching-shen ping*).

Only one of the more than one dozen barefoot doctors we interviewed admitted currently treating patients with mental illness or mental retardation. Most denied that they had encountered any depressed patients, but all had experience with treating neurasthenia. Miss Chen, our interpreter, had hardly any experience with mental illness during her two years as a barefoot doctor in Heilungkiang. These barefoot doctors reported being taught, however, to "calm" cases of acute psychoses with injectable chlorpromazine and then refer them to local hospitals. Again the interesting question for further research is to what extent these and other health care providers fail to diagnose depression, hysteria, anxiety neurosis, and other mental illness that are common in other Chinese communities.

In the suburbs of Sian, five members of our group strolled by ourselves into a farming brigade near our hotel where we encountered one patient with strange behavior; the neighbors told us he had a serious mental illness of many years' duration. This 46-year-old man had been hospitalized at least once in the provincial psychiatric hospital for a period of months. He is cared for by his children and wife, and the neighbors offer help from time to time. He has not been in the hospital in recent years. He was described by his neighbors as harmless, but they added that he frequently "says strange things and speaks in a strange voice and has strange thoughts." They claimed not to fear him, paid little attention to his exaggerated behavior with us, and eventually when he brought out a large pipe, put on a hat, and spoke in a high falsetto voice, one of his daughters drove him back to their home with a threatening voice and a few light slaps to his body. This patient's production team did not have a barefoot doctor nearby, but was close to a hospital. It was unclear how often he went for treatment, and we did not learn the kind of treatment he received. Nor did we learn if his work responsibilities were different from those of his neighbors. This was the only example we witnessed of a patient with chronic mental illness in a community setting.

Like commune and county hospitals, the traditional Chinese medicine hospitals we visited refer patients to psychiatric hospitals. The staff of the First Teaching Hospital of Hunan Provincial Medical School of Traditional Chinese Medicine reported that psychotic patients seen in the outpatient clinic were referred immediately and not treated as inpatients. Like their Western-style colleagues, these traditional doctors were familiar with the term "hysteria," but claimed to encounter patients with this problem only rarely and regarded it, like neurasthenia, as a physical, not a mental illness. Such cases would receive out-patient treatment with herbs and acupuncture.

At the San Yang Commune Hospital in Tao Yuan County, Hunan, we learned that each year this hospital, which serves a commune population of 22,900, sees three or four cases of psychosis (all schizophrenics). At the time of our visit two patients with schizophrenia who were being treated in the hospital were on leave to their homes. Both young men had been admitted for their first hospitalization for psychosis three months before our visit. Their families brought them to the hospital because of delusional thinking without consulting barefoot doctors. They did not exhibit violent behavior nor were they paranoid. But both were diagnosed as suffering from "excited schizophrenia" and were treated with chlorpromazine, trifluperazine, and traditional herbal medicines. If their symptoms were controlled they would return to live with their families and would be encouraged to continue to do farming. If they did not improve, they would have been referred to the provincial psychiatric hospital. Their families were said to want them back.

At the nearby Tao Yuan County People's Hospital, we learned that cases of psychosis referred from commune hospitals to the provincial psychiatric hospital would pass through this county hospital, where the diagnosis would be con-firmed. Psychiatric patients with severe excitement who were difficult to control would be sent directly to the psychiatric hospital. Cases without pathological excitement would be kept for two or three days to reassess the diagnoses given by the commune hospitals, and a decision would be made concerning referral. Like the commune hospital we visited, the county hospital might treat non-disruptive psychotic patients for up to three months. If no improvement occurred by then, patients would be referred to the psychiatric hospital. Each year the hospital treats three or four psychotic patients, but we were told that most cases of psychosis were treated in the 60 commune hospitals in this county of 880,000 people. Patients at the psychiatric hospital would be returned to their families eventually even if there was only partial improvement. If, however, there was no change in their symptoms and behavior, they might remain at the psychiatric hospital.

At the Chuan-shan Central Hospital in Kweilin, only two patients with psychosis had been seen during the past year in a commune with 18,600 people, despite the fact that this hospital provided technical support to three commune hospitals. One patient whose psychosis was described to us as severe was referred to the provincial psychiatric hospital. The other patient was treated in the internal medicine clinic with Western antipsychotic drugs. In all of Kweilin there are no psychiatrists, and the provincial psychiatric hospital is a considerable distance away.

EPIDEMIOLOGY OF MENTAL ILLNESS IN CHINA

In the Tao-hsu Commune Hospital, Heng County, Kwangsi, which serves a commune population of 56,923, our hosts reported that no cases of mental illness were seen in 1976 or 1977. (In 1977 there were 43,266 outpatient clinic visits and 523 inpatients.) Of the eight patients we interviewed in the outpatient clinic, however, one impressed one of the authors (A.K.)[2] as a case of somatization owing to Briquet's Syndrome (hysteria). Heng County Hospital itself, which has 145 beds and has 150,000 outpatient visits and 4,000 inpatients annually, serving a population of 780,000, treated only three cases of mental illness in the previous three years. These cases included one patient with schizophrenia, another with depression, and a third with organic psychosis following a head injury. Because the World Health Organization (WHO) reports the prevalence rate of schizophrenia for a variety of Western and non-Western societies as ranging from two to ten per 1,000 (Sartorius and Jablensky 1976), including Chinese populations in Taiwan, one would expect a much greater number of schizophrenic patients being seen at the Heng County Hospital and similar institutions. The low reported prevalence of mental illness in the PRC deserves careful study. In the absence of population-based surveys, hospital-based data like this may lead to gross underassessment of the actual magnitude of schizophrenia and other psychiatric disorders, which in turn may undervalue the need for rural psychiatric services. (Of the 16 patients we interviewed in the outpatient clinic at this hospital at least one and possibly a second impressed A.K. as cases of somatization of psychiatric disorder.)

The only psychiatric epidemiological data we saw in China were at the psychiatry department of the #3 Affiliated Hospital of the Peking Medical College. We visited the department's inpatient and outpatient facilities, interviewed and observed treatment of several inpatients, and spent about three hours talking with Dr. Hou Yi, Deputy Head of the Department, and Dr. Lo Huo-chun, Attending Psychiatrist. The psychiatric service was founded in 1951 as the center for clinical psychiatric teaching and care at Peking Medical College. This department works closely with at least one suburban county of Peking, where they carry out periodic surveys of the number and types of patients with mental illness, consult with and supervise doctors in commune hospitals and barefoot doctors who care for the mentally ill, give speciality treatment to selected patients, and teach prevention.

In this suburban county they have conducted mass surveys in different communes yearly since 1974. The surveys are conducted in the following manner: first local barefoot doctors were trained to identify mental disorders; then, based on their knowledge of the local population, they decided on cases whom they "presumed" to be suffering from mental illness. (There have been no community-wide surveys in which psychiatrists or physicians conduct household surveys). Each "presumed case" of mental illness is reevaluated by a psychiatrist from this department to determine the "cases" listed in Table 1. Drs. Hou and Lo cautioned that these were crude statistics that should not be regarded as having true epidemological significance. We agree with them on this point, but they are the only survey data we obtained during our visit in spite of our repeated attempts

TABLE 1

Survey of Certain Types of Mental Illness[a] in One Suburban County of Peking

Commune	Population	No. of Brigades	Date of Survey	No. of Local Barefoot Doctors	Cases Treated in Home Total Cases / Beds[b]	Schizophrenic Home Patients / Beds	Epilepsy Home / Beds	Mental Retardation Home / Beds	Other Psychoses[c] Home / Beds
1	14,807	8	7-10-74	24	163 /	/ 24	/ 15	/ 9	/ 15
2	13,514	10	3-24-75	11	128 / 52	27 / 23	41 / 15	49 / 6	11 / 8
3	18,158	4	7-14-75	71	206 / 113	59 / 54	50 / 25	76 / 13	21 / 21
4	43,129	14	10-20-75	24	335 / 137	61 / 36	98 / 37	141 / 35	35 / 29
5	15,230	8	2-23-76	12	122 / 82	28 / 25	39 / 16	42 / 36	13 / 5
6	19,481	7	4-19-76	12	/ 56	-1 / 16[d]	/ 17	/ 17	/ 6
7	8,396	7	7-19-76	12	60 / 29	/ 6	/ 14	/ 8	/ 1
8	12,837	9	—[e]	10	80 / 42	26 / 24	18 / 6	18 / 9	18 / 3
9	1,978	4	—	3	/ 33	/ 18	/ 5	/ 2	/ 8
10	12,999	10	—	24	83 / 45	19 / 19	36 / 25	18 /	10 / 1
11	17,694	—	—	36	85 / 57	23 / 19	24 / 23	28 / 11	10 / 4
12[e]	—	—	—	—	—	—	—	—	—
Total	189,915	—	—	247	/ 787	/ 292	/ 221	/ 159	/ 115

[a] This survey was restricted to patients suffering from psychoses, epilepsy, and mental retardation. Cases of neurosis and other psychiatric problems are not included.

[b] "Home beds" are defined as patients treated in their own homes by visiting nurses and barefoot doctors working with families.

[c] "Other psychoses" include reactive (psychogenic or atypical) psychoses and manic-depressive psychosis.

[d] We did not learn what "-1" meant.

[e] Kleinman failed to record these data.

Note: It was not clear to the authors if this data collection involved doctors working in commune hospitals as well as barefoot doctors. Lu (1978), reporting on these surveys, indicated that the initial identification of cases was made by the barefoot doctors.

to discover what was known about the prevalence of mental illness at national, provincial, county, and commune levels. We thus present the data recognizing full well their serious limitations. We were unable to clarify a number of questions raised by the findings, such as why "total cases treated" are not reported for certain communes or the significance of absent numerators under "epilepsy," "mental retardation," "other psychoses," and "schizophrenic patients." Nor were we able to discover why the number of local barefoot doctors or numbers of reported cases varied so much for some of the communes. It is of interest that the numbers of schizophrenic patients in each commune are much higher than the anecdotal material reported to us in rural communes, even though these numbers still are very low when compared to the figures of two to ten schizophrenia cases per 1000 population cited by WHO as the best available epidemiological estimates from a number of international surveys. Of course, it is to be expected that the Peking statistics significantly underestimate actual number of cases because of the relatively casual way cases were determined, without scientific sampling or house-to-house surveys.[3]

In addition to these data, other data were illustrated on wall charts describing the department's suburban catchment area of approximately 190,000 people. Patients in home beds in 1977 were classified in terms of clinical improvement on an A to D system with "A" representing clinical recovery and "D" no effect. Of the schizophrenic patients, 102 of 232 were classified as clinically recovered, clearly an impressive statistic for such a difficult patient population! Further questioning, however, revealed that patients who had a remission of symptoms for one month are classified as clinically recovered, and that they continue in the "A" group even if their symptoms recur. This is less impressive, and it would have been a disservice to have reported the superficial findings uncritically. The doctors at the hospital seemed sincere, and certainly we found no evidence of a desire to mislead us. If one persisted in asking the right questions, issues could be clarified, but this is difficult under the conditions of such a delegation visit.

PSYCHIATRIC THEORIES AND PRACTICES

Because most of what we learned about psychiatric theories and practices in China resulted from meetings with psychiatrists and neurologists at hospitals in Peking, Changsha, and Kwangchow, we shall describe these discussions in detail. Before we do so, however, some relevant background information needs to be reviewed.

Our trip to China occurred at a time of great political change. This manifested itself in part in somewhat more freedom to explore psychiatric and psychosocial issues than prior groups had experienced. But since our mandate was to study rural health care, psychiatric services were viewed by our hosts as a somewhat marginal interest, and hence we did not get to spend as much time studying psychiatric care as we would have liked. While we were in China, however, psychology was being rehabilitated. The June 26, 1978, issue of *Kuang-ming jih-pao* (the leading newspaper for intellectuals) reported the results of a national psychological convention that was held in Hangchow on May 8–15, 1978. This convention asserted the importance of psychology and detailed part of the content of an eight-year plan for national psychological research. The "Gang of Four" was blamed for the "mutilation" of professional psychology. Chairman Hua was praised for giving the profession "new life" so that it could go on to make important teaching and research contributions. Developmental psychology was discussed at the convention, and the nature and purposes of this discipline were described to the paper's readers in terms educated laymen could understand. The practical educational significance of this field of psychology received particular stress. After a view of the historical development of psychological research beginning with the work of William Wundt, readers of the article were informed that the conference participants were unanimous in agreeing to "actively promote teaching and research work in psychology" so as to contribute to the Four Modernizations Movement and to the strengthening of our "grand, socialist nation." Subsequent issues of *Kuang-ming jih-pao* have introduced other aspects of psychology to readers. Although this dramatic change in the fortunes of psychology in China occurred while we were in the PRC, we saw little evidence of it. It is, however, reasonable to surmise that this development and many related changes portend significant alterations in the role and functions of psychiatry in China. Thus special caution should be attached to this concluding section of the chapter, because what we learned may be more representative of the past than predictive of the future.

The first psychiatric department visited was at Peking's #3 Hospital. The department has 24 doctors and 15 nurses, and maintains 100 beds, divided into separate wards for men and women. The outpatient clinic has approximately 100 patient visits each day. Most of the 100 outpatients in this clinic, we were told, were suffering from psychosis. The next largest group suffer neurasthenia and other neuroses. (Unlike their medical colleagues in the county and commune hospitals we visited, the psychiatrists in this hospital labeled neurasthenia a neurosis.) Most of the patients with psychosis are discharged patients who return once every two weeks or month for follow-up care. We were told that whereas most neurotic cases are self-referrals to the clinic, most psychotic cases are brought to the clinic (occasionally against their will) by family or co-workers. Neurotic patients by and large are not released from work obligations, whereas psychotic patients routinely are for the period of time they are actively psychotic. Treatment of both neurotic and psychotic patients may involve family, neighbors, and co-workers, who help in the resolution of practical problems involving the patients. Somatization was recognized by Drs. Hou and Lo as a common manifestation of both neurotic and psychotic disorders, usually not recognized as such by local doctors.

Psychotic patients, who frequently are admitted to one of the inpatient wards when first brought to the clinic, are treated first with antipsychotic medications (e.g., chlorpromazine or haloperidol) along with milieu therapy and small group discussions (having both political and therapeutic functions), participation in structured patient activities (exercises, athletic games, singing), occupational therapy, and so forth. If patients are refractory to these interventions, insulin shock therapy is used. Roughly 16 percent of all inpatients were estimated to receive insulin shock therapy. This is usually used in such a way as not to produce coma. Electro-convulsive therapy (ECT) is not used in this department because its early use was associated with untoward effects that frightened patients and families. This was reported as a local problem, because Dr. Hou remarked that ECT was used in other psychiatric hospitals. Long-acting injectable phenothiazines are increasingly being used in the treatment of chronic schizophrenia.

All patients who attend the psychiatric clinic pay a registration fee of ten cents. Some pay only this fee, but most may pay more. If the patient's visit is not paid for out of cooperative insurance system funds, then the patient may have to pay himself for medication. This may involve as much as two to three yuan. People who visit the clinic who are not part of a cooperative insurance fund may be covered by a certificate saying they cannot pay, in which case the government pays the hospital. Inpatients pay one yuan per day as a basic fee for room, but not including medication or food. Patients with severe chronic mental disorders that do not respond to treatment in this hospital are sent to the Stability Hospital (the municipal psychiatric hospital) for long-term care.

Besides patient care, the department of psychiatry has research and teaching activities. Although there is presently no active research program, future plans include mass surveys and biochemical studies of the mechanisms of schizophrenia. During the current five-year medical school curriculum, sixty hours of neurology and psychiatry lectures are given. No clinical training in psychiatry is provided to medical students, but there is a three-year postgraduate training program to train psychiatrists.

We were told that psychoanalytic approaches had no objective basis and put too much emphasis on sex. Instead, Drs. Hou and Lo supported a dialectical materialist approach, which used the doctor-patient relationship to bring the initiatives of the patient into full play. We were told that the acceptance of the therapy by the patient depends on the doctor's outlook and on the quality of doctor-patient relationships. In such therapeutic relationships, the patient is taught to take an optimistic view of his illness and its treatment. For example, they teach schizophrenic patients, who are frightened by the seriousness of their disorder, that it can be cured and that a good attitude can lead to a better outcome. Patients with neurasthenia are told that their insomnia and anxiety are caused by "a functional disorder of the brain nerves." If the patient can tell the doctor about the "mental factors" contributing to this disorder, they are told their doctors will then be better able to cure them. For example, if the patient is a daughter-in-law who is having regular conflicts with her mother-in-law, they tell the patient that such conflicts are "normal" and widespread. The patient must "face up to them and solve them." These conflicts can be examined in terms of their concrete contradictions. These in turn can be analyzed from a dialectical materialist position. Then the patient can take a "correct attitude" toward her mother-in-law. If they cannot solve their problems among themselves, which is encouraged, then neighbors, family members, friends, and co-workers may be asked to help resolve the conflict.

They claim not to have problems with confidentiality. Dr. Hou told us that "mental illness is a public problem." Hence it is important to share information about the patient's problem with family, neighbors, and co-workers. But some limitations are placed on such communication, and information is shared with others primarily when it serves a therapeutic purpose.

We were told that they do not see cases of sexual neurosis (common in Taiwan, Hong Kong, and in overseas Chinese communities) or homosexuality or alcoholism (also uncommon in other Chinese populations). Suicide also is reported as uncommon. Though they recognize that cases of depression are frequently masked by somatic symptoms, they do not see many cases of somatized depression, most of which they believe are treated in medical clinics. They have only limited experience using antidepressant drugs. Their consultation-liaison service is limited to consultation on psychotic patients who are on other services in their hospital. They do not consult on questions concerning psychosocial concomitants of physical disease or death counseling.

We observed three female patients in their early twenties receive insulin shock therapy for catatonia. We also met one middle-aged man who had developed drug dependence on a tranquilizer.

Drs. Hou and Lo were looking forward to what they said would be the first publications of the *Journal of the Chinese Society of Neurology and Psychiatry* since the Cultural Revolution.[4] The society, they reported, was debating whether to become active again.

The second psychiatric facility we visited was the department of mental disease of the #2 Teaching Hospital, Hunan Medical School – the only psychiatric unit in that medical school and the only academic psychiatry faculty in the province. The department's senior staff includes Professor Ling Ming-yu, Lecturer and Deputy Director Shen Chi-chieh, and Associate Professor Young Der-son (Yang Te-shen).

The department of mental disease has a staff of 20 doctors, including postgraduate trainees, oversees 65 inpatient beds, and sees between 100 and 150 outpatients each day. The department trains psychiatrists for specialty and general hospitals in the province. Until recently, the postgraduate training program in psychiatry had been reduced to a single year's course as a direct result of policy mandated during the Cultural Revolution. Our hosts indicated hopes of returning to a longer program that they feel will produce better-trained psychiatrists. They are hesitant to call the graduates of their one-year course "psychiatrists" because of their limited training. Of the 300 to 400 "psychiatrists" they estimated were practicing in Hunan Province (estimated population in 1976: 49,000,000), most received their training in this department. The input into the general didactic and clinical clerkship program for medical students is limited to just a few hours devoted to a brief review of schizophrenia and a few other psychiatric disorders and their treatment. The one-year postgraduate course, which will be expanded to several years, includes lecture-demonsration series on biological aspects of psychiatry, descriptive psychiatry, psychopharmacology, and psychotherapy. Each trainee engages in supervised clinical work with inpatients and outpatients, including experience in what the staff call "individual psychotherapy."

In 1958 they founded a psychiatric research group, but all research stopped in the Cultural Revolution. Only in the last year have they begun again to conduct clinical studies after a hiatus of about a decade. At present twelve of their 65 inpatient beds are devoted to the experimental use of various traditional Chinese medicines in the treatment of psychoses particularly. They believe that several of these indigenous medicines may be effective sedatives and anti-anxiety agents. The protocol they follow is to treat selected patients for one month with indigenous medicines. If at the end of that period the patients are not improved, then they switch to Western-style medication. They intend to start research in several other areas, and are particularly interested in standardizing and validating behavioral assessment scales and psychometric tests in order to conduct rigorous clinical studies. Professor Ling was trained in psychiatry by Dr. Lyman at Peking Union Medical College, and he in turn trained his two younger colleagues.

Their patients all come from Hunan Province. Sixty to seventy percent of inpatients carry the diagnosis of schizophrenia. They estimate that one-fifth of the schizophrenic patients they treat have "excited" schizophrenia, while four-fifths have depressed or "retarded" schizophrenia. Approximately 30 percent of inpatients suffer from various types of organic brain syndromes. They see few patients with manic-depressive psychosis, psychotic depression, or psychogenic psychosis. At least half the patients in the outpatient clinic suffer from neuroses. Of these patients, roughly 80 percent are diagnosed as neurasthenic, more than 10 percent have hysteria, but only a few patients are diagnosed as suffering from obsessive-compulsive neurosis, phobic neurosis, or anxiety neurosis. They see virtually no cases of homosexuality, alcoholism, or drug abuse. Professor Ling noted that although they see few cases of reactive depression, vegetative symptoms of depression are common among neurasthenic patients which they believed may represent "masked depression." Most of the other patients in the outpatient clinic suffer from schizophrenia, which they diagnose as a chronic psychosis associated with thought disorder, apathy, ambivalence and "loss of will," and obsessive symptoms.

In addition to antipsychotic medications similar to those used in America, they treat patients with lithium, hypnotics, and sedatives. Although they have read widely about antidepressive medications, they have used them infrequently.[5] (We could not determine if the limited use of antidepressants in the institutions we visited reflected unavailability because of economic reasons or other factors.)

Patients can stay on the inpatient service of this department for up to three months. Thereafter they are referred to the provincial psychiatric hospital, where they may stay up to six months, or to district hospitals, where patients may stay for several years. Most chronic patients are sent home after that time and are treated as outpatients, but some may stay for years in sanataria associated with factories and large state enterprises. This department participates in an informal "psychiatric network," including specialty and district hospitals. In this province there are ten "district hospitals," which are at the prefectural level between provincial and county hospitals. Each of these has a psychiatric service and treats inpatients for long periods of time. Changsha has a municipal psychiatric hospital with 200 beds and a provincial psychiatric hospital with more than 300 beds.

Although Dr. Ling and his staff admitted that mental illness was still heavily stigmatized in China, they noted that there were ongoing health education campaigns involving barefoot doctors and other production brigade members aimed at convincing peasants "not to look down on such patients." They point out to patients' families that because schizophrenia occurs worldwide and has a biological cause, it is like any other disease.

Professor Ling and his staff rarely see sexual neurosis or the culture-bound disorders well described for overseas Chinese communities. But they admitted that "perhaps our patients do not find it easy to talk to us about such things." They tell patients who have concerns about masturbation that "though it is wrong and they should try to stop, if they cannot stop it will not hurt them."

They and their staff provide some psychotherapy within the limitations of ten- to fifteen-minute outpatient interviews. They emphasize "the therapeutic relationship," "heart to heart talks," practical advice and support, and moral exhortation in the context of Maoist values. Dr. Ling and his colleagues expressed deep frustration with the effects of the Cultural Revolution, which they blamed for making their academic activities come to a halt for a decade. Although they now receive about twenty foreign psychiatric journals, for a period of time during and immediately following the Cultural Revolution they received no outside publications.[6] Thus Drs. Ling, Shen, and Young feel that they and their psychiatric colleagues throughout China need to catch up with recent technical developments in the West, raise significantly their level of clinical work, and initiate relevant research. Significantly, they look toward the West for a model of the way to proceed in these undertakings.[7]

Dr. Ling and his colleagues were acquainted with developments in biological psychiatry, and were particularly interested in competing ideas about the effects of drugs on brain processes, particularly the dopamine hypothesis. They believed that schizophrenia was a genetic vulnerability triggered by social and psychological factors. They seemed less acquainted with findings in social epidemiology and seemed unaware of studies linking social class to the prevalence of schizophrenia or sex to depression. They had the impression that women were more frequent psychiatric outpatients but had no supporting data.

At the Chung-Shan Medical College in Canton there is no psychiatry clinic at the medical school's main campus. The psychiatry department is located at the large provincial psychiatric hospital which we did not visit. Instead we visited the school's neurology outpatient clinic with Dr. Liang Hsui-chen, head of the department of neurology, and spoke with her and Dr. Leung Shiu-ling, head of the neurology clinic.

The department of neurology has six senior neurologists and eight junior staff members and trainees. Two of the senior staff are neurologists with special training in psychiatry. Each day in their outpatient clinic they see 80 to 100 patients. Roughly 10 percent have acute illness and 90 percent chronic illness. Approximately 20 percent of these patients are visiting the clinic for the first time. More than half of these patients are thought to be suffering from neuroses. Each day at least ten cases are diagnosed as suffering from neurasthenia, and each month 50 to 60 cases of hysteria are diagnosed. The staff recognize very few cases of depression. They do not think neurasthenia patients are suffering "masked depression." (Neurasthenia was viewed by Drs. Liang and Leung as the result of "decreased cerebral function," thought by them to affect primarily "brain workers" under a heavy load of intellectual work, and associated with symptoms such as headaches, insomnia, dizziness, and memory problems in the absence of "organic disease.") They see one or two schizophrenic patients each day. Unlike the Hunan Medical School, where many cases of epilepsy are treated in the psychiatry clinic, the neurology clinic at Chung Shan Medical College sees most cases of epilepsy. They also treat a wide range of other neurological problems.

Severe cases of schizophrenia are referred to the provincial psychiatric hospital in Kwangchow, while mild cases are treated in the clinic. Associated with the provincial psychiatric hospital is a special 1000-bed sanatarium where chronic patients (mostly patients with schizophrenia) stay who have proved intractable to treatment. Unlike the departments of psychiatry we visited in Hunan and Peking, this clinic (a) does not use the "excited/depressed or retarded" classification of schizophrenia[8] and (b) does not report a small percentage of paranoid symptoms for schizophrenic patients (roughly 50 percent of the schizophrenic patients they treat were said to be paranoid).

Each patient in the clinic is first seen for about fifteen minutes by a resident who then presents the patient briefly to one of the attending neurologists. No antidepressant medications are used in the clinic. Phobias are treated with talk therapy, as well as sedatives and chlorpromazine. Acupuncture is used to treat hysteria. Intravenous calcium bromide or calcium chloride and occasionally ether are used to treat the symptoms of "acute hysterical attacks."

While at the Chung Shan Medical Library, Kleinman asked to see the textbook of psychiatry written by this school's faculty (each of the departments of psychiatry we visited had compiled its own textbook for its students), but it could not be located. The school's textbook of neurology contained virtually no information on psychiatry, except for psychiatric problems associated with central nervous system disorders, like trauma and tumors. The textbook of internal medicine, which contained more than 800 pages, had 36 pages that were devoted to neuroses, including neurasthenia, hysteria, and immature personality. Depression was discussed in a single page.

In the library catalogue there were between 75 and 100 entries on psychiatric books. Most of these had been published prior to 1949. Only a few textbooks were listed with publication dates from the 1950s or later. There was no listing for Freud under psychology or psychiatry. The only psychiatric journals we saw on the periodical shelf were the *Journal of Nervous and Mental Disease, Acta Scandinavica Psychiatrica,* and *Excerpta Psychiatrica.* Whereas the psychiatry staffs in Hunan and Peking received the *American Journal of Psychiatry* and the *Archives of General Psychiatry,* these journals were not present here. The journal of psychiatric excerpts was from Japan. It contained brief abstracts of papers from the Western psychiatric literature. Roughly three-fourths of citations were biologically oriented, and most of the rest had a social or community psychiatry orientation. The periodical shelves, on the other hand, displayed a great many Western and Chinese journals of internal medicine.

We were told that in this medical school curriculum 24 hours of classroom lectures were devoted to general psychiatric topics such as major psychiatric disorders, their treatment, and prevention. In addition, there was a clinical clerkship in psychiatry for 26 hours.

CONCLUSION

We were able to observe only limited aspects of the treatment of mental illness in this vast country. Although we had greater access than previous visitors to some aspects of the system, we were able to learn almost nothing about how mental illness is identified, conceptualized, and dealt with at the family, production team, and production brigade levels. We had no opportunity to explore the way social controls in the primary group contributed to the containment of symptoms and social disruption and affected pathways into treatment. With the growing access to all aspects of Chinese institutions and the possibilities of long-term research in China, we conclude this paper with some suggestions for future research.

In considering the epidemiology of mental illness in China, it is essential to differentiate between incidence, prevalence, and help seeking, and to apply the same rigorous research criteria for case finding used by the World Health Organization in other countries. It would be worth investigating whether the incidence of mental illness in the PRC is lower than among other Chinese living groups and, if so, the determinants of such a difference. The incidence of mental illness (i.e., new cases that develop during a specified interval) may be the same in China as elsewhere, but not recognized because of cultural patterns of illness expression and illness behavior, because family members and other kin may avoid such definitions, because agricultural life allows the containment of deviance, or because a tight-knit social system and strong expectancies may minimize the most aggressive and bizarre manifestations of psychotic behavior. Barefoot doctors and most doctors at the commune level are untrained to recognize anything but the most blatant and obvious pathology, and if the manifestations of psychosis are masked or restrained because of social conditions, they may not be recognized. This inattention is reinforced by national health policy which defines mental illness as a low priority.

Even if the incidence of mental illness in the PRC is no different than elsewhere, its prevalence may be lower. The Chinese have a strong family and social system, a vital sense of determination and purpose, and a pronounced sense of interdependency. Because such a system offers a variety of economic and social supports, and because the Chinese are pragmatically ingenious in social management despite their rejection of social factors as significant causes of mental illness in the PRC, it is possible that the course of illness varies from that in other Chinese populations. If available supports and controls work to shorten the acute course of mental illness, then the prevalence rate may be lower. Rural China offers a fascinating laboratory to examine the interaction between psychobiological factors and social organization.

Our discussion of the organization of mental health services and the relationships between psychiatric and general medical care services reveals the fragmentation of our knowledge. Many of the relevant reactions and definitions we would like to understand occur in the production teams and communes prior to the provision of care, and we have almost no information as to what actually takes place. We have no notion of how many people in the community who can benefit from existing knowledge and interventions are never defined as mentally ill. Moreover, we have only the most vague notions of mental health care in the mainstream of mental health institutions in China, although we have some sense of current thinking in the teaching hospitals.

Perhaps most fascinating is the discordance between the "social psychiatric aspects" of Chinese life and the treatment of mental disorder and the insistence by Chinese psychiatric specialists that psychiatry is a biological discipline. It remains to be seen to what extent this changes with greater academic freedom and contact with the outside. The fact is that despite China's ingenuity in manipulating social structure, the practice of clinical medicine is bereft of concern for the impact of familial or psychosocial events on the occurrence or course of illness. This duality requires further examination.

Over the next few years it is reasonable to expect that the Chinese will themselves answer some of the questions we have raised with the release of further data on the epidemiology and treatment of mental illness. It is also to be hoped that visitors will be able to report on chronic psychiatric hospitals and other aspects of China's mental health delivery system that we were unable to observe. But, most important, perhaps there will be opportunities for collaborative cross-cultural research on clinical epidemiology of psychiatric diseases and illness behaviors that will provide new information about universal and culture-specific dimensions of mental illness among Chinese and that will assess the impact of

China's immense sociopolitical change on social deviance and psychopathology. Such research should be able to tell us much more about the obvious achievements of China's psychiatric care system as well as about the problems it still faces, with the expectation that such knowledge should be of practical use in developing more effective psychiatric treatment systems in China and among Chinese populations elsewhere.

NOTES

1. Certain of the materials presented in this article are reprinted from Arthur Kleinman and David Mechanic, The Treatment of Mental Illness in China, and David Mechanic and Arthur Kleinman, Patient Self-Care and Utilization of Ambulatory Medical Care Services, chapters in the forthcoming Report of the Rural Health Care Systems Delegation to China, Committee on Scholarly Communication with the People's Republic of China, National Academy of Sciences; and from Arthur Kleinman and David Mechanic: Some Observations on Psychiatry in the People's Republic of China, Journal of Nervous and Mental Disease 167: 267–274, 1979.
2. Because we often had limited interviews, did not have detailed personal and family histories or psychological test results, and were not in a position to conduct further medical tests, our impressions could not be substantiated in most cases. Therefore, readers should regard these impressions as unsupported and tentative. Because we did not make the diagnosis of somatization if there was any evidence of specific organic disease – and we selected only those cases with chronic or subacute complaints that had undergone medical workups that had not turned up positive findings – we believe that our overall assessment is a conservative estimate of prevalence of somatization in our sample. But our diagnosis of individual cases could well be off the mark.
3. As noted in Lin et al. above, psychiatrists from the People's Republic who recently visited the United States as part of an American Psychiatric Association sponsored group unofficially reported the results of unpublished epidemiological surveys indicating that the prevalence rate for schizophrenia in urban areas in China is 3 cases/1000 population and in rural areas is closer to 2 cases/1000 population. It was also informally reported that the prevalence rate for all psychosis is 5 to 7 cases/1000 population (Dr. Young Der-son personal communication).
4. Subsequently, this journal has begun to be published again. Copies in Chinese with Table of Contents in English can now be obtained from the Chinese Medical Association in Peking. The March 1980 issue published psychiatric epidemiology data.
5. During his visit to the Department of Psychiatry, University of Washington, in May 1979, Dr. Young Der-son noted that in the one year since this visit took place he and his colleagues had gained more experience in using antidepressant medications. He reported informally his clinical impression that the response of neurasthenic patients to these medications was not as good as had been hoped.
6. Their department publishes a journal of translations of foreign psychiatric articles and abstracts into Chinese called the *Referential Journal of Foreign Psychiatry*.
7. Though in research and service delivery they look toward the West, they make clear their attitude is to develop their own approach to psychiatry, appropriate for their Chinese environment. Dr. Young, for example, has developed his own theoretical model of psychiatric disorders that integrates German descriptive psychiatry with Russian neuro-psychiatry. See Young Der-son: The Relationship between Etiology and Symptomatology in Psychiatry. *Culture, Medicine and Psychiatry* 4(1), 1980.
8. Subsequently, it has been reported that the Chinese Society of Neurology and Psychiatry is in process of developing a new system of psychiatric classification which will eventually

be used throughout China to standardize psychiatric concepts and terms (Dr. Young Der-son, personal communication).

REFERENCES

Chin, R. and Chin, A. L. S.
1969 Psychological Research in Communist China, 1949–1966. Cambridge, Mass.: M.I.T. Press
Gaw, A. C.
1975 An integrated approach in the delivery of health care to a Chinese community in America: The Boston experience. *In* A. Kleinman et al., eds.: Medicine in Chinese Cultures. U.S. Government Printing Office for Fogarty International Center, N.I.H.; pp. 327–350.
Ho, D. Y. F.
1974 Prevention and treatment of mental illness in the People's Republic of China. American Journal of Orthopsychiatry 44:620–636.
Kety, S.
1973 Psychiatric concepts and treatment in the People's Republic of China. *In* Report of Medical Delegation to PRC, June 15–July 6, 1973. Washington, D.C.: Institute of Medicine, National Academy of Sciences; pp. 193–200.
Kleinman, A.
1975 Social, cultural and historical themes in the study of medicine in Chinese societies. *In* A. Kleinman et al., eds.: Medicine in Chinese Cultures. Washington, D.C.: U.S. Government Printing Office for Fogarty International Center, N.I.H.; pp. 589–658.
Kleinman, A.
1977 Depression, somatization and the new cross-cultural psychiatry. Social Sciences and Medicine 11:3–10.
Kleinman, A.
1979 Patients and Healers in the Context of Culture. Berkeley: University of California Press.
Lamson, H.
1935 Social Pathology in China. Shanghai: Commercial Press.
Lin, T. Y. et al.
1969 Mental disorders in Taiwan, 15 years later. *In* W. Caudill and T. Y. Lin, eds.: Mental Health Research in Asia and the Pacific. Honolulu: East-West Center Press; pp. 66–91.
Lin, T. Y. et al.
1978 Ethnicity and patterns of help seeking. Culture, Medicine and Psychiatry 2:3–14.
Lowinger, P.
1978 Psychiatric opinions in Peking. Psychiatric Opinion 15(5): 36–39.
Lu, Y.
1978 The collective approach to psychiatric practice in the People's Republic of China. Social Problems 26:2–14.
Murphy, H. B. M.
1959 Culture and mental disorder in Singapore. *In* M. Opler, ed.: Culture and Mental Health. New York: MacMillan.
Sartorius, N. and Jablensky, A.
1976 Transcultural studies of schizophrenia. WHO Chronical 30:481–485.
Sidel, R.
1973 Mental diseases and their treatment. *In* Quinn, J. R., ed.: Medicine and Public Health in the People's Republic of China. DHEW No. (NIH) 72–67. U.S. Government Printing Office; pp. 289–305.

Tseng, W. S.
    1975 The nature of somatic complaints among psychiatric patients: The Chinese case.
          Compr. Psychiatry 16:237–245.
Tseng, W. S. and Hsu, J.
    1969 Chinese culture, personality formation and mental Illness. Int. J. Soc. Psychiatry
          16:5–14.

18. SHEN-K'UEI SYNDROME:
A CULTURE-SPECIFIC SEXUAL NEUROSIS IN TAIWAN

INTRODUCTION

Shen-k'uei means "vital or kidney deficiency." In classical Chinese medicine, *shen* (kidney) is the reservoir of vital essence in semen (*ching*), and *k'uei* signifies deficiency. *Shen-k'uei* is a culture-specific disease that is described in classical Chinese medical texts and widely understood in Chinese communities. We shall refer to the *shen-k'uei* "syndrome" because it includes various symptom manifestations and illness behaviors. For example, Rin (1966) described two rare forms of this syndrome among Chinese male patients in Taiwan: *koro* and frigophobia. Both are recognized as culture-bound psychiatric syndromes among Chinese. In the one fear that the penis is shrinking and that its retraction into the abdomen will lead to death and in the other fear of cold owing to loss of seminal essence, which is believed to reduce the body's *ch'i* (vital essence) and through it the male component (*yang*) which produces an imbalance between hot/cold bodily constituents, relate to traditional Chinese cultural beliefs and rules concerning male genital sexuality. Although both conditions can be explained in terms of contemporary psychiatric concepts, their symptomatology and illness behavior are meaningful only in the context of Chinese culture. A third form of the *shen-k'uei* syndrome is a psychological condition popularly associated with excessive semen loss owing to frequent intercourse, masturbation, nocturnal emission or passing of "white turbid urine," which is believed to contain semen. It is this commonly occurring, but heretofore unstudied, sexual neurosis that we will discuss in this paper as the core *shen-k'uei* syndrome.

Adolescent or young adult males in Taiwan who believe they are suffering from *shen-k'uei* visit physicians in a state of marked anxiety or panic complaining of somatic symptoms, for which no organic pathology can be demonstrated, including: dizziness, backache, fatigability, general weakness, insomnia, frequent dreams, appearance of white hair, and physical thinness. Some patients also complain of sexual dysfunctions, such as premature ejaculation and impotence. Many fear that if the condition is not cured their physical health will be seriously damaged and infertility will result.

This characteristic sexual neurosis in Taiwan is frequently seen by general practitioners, urologists, and indigenous Chinese doctors, and much less frequently by psychiatrists, since patients focus on the somatic complaints and believe that it is a physical disorder. Because this disorder has not been extensively described and discussed in the biomedical literature, it is often misdiagnosed and inappropriately and ineffectively treated.

In the classical Chinese medical texts, the key conceptions of *yin/yang* and

357

A. Kleinman and T.-Y. Lin (eds.), Normal and Abnormal Behavior in Chinese Culture, 357–369.
Copyright © 1980 by D. Reidel Publishing Company.

the harmonious relationship between microcosm and macrocosm are elaborated in terms of correspondences between the five viscera (liver, heart, spleen, lungs, and kidneys), five emotions (anger, joy, worry, sorrow, and fear), five climatic factors (wind, heat, humidity, dryness, and cold) and the Five Elements or Phases (*wu-hsing*) — wood, fire, earth, metal, and water (Tseng 1973). *Shen* (kidney) is viewed as the major site for storage of *ching* (seminal essence) which contains *ch'i* (vital essence) whose normal amount and free flow through the body's channels is the source of health and whose loss and inability to flow through blocked channels is the source of disease, infertility, and physical and mental debility. It is believed that *ch'i* derived from *ching* stored in the kidney is mobilized when the body is in need of increased vitality and that the bone marrow and brain, among other organs, are sustained from this source. Not only mental functioning is held to be directly affected by the condition of the kidneys, but the ears, hair and other organs are also dependent on normal kidney functioning. If the kidneys are in good condition (i.e., full of *ching*), the individual will be healthy, strong and intelligent, and will live a long life. But if there is "weakness" or "deficiency" of the kidneys due to excessive loss of *ching,* the individual will become weak, thin, and infertile; he will experience a decrease in his mental functioning, and hearing and normal growth of hair will be disturbed.

This culture-specific illness category is fully described in contemporary Chinese medical texts published in Taiwan (Hsieh 1977; Ku-Wu-Chen 1939). For example, in a text written by a traditional Chinese physican, Ku-Wu-Chen, in 1939, nocturnal emission, emission on sight of sexual objects, *koro* (shrinking penis), hypersexuality as a cause of death, premature ejaculation, and impotence were all included under the category of sexual diseases where their pathogenesis was said to be either directly or indirectly related to *shen-k'uei.* The etiology of premature ejaculation was ascribed to hypersexuality, masturbation and sodomy leading to deficiency of *"ching."* These traditional notions are still widely believed in Taiwan's popular culture, where they are routinely supported by the explanations for sickness given to patients (and written in books and newspaper articles) by traditional Chinese physicians and other folk healers. In addition, popular culture draws on China's rich literary tradition as a source of traditional notions about sexuality. For example, the famous indigenous sexual manual, *The Art of the Bed Chamber,* which still is popular among Chinese in Taiwan, cautions that men should prevent emission of semen during intercourse in order not to diminish their limited supply of *yang ch'i,* but at the same time encourages frequent intercourse in order to strengthen men's vitality through the absorption of women's *yin ch'i* (cf. Ku-Wu-Chen 1939; Weakland 1956; Tu 1974). For the same reason, the Taoist writings on sex advise the benefits of retrograde ejaculation.

Yap (1965), who worked with Cantonese patients in Hong Kong, reported *shen-k'uei* as a neurasthenic state associated with sexual excess and including such symptoms as giddiness, physical and psychological debility, perineal aching, and shivering at the end of micturition. Rin (1965), writing about *koro*, noted that neurotic or psychophysiological symptoms manifested by male patients were often regarded as manifesting deficient vitality in terms of the traditional illness belief described above. Tseng (1973) said of *shen-k'uei*:

Since semen was thought of as the essence of energy and the excretion of it was believed to result in a loss of vital energy, nocturnal ejaculation was an illness attributed to poor mental control over sexual desire. This misconception has had an effect upon young men even today, who fear that, due to excessive nocturnal ejaculation, they might suffer from vital insufficiency, or neurasthenia, a western medical term introduced at the beginning of the 20th century.

Clyne (1964) described a syndrome similar to *shen-k'uei* among Bangladeshi men living in the East End of London, which he labeled the Bangladeshi Syndrome. His patients complained of urethral discharge and penile pain, but there was no evidence of sexually transmitted disease. They frequently insisted that sperm was being lost in their urine. This indeed was happening owing to prostatovesicular overflow, a physiological consequence of sexual continence. These Bangladeshi patients also complained of weakness and chest or abdominal pain, among various other somatic complaints. Clyne noted that cultural taboos dictated that masturbation and frequent nocturnal emissions were harmful. These cultural beliefs generated anxiety among his patients who were constrained not to masturbate.

In Indian culture, as among Chinese, semen is held to bestow physical and mental robustness, longevity, and even supernatural powers. Frequent involuntary or voluntary loss of semen is thought to be dangerous to health. Malhotra and Wig (1977) describe the *Dhat* syndrome in India as a culture-bound sexual neurosis occurring mostly in low-income and low-education individuals, in whom nocturnal emission leads to severe anxiety and hypochondriasis, often associated with impotence.

Rao (1978), in a general review of psychiatry in India, also mentions the *Dhat* syndrome but discusses as well the ascetic syndrome. It occurs in adolescents and young adults as a morbid preoccupation with control of sexual impulses. The sufferer becomes withdrawn, sexually abstinent, and loses weight. Rao further describes an attenuated form of *koro* characterized by impotence and hypochondriacal preoccupation with the size and shape of the penis and the quantity and quality of semen. In the popular viewpoint, the syndrome is invariably attributed to masturbation.

Obeyesekere (1976), writing about the impact of Ayurvedic ideas on culture and the individual in Sri Lanka, describes a class of culture-bound diseases dealing with loss of *dhatu* (vital components of the body), particularly loss of semen, *Prameha* disease. There are twenty types of *Prameha* disease caused by emission of semen in the urine, frequent night emissions, or when a "flour-like" substance of damaged semen is discharged with urine. Sexual excess, sexual misbehavior, or "bad living" are the most common causes of *Prameha*. "Bad living" includes illicit sexual relations, too frequent or prolonged sex, sexual fantasies, and the consumption of alcohol or opium. The common symptoms of *Prameha* are the passing of semen in the urine, the discharge of oily matter in the urine, nocturnal emissions, palpitations, tearing from the eyes, giddiness, "slowly dissolving kidneys," and backache. Swelling of joints, particularly the ankles, may result if *Prameha* is not treated. The symptoms are similar in men and women, except that the semen is believed to leave the vagina in the form of a white discharge (Ayurvedic physicians believe that females also secrete semen). Obeyesekere theorizes that anxiety regarding semen loss is caused by the Ayurvedic belief that semen is the most important *dhatus* (vital energy) of the body. Guilt and anxiety regarding sex are generated in Sri Lanka, Obeyesekere explains, because the expression of sexual and aggressive drives are radically circumscribed from very early childhood. Nocturnal emission and masturbation lead to guilt and anxiety, which in turn are expressed by fear of semen loss.

This traditional illness belief in the pathophysiological effects of semen loss and the culturally constituted sexual neuroses to which it gives rise is not limited to South Asian and Chinese cultures. Engelhardt (1974) demonstrates that masturbation came to be viewed in the West as a disease causing physical and psychological problems in the eighteenth and nineteenth centuries. Freud, Engelhardt reveals, believed that masturbation gave rise to neurasthenia. Medical commentators at the time claimed that because masturbation produced physical debility it was to be regarded as a physical disease requiring physical remedies. Engelhardt regards the "disease of masturbation" not as a historical example of a sexual neurosis in the West, but as an illustration of how medicine culturally constructs disease categories for behaviors that previously fit moral or legal categories. In the event, the point we wish to make is that while particular beliefs and behaviors associated with the *shen-k'uei* syndrome may be more or less specific to Chinese culture, there is considerable overlap with related disorders in other Asian and even Western societies. As a result, it is plausible to regard these disorders as a universally occurring *disease* (sexual neurosis) or group of diseases (e.g., anxiety neurosis, depression, hypochondriacal neurosis — all causing somatization) for which the *illness* behaviors, experiences, and beliefs are culture-specific. Indeed, this may be a way of categorizing most culture-bound disorders.

DESCRIPTION OF A CLINICAL STUDY:

Method and Subjects:

In the rest of this chapter, we will discuss the findings of a clinical study that we have carried out to better characterize the *shen-k'uei* syndrome.

In the Outpatient Clinic of the Department of Urology, National Taiwan University Hospital, there is a special clinic for patients with sexual problems. Each year between 300 and 400 new patients visit the clinic, almost all of whom are males. The majority of sexual problems involve such sexual dysfunctions as impotence and premature ejaculation. Patients with the *shen-k'uei* syndrome appear in the clinic commonly. As we have noted, patients with sexual problems in Taiwan do not usually go to psychiatry clinics. This is because of the stigma attached to mental illness and the associated negative attitudes toward psychiatry. As a result patients usually seek help initially from general practitioners and traditional Chinese physicians, many of whom claim to specialize in the treatment of sexual problems. If these treatments fail, patients then turn to the special clinic where this study was conducted.

From July to November 1977, 87 cases who visited the special clinic were investigated. Inclusion criteria for participation in the study were males, ages 18–50, who possessed at least 6 years of primary school education, who were not suffering from any major medical or neurological diseases (e.g., cardiovascular diseases, diabetes, hepatitis, asthma, renal or genito-urinary diseases), who were not suffering from endogenous depression or psychoses, and who had not been taking antipsychotic or other drugs known to affect sexual function for at least two months prior to entering the study. Only those patients who met these criteria and who completed the SCL-90 questionnaire during their first visit to the special clinic were studied.

The mean age of the patients in our sample was 28.8 ± 6.9; 45 percent came from the middle class, while 47 percent were from lower-class socioeconomic backgrounds. Seventy patients were Taiwanese, and 17 were Mainlanders. Thirty-one patients were married, and 56 unmarried. Most of the patients had some affiliation with Taiwan's syncretic folk religion, which contains a mixture of Taoist, Buddhist and Confucian elements.

A translated version of the Johns Hopkins Symptom Checklist (SCL-90) (Derogatis et al. 1973), an outpatient psychiatric self-rating scale, was administered to each subject to delineate psychiatric symptomatology. All patients were interviewed by a urologist, who included in his evaluation elicitation of patients' conception of their illness. Approximately one-third of the subjects were referred to and interviewed by the first author because they were diagnosed as neurotic and also had strong concerns about *shen-k'uei*.

Phenomenology:

In each case, the authors agreed on a diagnosis. Sixty-four cases (28 married, 36 unmarried) belonged to the sexual dysfunctions group: 32 suffered from secondary impotence, 31 premature ejaculation, and one retarded ejaculation. The remaining 23 cases suffered from sexual neurosis with *shen-k'uei* syndrome manifested as their primary problem. Each subject with *shen-k'uei* underwent a formal mental status evaluation by the first author.

Eighty-one percent of the patients with sexual dysfunctions (52/64) attributed the cause of their sexual disorders to too frequent masturbation, nocturnal emissions, or excessive sexual intercourse. They believed that too much loss of semen either would or already had produced "kidney or vital deficiency" and weakness in their nerves (sexual neurasthenia). These problems in turn were believed responsible for "weakening" the power of erection and ejaculation. The common symptoms this group presented included: emission of semen on the sight of erotic subjects; "flour-like substance" in the urine, especially at the end of micturition or defecation; frequency of urination; backache; weakness in the extremities or general weakness; dizziness; tinnitus; poor memory; difficulty in concentration; blurring of vision; and insomnia.

Most of the patients who didn't believe in the concept of *shen-k'uei* had higher socioeconomic status and were more likely to be married. These patients were frustrated, anxious and fearful of the possibility that they would be infertile and as a result have unhappy marriages in future.

The group of 23 patients with the *shen-k'uei* syndrome didn't suffer from sexual dysfunctions. Their ages ranged from 18 to 33 years with the mean at 24.4 ± 4.3. Eleven belonged to the middle class and 12 to the lower class. Only 3 were married, which comports with the clinical impression that married men rarely present with *shen-k'uei*. Of these 3 patients, two complained of postcoital low back pain and weakness in their extremities; another complained of loss of libido, fatigability, and insomnia. But psychiatric evaluation of these 3 patients revealed that the former two were experiencing psychophysiological disorders, while the latter had a neurotic depression with somatization which he had interpreted to be *shen-k'uei*.

Among the 20 unmarried patients, 7 were semiskilled workers, 7 were senior high school or college students, 5 were skilled workers, and one was a government employee. Only 5 had ever experienced sexual intercourse, all with prostitutes. Several of them had experienced impotence or premature ejaculation but only on one or two occasions.

All the *shen-k'uei* patients reported masturbation and/or nocturnal emission. Most deeply regretted these behaviors and were trying unsuccessfully to stop. One patient was in such a panic over the feared consequences of masturbation that he tied both of his hands at bedtime in order to restrain himself from masturbating. Another patient so feared his nocturnal emissions would lead to *shen-k'uei* that he attempted to prevent them by blocking the urethral pathway by tying a bandage around the shaft of the penis. Although the symptoms of these patients were similar to those listed above for the patients with sexual dysfunction, the *shen-k'uei* patients were more anxious, depressed, and hypochondriacal (see Figure 1). Some younger patients had additional complaints, including thinness of body stature, loss of hair, premature gray hairs, deepened yellowish color of skin or urine, and an oily layer on the surface of their urine.

The SCL-90 symptom profile of each of the groups of sexual dysfunction, *shen-k'uei* syndrome, neurotic and non-neurotic psychiatric outpatients, and normal controls is presented in Figure 1. The symptom distress index of each subscale (I: somatization; II: obsessive-compulsion; III: interpersonal sensitivity; IV: depression; V: anxiety; VI: anger-hostility; VII: phobic-anxiety; VIII:

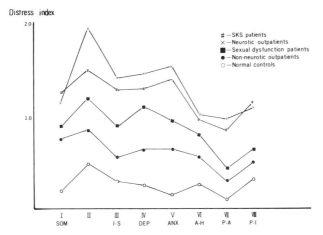

Fig. 1. SCL-90 symptom profile of SKS, neurotic, sexual dysfunction, non-neurotic 7 normal control groups.

paranoid ideation) is roughly the same for the *shen-k'uei* syndrome (SKS) group and the neurotic group. Student's t-test is statistically nonsignificant for these two groups, though the neurotic group has a severer obsessive-compulsive score (P < 0.10). The sexual dysfunction group has significantly lower scores in all the subscales, except anger-hostility, than the neurotic group (P < 0.05). Fig. 2 shows the mean profile for the 23 SKS males. It is plotted against a norm developed for neurotic psychiatric male outpatients. In general, the profile fluctuates between 0.5 and –0.5 standard deviations around the outpatient mean, except for the phobic-anxiety subscale. The pattern of the profile for the SKS group shows elevations on somatization and paranoid ideation above the average level of the neurotic outpatients. Thus, the psychopathology of the SKS

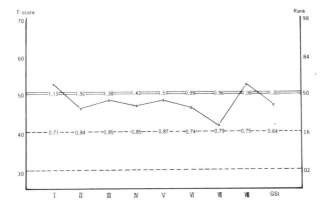

Fig. 2. SCL-90 Symptom Profile of SKS patients (The mean profile for SKS males plotted against a norm developed from neurotic psychiatric male out-patients.)

patients reaches the level exhibited by full blown neurotic outpatients seen in the psychiatric department's clinic at National Taiwan University Hospital. Three of the SKS patients, who presented pan-neurotic symptoms, were thought to be suffering from the Borderline Syndrome. Almost all of the SKS patients, and those who had sexual dysfunctions along with *shen-k'uei* belief, showed traits of introversion, psychosexual inhibition, passivity, and inferiority.

The treatment of the patients in this study was rather difficult, because of their pronounced hypochondriasis. Predisposing and concurrent psychosocial stresses were somatized. Patients demanded physical and laboratory examinations, especially a urological work-up, because they believed they were suffering physical disorders and therefore wished to have renal function, semen abnormalities, and problems with their "sexual nerves" evaluated. Some patients asked the doctors to check their brains and spines to see whether there were any pathologic changes. Many rejected the doctor's use of psychologic explanations. Most patients had already taken various tonics and traditional herbs before they had come to the special clinic, and expected additional somatic treatment. Prognosis was generally rather poor. About seventy percent of the SKS patients failed to experience improvement of their symptoms, most of which had lasted for more than 3 years. However, all of the 7 students with *shen-k'uei* syndrome, who were adolescents or young adults, changed their concepts of sexuality and gave up the belief that they were suffering from *shen-k'uei* after they received instruction in modern concepts of human sexuality along with psychological reassurance from their doctors. The SCL-90 scores decreased considerably in 5 of these cases in which the diagnoses were transient anxiety attacks and anxiety neurosis; but the two students suffering from hypochondriacal neurosis did not achieve the same improvement. Table 1 lists the diagnoses for all the patients in the *shen-k'uei* group.

TABLE 1

Classification of SKS Patients According to Psychiatric Diagnosis

Diagnosis	Number of cases
Transient anxiety state	6
Anxiety neurosis	6
Hypochondriacal neurosis	5
Borderline personality disorder	3
Psychophysiological disorder	2
Reactive depression	1
Total	23

When compared with studies of sexual neuroses from other Asian cultures, *shen-k'uei* syndrome appears similar to Bangladeshi syndrome, Indian *Dhat* syndrome, and *Prameha* disease in Sri Lanka. Because Obeyesekere's extensive and detailed study of *Prameha* disease, both from anthropological and psychiatric

TABLE 2

Comparison between *shen-k'uei* syndrome in Taiwan and *Prameha* disease in Sri Lanka

	Shen-k'uei Syndrome	*Prameha* Disease
Cultural beliefs	Chinese traditional medicine: Theories of *Yin* and *Yang*, the Five Elements of the universe, the Five Viscera (Kidney, the organ that stores vital essence, *ching* or semen).	Ayurvedic medicine: Theories of the Five *Bhutas* (basic elements of the universe), Three Humors, the Seven *Dhatu* (the Seven Components of the body), of which semen, the most important one, is the source of vital energy.
Symptomatology	Primary complaint: excessive loss of semen (*ching*) via urine, masturbation, nocturnal emission, etc. Secondary complaints: 1. Growth and reproduction: Fear of retardation of physical development and of lack of energy (weakness), and fear of infertility and impotence. 2. Nervous system: Dizziness, blurring of vision, concentration difficulty, memory disturbance, palpitations, cold sweating, insomnia, frequent and bad dreams, "sexual neurasthenia". 3. Bones and spine: Backache, weakness in limbs, deep pain in bones, fear of bone marrow drying up. 4. Hearing and hair: Tinnitus, grayish or whitish discoloration and shedding of hair. 5. Kidneys and urinary system: Flank pain, deep yellowish discoloration of urine, frequency of urination, pain in the groin.	Primary complaint: excessive loss of semen via emission of semen in the urine, masturbation, nocturnal emission, "bad living", etc. Secondary complaints: 1. Growth and reproduction: Loss of vital energy, effect on reproductive function not specified. 2. Nervous system: Dizziness, palpitation, tearing from the eyes. 3. Bones and spine: Backache, swelling of joints. 4. Kidneys: "Slowly dissolving".
Sex difference	Rare in females.	Common in females.
Psychopathology	Psycho-sexual inhibition, sexual abstinence, guilt, anxiety and hypochondriasis.	Guilt, anxiety and hypochondriasis.
Concurrent psychosocial and cultural factors	Inhibition of sexual and aggressive drives; lack of sex education; found among middle and lower classes.	Inhibition of sexual and aggressive drives; lack of sex education; found among middle and lower classes.

points of view, provides an especially interesting comparison, we have summarized his findings and ours for *shen-k'uei* in Table 2. Both disorders are culture-bound psychiatric syndromes that contain as their core pathology symptoms and illness behavior organized around deficiency of vital essence. Hence their pathogenesis is based on similar culturally constituted illness beliefs. Their symptomatology, moreover, also is similar. The major difference results from the emphasis, in Chinese culture, on the role of the kidneys in reproductive, sexual and nervous functions. Whereas tinnitus and premature whiteness of hair are associated with *shen-k'uei*, they are absent from the Sri Lanka syndrome. Another difference concerns sex of the patient. *Prameha* disease is frequently seen in females; only one female patient with *shen-k'uei* syndrome has been seen by the first author. In both cultures, vaginal discharge at times of sexual arousal is regarded as vital essence. The reason why female cases are rarely seen in Taiwan is not known and deserves further study.

CASE ILLUSTRATIONS

To better illustrate *shen-k'uei,* we briefly describe two cases.

Case 1: Mr. Wang is a 19-year-old unmarried Taiwanese from a rural peasant family who is an only son and youngest child with 6 sisters. He was overprotected and indulged in his family. After graduation from junior middle school, he worked as a semiskilled machine operator in a factory. He was referred by a urologist to the outpatient psychiatry clinic at National Taiwan University Hospital with a chief complaint of excessive nocturnal emission which the patient believes has caused loss of physical strength, small muscle bulk, weakness in limbs, palpitations, cold sweats, dizziness, blurring of vision, low back pain, frequency of urination, deep yellowish discoloration of urine, and loss of libido and lack of orgasm during masturbation. The symptoms have lasted for two years. Mr. Wang attributes the cause of his problem to *shen-k'uei* which he learned about from commercial advertisements of a traditional Chinese medicine reputed to cure it. He has masturbated regularly since age 9, but stopped as soon as he began to suffer the symptoms he believed resulted from excessive loss of semen. He also believed that *shen-k'uei* produced the "sexual neurasthenia" which he held responsible for his loss of libido and absence of orgasm during masturbation. Initially, his mother treated him with special foods such as ginseng and snake meat. Later he visited traditional Chinese doctors and received various herbal drugs for the purpose of increasing his *ching* and strengthening his kidneys. He also visited several Western doctors who gave him injections and oral preparations of vitamins. Because his nocturnal emission did not cease, he visited the special clinic at National Taiwan University Hospital.

The patient has never experienced sexual intercourse. He fears entering an intimate female relationship because of the threat of impotence. Psychiatric evaluation revealed a psychosexually overinhibited adolescent who had transient anxiety and hypochondriacal complaints but was not psychotic. Mr. Wang was felt to be suffering from an adolescent adjustment reaction. He was treated with thioridazine, 25 mg. at bedtime, which stopped the nocturnal emission. The patient was also given sex education and counseling. One month after his initial assessment in the special clinic, he appeared much more relaxed and had given up the idea that he was suffering from *shen-k'uei.*

Case 2: Mr. Chou is a 26-year-old Taiwanese, unmarried, university student. His problems began with an involuntary emission of semen at age 16, about which he felt deeply guilty and blamed on masturbation. He became fearful that this experience would lead to impotence. When masturbating he felt that his erection was not as firm as before and that he was unable to experience the same degree of sexual arousal as in the past. At this time, he developed anxiety attacks characterized by palpitations, tremor, dizziness, headaches and a painful precordial sensation. He thought that these were symptoms of *shen-k'uei* brought on by semen loss. When his symptoms did not improve, he visited Western and traditional doctors, demonstrating increasing hypochondriacal preoccupation. His academic performance declined and he failed the college entrance examination. He became depressed, believed that he had let his family down at a time when their aspirations centered on him as the only family member with the chance to enter college, and feeling helpless and hopeless made a suicide attempt by ingesting an overdose of sleeping pills. Subsequently he entered the army, performed well, repeated and this time passed the college entrance examination, and is now doing well academically.

Although he no longer believes he is suffering from *shen-k'uei,* he is still preoccupied with the quality of his erections and sexual arousal during masturbation, which he fears are inadequate and possibly an early sign of impotence. He has never had sexual intercourse, and avoids experiencing it lest his fears of impotence come true. Relevant history includes the patient's resentment of his dominant mother and weak father, and his ambivalence about the high expectations they placed on him to succeed on behalf of the family. These issues were particularly forceful in late adolescence when he was attempting to cope with the severe stress of the college entrance examination by resorting to the maladaptive coping strategy of displacing and isolating his anxiety on his somatic symptoms and guilt over masturbation. Psychiatric evaluation was consistent with the diagnosis of somatization owing to hypochondriacal neurosis.

These two case vignettes illustrate the kinds of psychological and social problems associated with the *shen-k'uei* syndrome. We believe that both cases along with the findings from our clinical study fill in our picture of this culture-bound syndrome. They suggest that culture works to provide culturally-constituted illness categories and socially-sanctioned behavioral norms which in turn create common behavioral pathways along which are channeled psycho-pathological and deviant behavior of many different kinds with the result that similar patterns of culturally-specific illness behavior are manifested by different, universally-occurring psychiatric diseases (cf. Carr 1978; Kleinman 1978). We suggest that this model of *shen-k'uei* as a culture-bound syndrome can be generalized to the entire class of culture-bound syndromes.

SUMMARY

In this paper *shen-k'uei*, vital or kidney deficiency, a culture-specific disease that is described in classical Chinese medical texts and widely known in Chinese communities is introduced. *Shen-k'uei* syndrome is a pathological condition particularly associated with excessive semen loss owing to frequent intercourse, masturbation, nocturnal emission, etc., and it is this commonly occurring sexual neurosis that we refer as the core *shen-k'uei* syndrome. Various categories of sexual behavior and diseases are described in contemporary Chinese medicine texts where their pathogenesis is related to *shen-k'uei.* Hence, *shen-k'uei* syndrome is a culture-specific illness that includes *koro* and frigophobia, which have been previously reported among Chinese patients. Similar types of culture-specific sexual neurosis have been recognized in other Asian countries, such as

Bangladesh, India, and Sri Lanka. In this paper, *shen-k'uei* syndrome is contrasted to *Prameha* disease indigenous to the Ayurvedic culture of Sri Lanka, demonstrating the fundamental belief in both cultures that semen is the most important vital energy of the human body and that loss of it causes a wide range of physical problems. It is plausible to regard these disorders as a universally occurring *disease* (sexual neurosis) or group of diseases (e.g., anxiety neurosis, depression, hypochondriacal neurosis) for which *illness* behaviors, experiences, and beliefs are culture-specific. This may be a way of categorizing most culture-bound disorders.

Eighty-seven male patients, of whom 64 belonged to the sexual dysfunction group and 23 suffered from the core *shen-k'uei* syndrome, were studied. Eighty-one percent of the patients with sexual dysfunctions adopted the notion of *shen-k'uei* as the cause of their problems. Psychopathology as manifested on the SCL-90 symptom profile for the *shen-k'uei* syndrome group reached the level exhibited by full-blown neurotic outpatients seen in the psychiatric clinic. The underlying psychiatric diagnosis of *shen-k'uei* patients was discussed, and two cases of *shen-k'uei* were presented.

ACKNOWLEDGEMENT

The authors wish to thank Dr. King-Tsu Chen and Miss Yin-Yuh Lee for their help in conducting the study, and Dr. Arthur Kleinman for his editorial comments on an earlier version of this chapter.

REFERENCES

Carr, J. E.
    1978 Ethno-behaviorism and the culture-bound syndromes: The case of *Amok*. Culture, medicine and Psychiatry 2: 269–293.
Clyne, M. B.
    1964 Indian patients. Practitioner 193: 195–199.
Derogatis, L. R., et al.
    1973 An outpatient psychiatric rating scale – preliminary report. Psychopharmacol. Bull. 9: 13–28.
Engelhardt, H. T.
    1974 The disease of masturbation: Values and the concept of disease. Bulletin of the History of Medicine 48: 234–248.
Hsieh, K.
    1977 Dictionary of Chinese Medicine. (In Chinese) Taipei: Commercial Press.
Kleinman, A. M.
    1978 Three faces of culture-bound syndromes: Their implications for cross-cultural research. Culture, Medicine and Psychiatry 2(2): 207–208.
Ku-Wu-Chen, D.
    1939 A Clinical Text of Chinese Medicine. (In Chinese) Taipei: General Press. (Reprinted 1976).
Malhotra, H. K. and Wig, N. N.
    1977 Dhat syndrome: a culture-bound sex neurosis of the orient. Transcultural Psychiatric Research Review 15: 56.

Obeyesekere, G.
  1976 The impact of Ayurvedic ideas on the culture and the individual in Sri Lanka. *In* Asian Medical Systems: A Comparative Study, ed. Leslie, C. Berkeley: University of California Press; pp. 201–226.
Rao, A. V.
  1978 Some aspects of Psychiatry in India. Transcultural Psychiatric Research Revew 15: 7–38.
Rin, H.
  1965 A study of the etiology of koro in respect to the Chinese concept of illness. International J. Social Psychiatry 11: 7–13.
Rin, H.
  1966 Two forms of vital deficiency syndrome among Chinese male mental patients. Transcultural Psychiatric Research Review 3: 19–21.
Tseng, W. S.
  1973 The development of psychiatric concepts in traditional Chinese medicine. Arch. Gen. Psychiatry 29: 569–575.
Tu, W. T.
  1974 Traditional Chinese Sexology. (In Chinese) Taipei: University Press Inc.
Weakland, J. J.
  1956 Orality in Chinese conceptions of male genital sexuality. Psychiatry 19:237–247.
Yap, P. M.
  1965 Koro – a culture-bound depersonalization syndrome. Brit. J. Psychiat. 111: 43–50.

19. CULTURE-BOUND SYNDROMES AMONG OVERSEAS CHINESE

> *By nature men are nearly alike; by practice, they get to be wide apart.*
>
> Confucius, Analects, bk. xvii. c. ii.

There are about twenty million Chinese living outside of China, compared with about nine hundred million living on the mainland and about seventeen million on the Island of Taiwan. Of these twenty million, about fifteen million are distributed throughout the countries of Southeast Asia and the remainder are scattered over the rest of the world.

Like the Hakkas, who were the gypsies of China and who, in their wanderings from place to place, starting from the north and traveling down to the southern provinces, always carried with them the bones of their ancestors in earthenware urns together with the rest of their possessions, the overseas Chinese have carried their culture and ethnic idiosyncrasies with them wherever they went. For most, there is some degree of assimilation with the community into which they have settled. The extent of the assimilation will depend on a number of factors. These include the size of the Chinese group in the community, the smaller the group the faster its assimilation, and the political pressures imposed upon the emigré Chinese to assimilate. To some extent, assimilation is a function of the number of generations a particular family has been away from China. The personality dimension of the individual is also an important determinant of the speed with which he assimilates into the host community.

These overseas Chinese, or *hua ch'iao* as they are called, tend to retain certain of their traditional folkways no matter to what degree they have assimilated into the host society and tend to make use of these, even though the same practices have evolved into something else or have been abandoned in the mother country.

CONCEPT OF DISEASE

In the People's Republic of China, rural peasants now go to barefoot doctors and doctors at commune hospitals for treatment of their illnesses who may use traditional herbal and acupuncture therapies, but whose conceptual orientation is essentially that of biomedicine. In urban areas in China, patients most often see formally trained Western-style doctors, who may attempt to use traditional Chinese medical beliefs, but whose general framework is biomedical. Even the traditional Chinese-style doctors they visit often possess some training in the ideas and approaches of Western medical science and may present their ideas to patients in an idiom that combines traditional and modern notions. Temple mediums and other folk healers no longer are allowed to practice in the People's

371

A. Kleinman and T.-Y. Lin (eds.), Normal and Abnormal Behavior in Chinese Culture, 371–386.
Copyright © 1980 by D. Reidel Publishing Company.

Republic, and the traditional cosmological beliefs they use are not sanctioned by China's health care system. Modern medical concepts are widely spread and enforced through schools, mass media and political campaigns.

In contrast, overseas Chinese in Southeast Asia still frequently visit traditional Chinese-style doctors, temple mediums and other folk healers who know little of Western medicine and who present their ideas in the same classical form in which they were used in China in the past. Traditional Chinese illness beliefs (both secular and sacred) are still strongly sanctioned by the communities within which these practitioners practice. In these overseas Chinese communities, resort may also be made to native healers of the host culture, and indigenous beliefs may be integrated with or at least supported by traditional Chinese beliefs. Biomedical ideas and practices are poorly understood and misapplied, and are not systematically integrated with traditional ones. This cultural conservation of many overseas Chinese communities with respect to their illness beliefs and practices also is reflected in the symptomatology of their culture-bound syndromes. Knowledge of these syndromes and of the cultural belief system they are based upon is transmitted, reaffirmed, and put to practical use in the family and social network.

Although there is no set of beliefs held universally by the *hua ch'iao* Chinese, in general these involve the concept that disease is caused by an excess or deficit of *yin* or *yang* principles. To varying degrees they have also retained or acquired anew from indigenous communities in which they live the belief that their illnesses may be caused by malevolent spirits, including those of one's dead relatives, one's enemies or those called from the nether-world at the invocation of various agencies such as shamans.

YIN AND YANG

Diseases in the traditional Chinese conceptual system, in their simplest and most fundamental characterization, are thought of as being due to an imbalance of the *yin* or the *yang* principles in the body. *Yin* is thought of as the female, the cold, the negative aspect of nature, while *yang* is conceived of as the male, the hot and the positive component. The body's vital essence (*ch'i*) is thought to possess both *yin* and *yang* types. Conditions such as impotence are thought to be due to an excess of the *yin* principle, whereas a headache or a rash may be believed due to an excess of the *yang*. An upper respiratory tract infection may be thought of as a combined excess of both *yin* and *yang*. Of course, traditional Chinese medical beliefs are much more complex and sophisticated than this crude outline, but these are core popular culture concepts guiding the illness behavior of overseas Chinese.

When an illness is thought to be due to *yin-yang* imbalance, the patient or his family will first attempt to remedy it with diet and special foods, but if the problem does not improve they will consult a traditional Chinese-style herbal physician for a cure. The treatment will be based essentially on the precepts of the ancient masters of herbal medicine which have been handed down through the vast classical Chinese medical literature. The prescription will be for a medicament which will either reduce an excess of or make up for a deficit in the principle involved. The interaction which takes place during the consultation is usually an educational experience for the patient and his relatives. It is through this means that traditional concepts of disease causation and consequently of the culture-bound syndromes are reinforced and perpetuated, despite social changes in the secular lives of these *hua ch'iao* Chinese. Participation in religious rituals, family-based socialization experiences, and the community-wide system of norms will also strengthen these concepts and legitimize their application to particular illness episodes.

TEMPLE MEDIUMS

While traditional Chinese medicine is based largely on an empiricism accumulated over many centuries of experience and rationalized in a formal, literate theoretical system, albeit one quite different from the Western tradition, temple mediums, by contrast, function on the basis of an oral folk tradition and its rituals. This tradition still retains a sizeable following among the more traditionally-minded section of the *hua ch'iao* population, particularly older females. Also, in contrast to Chinese-style herbal physicians who tend to address themselves to the recognition and treatment of somatic symptoms, temple mediums tend to deal with psychosocial problems and the misfortunes and vicissitudes of life, but treat them in a cosmological idiom based on traditional beliefs in gods, ghosts and ancestors. Both Chinese-style physicians and temple mediums and other sacred folk healers endeavor to reinforce concepts which are congruent with their patients' indigenous belief systems, and by so doing they perpetuate the occurrence of the same culturally constituted clinical states which we regard as culture-bound syndromes. Of course, primary socialization in Chinese families also involves a similar process of learning culturally approved patterns of behavioral deviance.

CULTURE-BOUND SYNDROMES

While there is a fairly wide variety of conditions which can be described as culture-bound syndromes found among the overseas Chinese in Southeast Asia, these can be classified into three major groups:

(1)   psychosexual problems;
(2)   possession states; and
(3)   other conditions.

Broadly speaking psychosexual problems are often conceived of as being due to a disturbance of the *yin-yang* balance and therefore usually are treated by traditional Chinese-style physicians, while possession states may arise either from Chinese concepts of spirit possession or from concepts of spirit possession belonging to the indigenous population among whom the overseas Chinese live. Depending on what is believed to be the causative agent, the patient may be brought to either a Taoist temple medium or a native shaman in the hope of obtaining a cure. However, a sharp distinction between these two types of conditions cannot always be maintained, and not infrequently traditional Chinese-style physicians are called upon to treat possession states, while psychosexual problems may be brought to temple mediums or indigenous shamans.

It was found that of a sample of patients referred to a university psychiatric clinic in Malaysia, 31% had been to an indigenous healer of one description or another for treatment before they were brought for psychiatric evaluation (Teoh, Kinzie and Tan 1972). Of this sample, if one took only those patients suffering from culture-bound syndromes, the proportion who had consulted indigenous healers before coming for psychiatric evaluation was very much greater.

While such syndromes are more often seen among patients of the lower socio-economic class and in families in impoverished social situations, this is so largely because of the lesser likelihood that such patients have acquired a Western orientation in their attitudes and values concerning illness. Culture-bound syndromes are not uncommonly seen among educated Chinese patients from upper and middle socio-economic classes as well. The operative factor thus appears to be the adherence of the patient to traditional Chinese attitudes and values.

PSYCHOSEXUAL PROBLEMS

In a study of the symptomatology of anxiety states, Tan (1969) reported a high incidence of complaints related to psychosexual function among Chinese patients presenting with symptoms of anxiety at the University of Malaya Medical Centre's Psychiatric Clinic. Complaints of psychosexual dysfunction ranged from guilt about masturbation and contact with prostitutes to impotence, premature ejaculation, nocturnal emission and spermatorrhoea. The preoccupation with sexual function as a manifestation of an underlying neurotic conflict is a phenomenon that is widespread among the various cultures in Asia. The beliefs that sexual excess can lead to emaciation and eventually death and that one drop of semen is derived from ten drops of blood and each drop of blood is derived from the eating of ten grains of rice are widely held in Indian and Chinese culture and are popular among the Chinese of Southeast Asia (Ngui 1969; Carstairs 1967). Tan (1970) reported that there is a sizeable industry in Southeast Asia generally, but in Singapore and Malaysia in particular, manufacturing patent cures purported to be effective for the relief of various deficiencies of sexual function. The advertisements promoting such products and the literature that is supplied with them are replete with statements reinforcing such beliefs and thereby help perpetuate the occurrence of culture-bound psychosexual problems among overseas Chinese populations to whom these products are sold.

KORO

Koro has been reported in most overseas Chinese communities. It consists of the sudden onset of patient complaints of the sensation of retraction of the penis into the body. The culturally held belief has it that when the penis is completely retracted into the abdomen, the man dies. With this in mind, the patient goes into a panic and clings to his penis for dear life. The converse to this belief is the scene often enacted in the pediatric wards of hospitals in Southeast Asia where the mother of a moribund Chinese boy will perform fellatio on him in the hope that as long as the penis is prevented from retracting completely into the abdomen the boy will stay alive.

Gwee (1968) traced the origin of this condition to imperial China, about the tenth century A.D., when castration was considered the penultimate form of punishment which could be meted out by the emperor or his surrogates for serious offences which did not quite merit punishment by death.

Various psychodynamic formulations have been advanced to help explain *koro*. Gwee (1963) regarded it as a hysterical dissociative state; whereas Yap (1965) regarded it as a "culture-bound depersonalization syndrome" which he thought was a variant of Roth and Harper's (1962) "phobic-anxiety depersonalization syndrome." In that there is the subjective somatic sensation of the retraction of the penis, there is a certain degree of depersonalization and distortion of the body image. The striking feature of this condition is the overwhelming anxiety of acute onset which amounts to a state of panic in the patient at his realization of the possibility of impending doom. While this condition is often, in the author's experience, associated with feelings of guilt related to some sexual misbehavior or other areas of the patient's life, one cannot escape the conclusion that this is a culturally-determined form of severe castration anxiety.

Example A forty-three year old Chinese food supplier was in the capital city to represent his company in bidding for contracts to supply food to various institutions. It had been a stressful day in which he had failed in some of the bids but had succeeded in some others, in spite of the high quotations from his firm over which he felt a bit guilty. After dinner that evening with some of his colleagues, he was entertained by a few call girls, an experience which the patient later said he did not fully enjoy because of his preoccupation with the happenings of the day. When he finally retired to his airconditioned hotel room, he stripped himself and as he sat naked on the cold sheets of his bed he felt an extremely cold sensation on his scrotum. In that instance he realised that his penis was shrinking into his abdomen and he went into a state of panic, realizing he might die. He sweated profusely and was at a loss as to what to do for some time before he could compose himself. He ordered a strong alcohol-containing drink, following which he went to sleep. He caught the first plane home the next morning and requested an emergency private psychiatric consultation.

This condition is not confined to males. Females have become panic stricken on experiencing the sensation that their nipples, breasts or labia were retracting (van Wulfften Palthe 1936).

Also, this disorder is not confined to the Chinese in Southeast Asia. In Malaysia where the influence of Chinese culture is reasonably widespread, Chinese ideas of disease causation, largely transmitted through the agency of the local Chinese-style herbal physician, especially in rural village communities, have helped to spread such ideas even to non-Chinese. Hence cases of *koro* are not uncommon among Malays and Indians. Indeed, the word *koro* is of Javanese origin, being a corruption of *kura* meaning tortoise, probably comparing the penile retraction with the retraction of the head of the tortoise into its shell. The Chinese term for the condition is *so yang* meaning the withdrawal of the male organ and *so yin* when it occurs in the female. Koro is considered by Chinese-style physicians as a prime example of excess of *yin* (Gwee 1963). Treatment is based on injunctions to abstain from food stuffs which contain an excess of *yin*, including cold drinks, fruits and vegetables, especially in the uncooked state, and prescription of medicaments such as the ginseng root, alcohol and lean meat, substances which are considered to be rich in *yang*. It has been the author's experience that when faced with a case of *koro* in the emergency room situation an intravenous injection of calcium gluconate which gives an immediate sensation of warmth running through the whole body is a very effective form of acute management. Having thus reduced the anxiety and the panic, the patient can then be sedated for the night and his conflicts can be dealt with on a psychotherapeutic basis the following morning.

SPERMATORRHOEA

Given the Chinese, and indeed the widespread Asian, belief that sexual dissipation and the excessive loss of seminal fluid can lead to emaciation and even death, it is not surprising that any condition in which there is an involuntary loss of seminal fluid is viewed with extreme gravity, generates marked anxiety and is considered one which has to be treated urgently.

In his study of patients with anxiety symptoms in Kuala Lumpur, Tan (1969) found that 44 per cent of males and 20 per cent of females, mostly Chinese, expressed their anxiety symptoms in terms of sexual dysfunction. Of these, more than a third of the male patients complained of spermatorrhoea or nocturnal emissions which were excessive and hence undersirable. It is usual for such patients to complain of multiple symptoms relating to their sexual function and to have other hypochondriacal complaints as well. A case report will illustrate the point.

Example: A twenty-six year old male Chinese came from a broken home. He was raised by his mother, his father having deserted the family when he was five years old. He had a primary school education in Chinese and after a series of odd jobs, worked as a delivery van driver for the last two years. He complained of general weakness, tiredness on exertion, breathlessness and bad memory for the last ten years. He admitted masturbating since his teens with fantasies of intercourse with women. He occasionally visited prostitutes. He complained of having "poor" penile erection for the last ten years or so, and in the last six years had had frequent nocturnal emissions, at the rate of three to four nights a week, sometimes twice a night. The reason the patient gave for seeking psychiatric consultation was his complaint of "leaking sperm". He complained of losing seminal fluid most of the time, whether asleep or awake, and his underwear was wet with seminal stain on examination. However, he complained that his seminal discharge was especially excessive when he engaged in physical exertion, whether it was straining in passing stools or carrying heavy loads at his job. This patient had consulted a wide variety of local Chinese-style herbal physicians and general practitioners before coming for a psychiatric consultation. Whereas he was mostly told by the general practitioners that there was nothing wrong with him, Chinese-style physicians told him that he was suffering from an excess of both *yin* and *yang*. The excess of the *yin* was purported to give rise to his inability to have a strong erection, while the excess of *yang* was believed to result in an excessive production of seminal fluid and the incontinence accompanying it. He was enjoined to abstain from further sexual activities until he was cured. This puts the patient in a quandary as he was under the pressure of his mother, being the eldest son of the family, to marry and produce sons to continue the family name.

The physiology of the flow of seminal fluid in the absence of sexual excitement or any overt sexual activity is rather obscure. Contemporary scientific literature has little to say on this topic. It has often been summarily dismissed as arising out of the patient's imagination. This sexual preoccupation contrasts with the rather ascetic and asexual tone of *hua ch'iao* Confucian philosophy which provides the behavioral norms guiding their conduct.

While it is a commonly held belief among *hua ch'iao* Chinese that excessive loss of seminal fluid is deleterious to a man's physical health, commercial advertisements on behalf of traditional and patent medicines strongly reinforce it, such as the statement found in the literature of a sample of tablets sold for the purpose of treating spermatorrhoea which says:

The different kinds of involuntary emissions are the only common ailments of youth, but they are as dangerous as other diseases. Even for the sake of begetting posterity few will indulge in the wastage of this precious fluid, not to say its actual loss through involuntary emission. And how dreadful would it be if the involuntary emission should continue uncured!

SPIRIT POSSESSION

Belief in possession by spirits, evil or otherwise, exists among the overseas Chinese. It has been called by different names in different cultures, depending on whether the possession state is viewed as beneficial or malignant, useful or destructive. Among the Chinese, if a patient's illness cannot be understood in terms of the *yin-yang* polarity and especially if his symptoms are bizarre, the conclusion is often reached that he is possessed by a spirit which is probably malevolent, especially if the person is severely disabled because of the disturbance. However, a person may be possessed by a benevolent spirit even though he has not voluntarily sought possession. In such an instance, the person will be viewed as having extraordinary powers, including the power of healing and sometimes also the power of divination which will be a great financial advantage. An example of this latter instance was reported by Kinzie, Teoh and Tan (1976) in which a young girl who was normally shy and withdrawn, at the urging of friends and relatives, attained a possession state in which she was able to divine lucky numbers for the national lottery in Kuala Lumpur. Where the person in the possession state claims to have healing powers, he will usually perform his healing rituals in a Taoist temple, thus becoming a temple medium.

In states of possession by malignant spirits, the person is frequently distressed by the experience, although he may not have full awareness of what has transpired during the state of possession. In terms of psychiatric phenomenology, possession states may range from severe hypochondriasis or histrionic overbreathing in hysteria to the catatonic excitement of schizophrenia. Of course such an experience need not have psychopathological consequences. Lin (1953) described a condition known in Taiwan as *hsieh-ping* and characterized by a trance state in which the patient identifies with a dead person and manifests symptoms of tremors, disorientation, clouding of consciousness and delirium, with visual or auditory hallucinations. Lin considered this a manifestation of neurotic illness.

Belief in spirit possession among overseas Chinese is highly colored by beliefs of similar conditions held by the local indigenous community among whom they live. Similarly, the treatment considered necessary for the relief of such possession states will be colored by ideas held by the indigenous community as well. Such Chinese patients might be taken to mediums in the local Taoist temple for exorcism, but if this fails or if the offending spirit is viewed as being of indigenous origin, they would then be taken to a native shaman for a cure as well.

Example: A sixty-five year old Chinese widow had multiple somatic complaints such as dizziness, listlessness, loss of appetite, sensation of numbness and tingling in the extremeties, flatulence, etc. She consulted Chinese herbal physicians and general practitioners about her complaints. She was told by the general practitioners that she had high blood pressure. However, the tablets they prescribed had no effect on her symptoms. The traditional physicians diagnosed her as having "an imbalance of *yin* and *yang*". The medicaments they prescribed were equally ineffective. About four months prior to being referred for psychiatric consultation, she had a severe exacerbation of her symptoms. In addition she had severe sleep disturbance, felt very low in her spirits, was often tearful over the slightest aggravation and indeed occasionally contemplated suicide, especially when she came into conflict with her daughter-in-law with whom she lived. On the advice of relatives and friends, she consulted a Taoist temple medium who diagnosed her as being possessed by a malevolent spirit which resided in a tree which the patient passed as she crossed a vacant lot to market several times a week. The temple medium conducted an exorcism ceremony which did not have any significant effect. As this was thought to be an illness caused by a local indigenous spirit the patient was brought to a local shaman, known in Malaysia as a *bomoh,* for a cure. The *bomoh* conducted a similar exorcism ceremony which partially relieved the patient's symptoms for a few weeks. However, there was a recrudescence of symptoms and the patient, at the suggestion of her son's friend who was a general practitioner, was brought for psychiatric consultation. She was diagnosed as suffering from endogenous depression with classical signs of profound depression including sleep disturbance, other biological symptoms, tearfulness and suicidal preoccupation. The present episode of severe depression seemed to have been precipitated by a conflict with her daughter-in-law who threw a veiled threat at the patient that she would persuade the patient's son to get the patient to live elsewhere because they could not get along. Ejection from the home would constitute a "loss of face" among her friends and her relatives, and also threatened the patient with social isolation and loss of contact with her grandchildren, with whom she had a close relationship, and with the friends she had come to know in the neighbourhood. At a deeper level, however, sending her to live away would constitute an unfilial act on the part of her son which in turn would reflect on her as an incompetent mother. The patient improved on medication with tricyclic anti-depressants and after a number of family therapy sessions involving the patient, her son and daughter-in-law.

In general, it can be said that spirit possession, when viewed as a psychiatric illness, is essentially an attempt to formulate a culturally-appropriate cause and behavioral category for a condition whose pattern of symptoms are otherwise incomprehensible to the Chinese in terms of their conceptualization of *yin-yang* imbalance and related secular illness beliefs from classical Chinese medical theory. The overseas Chinese in Southeast Asia have maintained some cultural contact with the mainstream of Chinese culture but such contact has not been uniform. Most of these Chinese are descendents of peasant migrants and there has been a large degree of "sequestration" of folk beliefs held by their ancestors. The fact that the indigenous population shares similar beliefs of spirit possession as a cause of illness, especially with psychiatric symptoms, would reinforce this tendency to view bizarre symptomatology as the effect of possession by a malevolent spirit.

OTHER CULTURE-BOUND CONDITIONS

Apart from psychosexual problems and spirit possession, a number of other culture-bound conditions have been reported among the overseas Chinese of Southeast Asia such as *latah* and *amok*. In contrast with *koro* which is a disease seen essentially among the Chinese but which has spread to the indigenous population through cultural contact, conditions such as *latah* and *amok* are states seen essentially among the indigenous population which have spread to the Chinese owing to cultural contiguity and assimilation.

LATAH

This is a dissociative state, provoked usually in the form of a shout, a loud noise or a prod in the ribs, associated with altered consciousness, coprolalia, echolalia, echopraxia and in the more severe cases "command automatism." This condition was described by Yap (1952) as that found mainly among middle-aged women of the Malay or other indigenous races in Southeast Asia. However, a number of cases have been described among males as well, some of them younger than middle-aged. It is also said to be not uncommon among the Chinese *nonya* women, who have been in Malaysia for several generations, most of whom no longer speak Chinese dialects and whose families have largely assimilated Malay culture. Chiu, Tong and Schmidt (1972) described a large series of cases of *latah* whom they came across in their psychiatric survey in East Malaysia and reported finding a case in a Chinese who was adopted by a Malay family. There were a few cases among the Ibans, though most were among the Malays.

This condition is usually not considered an illness among the local population of these regions but merely an eccentricity which indeed may have some social value. Subjects of *latah* are often in great demand on social occasions such as wedding feasts and circumcision ceremonies (during which lavish dinners are given by the fathers of Muslim boys), when they will provide comic relief by their inappropriate sexual utterances when provoked and startled by members of the gathering. The sexual content of the coprolalic utterances of the *latah* subject is considered by Yap to be a socially-sanctioned mode of vicarious sexual expression. Although there has not yet been any systematic scientific study of the *latah* phenomenon from a psychological viewpoint, the hysterical nature of the condition is inescapable to the psychiatric observer. The condition invariably occurs in the presence of an audience, the behavior of the subject has a marked theatrical quality about it, often provoking spasms of laughter among the audience, and the subject pleads amnesia for her buffoonery when she comes out of her altered state of consciousness. Yap (1952) sees *latah* as a culture-bound phenomenon similar to other "startle" or psychogenic "shock" states known by various other names in different parts of the world ranging from Siberia to the North American continent (Yap 1974:95).

AMOK

The earlier reports of this condition dating from the middle of the nineteenth century to the middle of the twentieth century are mostly of a literary nature. Contemporary psychiatric reports of running *amok* by Tan (1965), Burton-Bradley (1968), Westermeyer (1973), and Zaguirre (1957), all reported this condition as occurring mostly among the Malayo-Polynesian people of Southeast Asia. However, in a recent report, Carr and Tan (1976) reported the condition as having occurred in a number of Chinese subjects as well in their survey of a psychiatric hospital sample who were judicially detained for having committed homicide.

The remarkable feature of the recent literature on *amok* is the lack of agreement regarding the clinical nature of the phenomenon. Van Loon (1927) thought that some of his cases could be due to cerebral malaria; both Burton-Bradley and Westermeyer, apart from reporting that all their patients were transiently psychotic, did not attach diagnostic labels to any of their cases. Tan (1965) reported five cases in whom all were schizophrenics, while Carr and Tan (1976) found twenty-one cases in the forensic ward of a psychiatric hospital in Malaysia of whom the cases who had indisputably run *amok*, mostly Malays, were schizophrenics also. But they noted that the different kinds of deviance and psychopathology associated with this syndrome suggested that it was a culturally-constituted "final common behavior pathway." In contrast, however, Yap (1952) regarded *amok*:

an acute hypereridic state in which an abnormal degree of hostility is aroused and remains undirected so that suicidal behaviour is merged into homicidal furor.

EPIDEMIC HYSTERIA

This phenomenon is remarkable in the sensational way in which it affects a large number of people within a community. It has been described in most cultures as documented by Sirois (1974) in his review of the world literature on this topic. In the Malaysian setting however, it has largely been a Malay phenomenon occurring almost exclusively among young women, mostly residents of boarding schools with strict discipline and limited social outlets. A typical example of this phenomenon was described by Tan (1963): an outbreak of epidemic hysteria occurring among the girls of an Islamic boarding school in the south of peninsular Malaysia, where the girls over a number of weeks were fainting and screaming because they claimed to be afflicted by evil spirits of various descriptions. As one girl in the school succumbed to this affliction, other girls would follow suit and the condition would spread to still other susceptible girls within this restricted community. The occurrence was of great concern to the larger community around the school and attracted much public attention. Chew, Phoon and Mae-Lin (1976) reported an epidemic of hysteria occurring among a multiracial group of factory workers in Singapore in which only the female Malay workers were affected. One Indian girl was involved but none of the Chinese were affected at all. The epidemic was stopped by closing down the factory for a few days.

Teoh and Tan (1976) in another study of a different outbreak of epidemic hysteria in a secular girls' boarding school in West Malaysia, using sociometric methodology, concluded that the affected individuals in such an epidemic were usually the most neurotic individuals linked by strong emotional bonds. The epidemic was seen essentially as a socially sanctioned mode of expressing discomfort with the social position in which the subjects found themselves. There appeared to be no other available avenues for the sanctioned expression of discontent open to these girls. The sensation created by the epidemic drew public attention to the unacceptable social situation in which the girls lived and changes followed, even though it took many weeks of such disturbance before the desired effects were brought about.

If one takes a broader perspective, the epidemic of *koro* in Singapore reported by Ngui (1969) can be regarded as an instance of epidemic hysteria among the Chinese. In that epidemic a number of male Chinese presented with *koro* initially to the clinics of Chinese-style physicians. A rumor was spread around the city of Singapore that the outbreak of *koro* was caused by the eating of contaminated pork sold in the city. Soon many more male Chinese were affected and presented at the casualty department of the Singapore General Hospital. There were a few female subjects afflicted also. The sociodynamics of this outbreak were not elucidated but one might speculate that because it occurred on such a large city-wide basis the conflict might have been related to certain socio-political problems affecting the entire city at that time.

TRANSCULTURAL DIMENSION

The culture-bound syndromes described in this paper have attracted attention to a large extent because of the "exotic" nature (to Western eyes) of their sympto-matology. The fact that they are described here as occurring among the *hua ch'iao* Chinese of Southeast Asia does not necessarily imply that they are peculiar to this group of people. Syndromes like *amok* and *latah* are conditions seen essentially among the native communities of Southeast Asia which afflict the immigrant Chinese as a result of their cultural contiguity and assimilation. Conversely, conditions like *koro* and the spermatorrhoea syndrome are essentially disorders of the *hua ch'iao* Chinese which have been observed among the natives of this region following their culture contact with the immigrant Chinese. This underscores the importance of beliefs and norms in the genesis of these syndromes. Without the acceptance of such culturally-determined beliefs and behavioral norms the development of these culture-bound syndromes would probably not eventuate.

THE SIGNIFICANCE OF CULTURAL BELIEFS AND NORMS

Culturally-determined beliefs and norms are significant in the genesis of these culture-bound syndromes in that they provide the conceptual framework and value orientation upon which the behavior of the group in a given set of circumstances is based. Such behavior even though largely deviant when viewed by the psychiatric observer is sanctioned by the cultural group and may even be expected by it in certain situations. This conceptual framework determines how the symptoms of the culture-bound syndromes are expressed by the sufferer and perceived and labeled by the community. Reinforcement of such behavior is provided by witnessing it in others and thus developing one's own expectation of susceptibility. A strong reinforcement of culture-bound illness behavior is provided by the commercial promotion of various medicinal products purported to be not just for the cure of symptoms of these syndromes but for their prevention as well. This process closely parallels the expectation of various types of behavior arising from the advertisement of certain consumer products in the mass media in Western society and further serves to reinforce the likelihood that this behavior will occur.

EQUIVALENT PSYCHIATRIC CATEGORIES

If one disregards the superficial manifestation of these culture-bound syndromes which are expressed in forms of behavior and feelings more or less specific to the culture in which they occur and considers instead the underlying psychodynamic implications of the symptoms themselves, it is usually clear to the observer that the basic emotional conflicts expressed are universal ones, well recognised in clinical practice. *Koro*, the spermatorrhoea syndrome and *latah* are manifestations of various types of neurotic disorders, while *amok* and spirit possession are behavior seen in psychotic states.

Such equivalence has a one-to-one correlation in the case of *koro*, the spermatorrhoea syndrome and *latah*, the equivalent diagnostic categories being acute anxiety neurosis, hypochondriacal neurosis and dissociative hysteria, respectively. In my own experience, *amok* is a manifestation of schizophrenia (Tan 1965), though this has not been the experience of other workers. The one-to-one correlation breaks down further in the case of spirit possession. Certainly they all resemble psychotic states. In some instances they are cases of depressive illness with bizarre delusions and hallucinations. Many are cases of schizophrenia. These possession states can be seen in personality disorders and hysterical reactions of the more bizarre kind. In the instances of epidemic hysteria referred to earlier, they are in fact culturally learnt coping behavior with stress (Table 1).

TABLE 1

Culture-Bound Syndromes and their Equivalents

Culture-Bound Syndromes	Psychiatric Diagnosis
Koro	Acute anxiety state
Spermatorrhoea Syndrome	Hypochondriacal neurosis with sexual symptomatology
Spirit possession	Mostly psychotic states
Latah	Dissociative hysteria
Amok	Schizophrenia

The universal occurence of epidemic hysteria further illustrates this point. As is obvious from Sirois' (1974) review of the subject, while these epidemics take the form of seeing ghosts and being possessed by evil spirits in Southeast Asia, in Western countries victims of such epidemics suffer from fainting attacks and gastrointestinal symptoms.

If this concept of diagnostic equivalence is accepted, one can conclude that these culture-bound syndromes are variants of universally occurring psychiatric disorders modified in their manifestation by culturally-determined modes of expression. If psychiatric symptoms are viewed as communications by the patient to the society around him of his emotional and psychic "dis-ease," it is not difficult to understand that this communication has to be made in forms and behaviors recognizable to, and understood by, the social group. Hence culturally-held beliefs and norms have the role of determining the forms in which the underlying psychiatric disorder manifests itself, i.e., these beliefs and norms have a *pathoplastic* rather than a *pathogenic* role in the manifestation of the symptoms of the culture-bound syndromes (Yap 1974).

I am in agreement with Yap that these culture-bound syndromes are "forms of psychopthology produced by certain systems of implicit values, social structure and obviously shared beliefs indigenous to certain areas . . . these are only a typical variance of generally distributed psychiatric disorders" (Yap 1969).

In the case of the spermatorrhoea syndrome, the physiological mechanism of the loss of seminal fluid in the absence of sexual arousal is obscure and further research is necessary for its elucidation.

CONCLUSION

It can be expected that with cultural change among the overseas Chinese, perhaps in form of Westernization and/or acculturation into the host communities of the region in which they live, there will be modification of these culturally-constituted beliefs and consequently some change as well should be expected in the mode of manifestation of these culture-bound syndromes. However, these modifications will not be radical as long as the agencies responsible for perpetuating and sanctioning the relevant cultural beliefs and behavioral norms continue to function. One suspects that it will take a massive social upheaval to eradicate these socially-sanctioned agencies, such as the revolution in China, which led to the integration of Chinese-style physicians with Western-style doctors while suppressing temple mediums and all other sacred folk practitioners, and apparently the system of cultural beliefs and practices with which they are associated. It would be important to learn if Chinese culture-bound syndromes still exist or have undergone significant modification in modern China.

REFERENCES

Burton-Bradley, B. G.
    1968 The amok syndrome in Papua and New Guinea. Medical Journal of Australia i: 252–256.
Carr, J. E. and Tan, E. K.
    1976 In search of the true amok. American Journal of Psychiatry 133: 1295–1299.
Carstairs, G. M.
    1967 The Twice-Born. Bloomington: Indiana University Press.
Chew, P. K., Phoon, W. H., and Mae-Lin, H. A.
    1976 Epidemic hysteria among some factory workers in Singapore. Singapore Medical Journal 17: 10–15.
Chiu, T., Tong, J. E., and Schmidt, K. E.
    1972 A clinical survey study of latah in Sarawak, Malaysia. Psychological Medicine 2: 155–165.

Gwee, A. L.
1963 Koro – a cultural disease. Singapore Medical Journal 4: 119–122.
Gwee, A. L.
1968 Koro – its origin and nature as a disease entity. Singapore Medical Journal 9: 3–6.
Kinzie, J. D., Teoh, J. L., and Tan, E. S.
1976 Native healers in Malaysia. *In* Culture-Bound Syndromes, Ethnopsychiatry and Alternative Therapies. W.P. Lebra, ed. Honolulu: University Press of Hawaii.
Lin, T. Y.
1953 A study of the incidence of mental disorders in Chinese and other cultures. Psychiatry 16: 313–336.
Ngui, P. W.
1969 The koro epidemic in Singapore. Australian and New Zealand Journal of Psychiatry 3: 263–266.
Roth, M. and Harper, M.
1962 Temporal lobe epilepsy and the phobic anxiety-depersonalization syndrome, Part II. Comprehensive Psychiatry 3: 215–226.
Sirois, F.
1974 Epidemic hysteria. Acta Psychiatrica Scandinavica, Supplement 252.
Tan, E. S.
1963 Epidemic hysteria. Medical Journal of Malaya 18:72–76.
Tan, E. S.
1965 Amok: A diagnostic consideration. Proceedings, Second Malayan Congress of Medicine, Singapore. pp. 22–25.
Tan, E. S.
1969 The symptomatology of anxiety in Malaysia. Australian and New Zealand Journal of Psychiatry 3: 271–276.
Tan, E. S.
1970 Sexual symptoms of anxiety. Proceedings of the Fifth Malaysia-Singapore Congress of Medicine 5: 146–148.
Teoh, J. I., Kinzie, J. D., and Tan, E. S.
1972 Referrals to a psychiatric clinic in West Malaysia. International Journal of Social Psychiatry 19: 301–307.
Teoh, J. I. and Tan, E. S.
1976 An Outbreak of Epidemic Hysteria in West Malaysia. *In* Culture-Bound Syndromes, Ethnopsychiatry and Alternative Therapies. W.P. Lebra, ed. Honolulu: University Press of Hawaii.
van Loon, F. H. G.
1927 Amok and latah. Journal of Abnormal and Social Psychology 21: 434–444.
van Wulfften-Palthe, P. M.
1936 Chapter on Neuropsychiatry. *In* A Clinical Textbook of Tropical Medicine. C.D. de Langen and A. Lichtenstein, eds. Batavia: Kloff & Co.
Westermeyer, J.
1973 On the epidemicity of amok violence. Archives of General Psychiatry 28: 873–876.
Yap, P. M.
1952 The latah reaction: Its psychodynamics and nosological position. Journal of Mental Science 98: 515–564.
Yap, P. M.
1962 Transcultural studies: A panel discussion. Acta Psychiatrica Scandinavica 38: 163–169.
Yap, P. M.
1965 Koro – A culture-bound depersonalization syndrome. British Journal of Psychiatry 111: 43–50.

Yap, P. M.
  1969 The Culture-Bound Reactive Syndromes. *In* Mental Health Research in Asia and
         the Pacific. W. Caudill and T. Y. Lin, eds. Honolulu: East-West Center Press.
Yap, P. M.
  1974 Comparative Psychiatry. Toronto: Toronto University Press for the Clarke
         Institute of Psychiatry.
Zaguirre, J. C.
  1957 Amuck. Journal of the Philippine Federation of General Practitioners 6: 1138–
         1149.

20. LOVE, DENIAL AND REJECTION:
RESPONSES OF CHINESE FAMILIES TO MENTAL ILLNESS

For Chinese people, the importance of the family, the institution which has patterned the entire social matrix, can hardly be overestimated. It is the bastion of their personal and economic security; it provides the frame of reference for personal and social organization; it controls all the behavioral and human relationships of its members through a clearly hierarchical structure and sanctioned code of conduct; it transmits moral, religious and social values from generation to generation through role modeling, coercion and discipline. It also offers a haven for safety, rest and recreation; it maintains the altar for ancestor and religious worship. The influence of the family on the lives of its mentally ill members is no less profound than it is for anyone else. The handling of the mentally ill in Chinese society cannot, therefore, be considered without taking family context into account.

THE FAMILY AND THE SICK

The loving care Chinese families give to their sick and handicapped members is legendary and common. Pearl Buck (1931) portrayed, through Wang Lung in *The Good Earth*, the tender concern with unfailing care and lifelong devotion of a father for his mentally retarded daughter. He even made all necessary provisions for her comfort after his death, including a coffin and a grave site next to his.

The grandparents of H.Y. exemplify a modern counterpart of Wang Lung. A 29 year-old Chinese male, H.Y. was "accidentally" discovered by a City Welfare Officer of Vancouver. He apparently had been suffering from hallucinations and delusions for over 12 years. The officer found this bizarrely behaving man living alone in the basement of a dilapidated, soon-to-be-demolished rooming house in Chinatown. Only the proprietor and the grandparents of this psychotic individual, who were also the tenants of the house, knew of his existence. In fact, the aged grandparents had been his sole custodians and providers. Out of their meager pension they had paid his rent, supplied his food, clothed him and taken care of his personal needs during his years of illness. During the interview, the old couple expressed concern only that it might not be possible for them to have H.Y. live with them any longer when they moved to a new rooming house.

He is such a nice boy . . . He smiles at us, you know, when he sees us bringing food down for him . . . It does not matter if we don't understand all he says . . . We tried everything to cure him – special food, the medicine and herbs from the old country, consulting the teachers and the priests, prayers and offerings at the temple." Question: "Why no Western doctors?" Answer: "Oh, they don't understand us. They may be good for other people, but

A. Kleinman and T.-Y. Lin (eds.), Normal and Abnormal Behavior in Chinese Culture, 387–401.
Copyright © 1980 by D. Reidel Publishing Company.

no good for us. They'll just take him away and put him into an asylum, and we'll never see him again . . . You see, he is happy with us . . . he never complains . . . he eats well, it is so important for a young man to eat well . . . Some day his sense might come back, as our ancestors and we have done nothing wrong . . . There is no reason to believe that this nice boy should be punished for his forefather's wrongdoings, if any . . . He'll be all right . . . we just don't want other people to know about him . . . They may think there is something wrong in our family . . . No, we don't have anyone in our family that had done anything wrong. I guess he was just born at a wrong time, under a wrong star . . . But, he was such a nice boy before he became like this . . .

The old couple talked on and on about H.Y. with tears in their eyes.

Wang Lung and H.Y.'s grandparents bear witness to the genuine concern for the well-being of family members — well or sick — which underlies the long-standing Chinese tradition of intrafamilial coping with stress, including the stress of mental illness.

CHINESE VIEW OF MENTAL ILLNESS AND ITS ETIOLOGY

Chinese family concern for conformity in the conduct of its individual members is deep-rooted in Confucian ethics and even further in ancient history. Psychiatric disorder, with its attendant irrational behavior, arouses familial responses of tender loving concern combined with attempts at correction.

The form which these attempts at correction assume stems from traditional views of mental illness, still widely held in Chinese communities. The multifaceted Chinese view of the etiology of mental illness includes moral, religious or cosmological, physiological, psychological, social and genetic factors. The weight of each component varies from one individual to the other; even for the same individual the weighting may vary over time, depending on changing circumstances. In most Chinese families living in contemporary societies, the various components usually coexist because of the mixed composition of the membership of the large family, each of whom holds his own view emphasizing one or two facets of the etiological factors.

The moral view, a commonly held etiology, emphasizes "misconduct" as a cause of mental illness; deviation from socially prescribed behavior especially in neglecting the respect due to ancestors. Mental illness is regarded as a punishment for violating Confucian norms governing interpersonal relations, especially filial piety. It is a widespread practice for the family, usually through the person of the male head, to lecture to or exhort the mentally ill individual often drawing upon Confucian teaching about the virtue of good conduct in the hope of correcting his misbehavior. Often, community leaders or teachers are called in to help the head of the family in preaching about proper conduct to the individual. The indigenous view is that, like other forms of immoral behavior, mental illness necessitates "correct" thinking and therefore requires "rectification" of personal errors (cf. Chapter 1 in this volume).

This moralistic view seems to dominate in the People's Republic of China. Recent visitors to its psychiatric hospitals are impressed by intensive "group therapy", almost solely relying on exhortation of Mao's thoughts as contained in the Red Book (Visher and Visher 1979). This is, in the writers' interpretation, a modern politicized version of the Chinese moralistic view in action, with Mao Tse-tung replacing Confucious as the holder of truth and standards of conduct for the Chinese.

The intensity of such exhortation is related to the degree of shame held by the family for their failure in controlling the behavior of their individual members. One effect of this preaching is that the patient is made to feel guilty about his own conduct, a factor which sometimes further complicates his problem. An extreme example of the guilty feeling resulting from failure to comply with expected norms governing filial piety can be seen in cases of *hsieh-ping* (Lin 1953). *Hsieh-ping* is characterized by a trance state plus identification with a dead person, usually a dead ancestor from the "after-life-world", for a period ranging from half an hour to several hours. The symptoms during such a state consist of tremor, disorientation, clouding of consciousness and delirium, often accompanied by visual or auditory hallucinations. The person becomes a different person, one from the "after-life-world" and imitates the manner of such a person. For example, he may say, "I am so-and-so, your grandfather who died many years ago. You should give me such-and-such offerings otherwise you will be punished" (Lin 1953).

Punitive consequences are also implicit in the religious or cosmological etiology of mental illness. It is regarded as the wrath, incurred by the patient or his family members, of gods and ancestors in either present or former lives. Clearly, then, Buddhist belief in reincarnation and Taoist as well as Buddhist belief in the supernatural spirit play an important part in the Chinese view of the etiology of mental and other illnesses. Prayers and offerings at Buddhist temples or calling of Taoist priests to perform shamanistic rites for curing mental patients are common practices engaged in by families (Tseng 1972). The healers, Taoist priests and shamans, engage in magical healing through expulsion of evil spirits, which are believed to have possessed the patient, and by divination. Acting as mediators between spirits and men, shamans enter autohypnotic trances, during which they are supposed to journey to the abodes of gods and demons, afterwards announcing the results of their meetings and conversations with the supernatural beings (Needham 1956:132).

Physiological or medical theory plays an important role in the Chinese view of both etiology and treatment of mental illness. This view has its roots in the *yin* and *yang* theory — all illness is caused by an imbalance of nature's opposing *yin* and *yang* forces. According to the *Nei-ching*, the Classic of Internal Medicine attributed to the Yellow Emperor (Veith 1966), mental illness is caused by five harmful emanations of *yin* and *yang*. These five disturbances are numbness (痺), wildness (狂), insanity (癲), disturbance of speech (瘖) and anger (怒). Excess or deficiency of physiological functions, e.g., breathing, eating, bowel movement, sexual activities including masturbation, physical exercise or exhaustion, can upset the *yin-yang* balance, thus leading to mental illness or rendering the person susceptible to forces that give rise to mental illness. Excessive sexual activity or abstinence are believed to be most harmful. Climatic changes also affect the above physiological functions, especially sexual functions, in causing harmful effects on the balance of *yin* and *yang*. For example, manic excitement is often called "peach blossom madness", as it is believed to occur frequently in the spring among the young and is manifested by hypersexuality. In China, peach blossoms symbolize sex and youth as well as the spring season (Lin 1953).

Popular belief in hormones, vitamins and brain dysfunction as the basis for behavioral or cognitive disorders is a modern addition to the somatic orientation of the Chinese to mental illness. A peculiar example of somatization among Chinese is *shen-k'uei* (defective or weak kidney) (see Chapter 18). It is one of the most commonly used terms referring to a condition characterized by general malaise, loss of interest, weakness, loss of appetite, insomnia, and loss of libido (sexual interest) which the Chinese attribute to defective functioning of the kidneys. The kidneys are regarded as the reservoir of vitality or physical energy for the whole body and essential for growth, procreation and mental functioning. Remedies are sought by the family, often in consultation with traditional herb doctors, for restoring the balance of *yin* and *yang* in the patient. This usually includes herbs and a special diet including visceral organs (brains, kidneys, spleens, etc.). Such popular medical treatment seems to offer a high degree of psychological relief to the family for their shame or guilt over the patient's mental condition, perhaps because it replaces negatively valued personal or family responsibility for the disorder with a sanctioned impersonal, organic etiology.

Chinese share views similar to Occidentals regarding the importance of psychosocial factors in the etiology of mental illness, e.g., failure in love affairs, finance and career, death and mourning, loss of face through public humiliation or failure in examinations, family break-up, etc. But they seem to give much more weight to the breakdown of the family relationship as a specific psychogenic factor than do other cultures. Conspicuously lacking in the statements of Chinese families of the etiology of mental illness is direct public reference to sex, probably due to their extreme sense of privacy in guarding their sex lives and their view of sex as a biological (physiological) function rather than an emotional (psychological) issue. Yet, in our clinical experiences, private Chinese concern about sex and its significance as a causative factor in mental illness is not less prevalent than Occidental concern. Not infrequently, arranged marriage is used explicitly or implicitly to cure mentally ill youth, based on the belief that sexual frustration is the cause of their illness.

Finally, there is not only a popular biological belief in genetic transmission, but also belief in the inheritance of the "disturbance" by virtue of parental/ ancestral "misconduct" that serves as a nucleus for future problems. This set of beliefs underlies the traditional marriage prohibition for those suffering mental illness, and sometimes even for their siblings. Genetic counselling often occupies a large amount of the time and efforts of a psychiatrist when dealing with questions commonly raised by the families of unmarried psychiatric patients: "Would the patient be able to get well enough to be married?", "Would marital life be good for the illness?", "Would his or her children have similar illness?". Underlying these questions are issues of heredity, prognosis and strong pressure on the family to marry off their children. Not infrequently, the psychiatrist finds himself being presented, against his advice, with an announcement of his patient's wedding and subsequently of the birth of a baby in a year's time. Worse still, the psychiatrist now has to treat the floridly psychotic patient with baby. The pressure on the family to arrange the marriage of a mentally ill youth is great indeed. However, it appears that a different psychology operates in the family's wish to arrange marriage for a mentally ill boy than a girl. In the case of a boy, the family wishes him to marry in order to produce a son and carry on the family name, hoping, or even believing, that his mental illness will not be passed on to the new born son. In the case of a girl, the dominant motivation seems to be getting rid of the potentially embarrassing and burdensome problem of keeping a psychiatric patient at home.

HIERARCHY AND PRAGMATISM: FAMILY'S CHOICE OF TREATMENT

As a rule the family, not the affected individual, makes the decision concerning treatment modality. It also assumes the whole responsibility of providing the necessary means and support to carry out the treatment. The process in reaching this decision seems to be determined by two major factors which are peculiar to the Chinese family; its intrafamilial hierarchy and pragmatism.

Each individual in the family has his or her own preferred treatment modalities for the sick individual, based on his or her views of the etiology. Sometimes these views coincide, but often they differ. The male dominated and age oriented family system, however, ascribes certain priority and weight to the view of particular individuals based on age, sex, ordinal position and role, social status, experience and knowledge. After weighing the pros and cons of the various views expressed, the head of the family assumes the responsibility for the final decision on the treatment modality and also for its implementation. The process of intrafamilial decision-making consists usually of informal discussion. Only in exceptional circumstances is a family council meeting considered to be useful in deciding on the competing views of the major figures of the family. Once a decision is arrived at all the family members participate in its implementation.

The pragmatism of the Chinese in dealing with their lives in general, and in everyday problem solving, also applies in the search for an effective treatment for the mentally ill family member. With utmost diligence and vigilence the head of the family and its members proceed with trial and error in carrying out treatments. If and when a treatment proves to be ineffective, then another round of selecting a treatment method starts in a similar fashion to the previous one with a renewed effort to implement it, always with the hope of obtaining satisfactory results. In this manner, the family applies all its efforts, resources, and time until it obtains the desired effect on the patient's illness. Only when they find that their own material or knowledge resources and skills have not proved effective in solving the problem, will the family bring in outsiders. However, this process of seeking outside help is a cautious one and expands in concentric circles to include relatives, elders of the community, officers of the Clan or Surname Association, school teachers and other trusted friends who the family regard as equal to their relatives. Their views on the etiology of mental illness are considered and their advice on treatment is valued. The weight of such consultation increases with time in selecting treatment modalities, in inverted relationship to the failure of the efforts of intrafamilial coping.

SHAME AND GUILT — A COMPLICATED MIX

The shame the family feels about the presence of a mentally ill member in its midst is, as a rule, intense and pervasive. This feeling is rooted in cultural views of the etiology of the mental disorder. The moral view implies that someone in the family has not behaved correctly, and thus the family should be ashamed of having failed in performing its duty of teaching or controlling its member's proper behavior. Similarly, but perhaps in somewhat lesser degree, the psychological etiological view of mental illness causes the family to feel ashamed. For failure in love affairs or business or other psychological difficulties of the individual that have presumably precipitated or caused the mental illness reflect the failure, in the minds of the family, of performing their duty in guiding or protecting the individual in order to avert such disaster. The religious etiology implicates the family as having had ancestors who committed some kind of misdeeds. According to the genetic theory, mental illness tarnishes the family name, making it difficult for its young people to marry, which of course brings extreme disgrace to all those connected with the family. Characteristically, it is the family, or the person(s) representing the family, either the head or someone in the similar position — and not the afflicted individual — who feels the shame of mental illness. *It is in this fear of the family exposing its own shame to outsiders that the origin of the stigma attached to mental illness in Chinese society can be found.* The stronger the wish of the family to protect its "disgrace" from being exposed, the more intense the stigma attached to mental illness becomes.

It cannot, however, be overlooked that an element of guilt plays an important role, albeit limited at the beginning, in emotional responses to mental illness. The fear that the family might not have fulfilled its duties in controlling the behavior of the afflicted member and, as a result, has tarnished the family name in the eyes of the outsiders, evokes a sense of guilt toward ancestors. Disgrace results from such an act against filial piety, a most essential virtue demanded of every Chinese family. The feeling of guilt of the family increases with time and with its repeated failure in attempting to restore the sanity of the afflicted

member. Recourse to religious healing becomes an increasingly frequent treatment modality during the protracted course of family coping with the mental
illness in its midst.

DENIAL AND SOMATIZATION

It is common experience of psychiatrists or social workers, even in the first interview, to be consulted by the family on detailed dietary measures, hormone
therapy, vitamins or herbs for the patient for either fortifying (*pu*) his *yin* or
cooling (*t'ui-huo*) his overheated *yang* in order to restore a proper balance. This
priority often totally frustrates the therapist in obtaining any meaningful
information on family history of psychosocial development. Here one finds a
tangible expression of a prevailing Chinese approach to mental illness: somatization and denial of psychological involvement of the family. The burden on the
family seems to be least when it views mental illness as medical or physiological
in nature and can treat it as such. It is easier for members to understand and
accept the cause or the mechanism of mental disturbance based on the age-old
yin-yang theory. The prescribed methods for restoring the sanity of the afflicted
individual are generally simple and concrete, mostly consisting of using herbs
or certain dietary measures which can be managed within the family without
the risk of exposing the patient to outsiders. Most significant of all, the medical
view implicates the family least and thus relieves it of the agonizing psychological burden of shame and guilt as well as the fear of the stigma of mental
illness.

The combination, and mutual reinforcement, of somatization and denial of
psychological-familial factors hardens Chinese patients' resistence to attempts at
psychotherapy or psychosocial intervention, especially by outsiders (including
professionals). To the Chinese, the family is a sacred bastion, to be shielded from
the eyes of outsiders, to be protected from the meddling of strangers. This is
particularly so, when it comes to mental illness if the quality of family control is
being questioned, its reputation and social status are at stake and the prospects
of marriage of the younger generation are endangered. Chen (1970) and Lee
(1973) reported that, while the "silent Chinese" do have a myriad of problems,
their strong sense of shame and pride have precluded and hindered their use of
community programs and services. Sue and McKinney (1975) also observed that
an admission of emotional problems and the inability to work out one's
problems would arouse shame and reflect poorly on the family name, all of
which results in the Chinese resistence to the use of professional services.

The process of somatization and denial of psychological-familial factors in
mental illness go even deeper in Chinese culture. With *shen-k'uei* as the prime
example, various disease conditions are ascribed to dysfunctioning of one organ
or the other. This even finds expression in daily usage: e.g., *kan-huo* (liver fire),
meaning an excess of hot energy in the liver, is popularly believed to cause dizziness, blurred vision, bad temper or fatigue. In the writers' clinical experiences,

many depressed patients' main complaints consist only of hypochondriacal symptoms, including the vegetative symptoms of depression, rather than the symptoms of mood change, low self-esteem, or guilt feelings as seen in the West. In a number of cases, these somatic symptoms of Chinese depressed patients become fixed as somatic delusions. These experiences are shared by Kleinman (1979:119—178).

LABELING AND REJECTION

The distinctive pattern of help-seeking behavior of the Chinese Canadians as identified in our Vancouver Study (Lin et al. 1978; Lin and Lin 1978) seems to depict the underlying familial forces at play in handling a mentally sick individual. Five phases can be distinguished in the course of help seeking from the onset of a psychiatric problem to the point when the afflicted individual ends up in a public institution or a mental health agency:

Phase 1. Exclusively intrafamilial coping.
Phase 2. Inclusion of certain trusted outsiders in the intrafamilial attempt at coping.
Phase 3. Consultation with outside helping agencies, physicians and finally a psychiatrist while keeping the patient at home.
Phase 4. Labeling of mental illness and subsequent series of hospitalizations.
Phase 5. Scapegoating and rejection.

The first three phases can be grouped together as a protracted intrafamilial and "pre-psychiatric" stage lasting from several to over 20 years. Dominant in its attempt to restore the sanity of the afflicted individual in this stage is the tender loving care of family members to the sick and their intense effort to mobilize intrafamilial resources with minimal assistance from outside resources. Strong feelings of shame and guilt contribute to, and sometimes dictate, shielding the patient from the outside world, except for a few trusted friends, community leaders or herbalists. Only when all these efforts have failed to effect changes in the behavioral pathology of the individual, does the family seek outside help — agencies or physicians, and, finally, a psychiatrist or other mental health workers — to assist in restoring the patient's mental condition. At this stage, attempts to help are still within family boundaries.

Labeling of the mental condition of the afflicted individual as mental illness seems to introduce a radical change in the family's attitude to the afflicted individual and its approach to intervention. To the family the notion of mental illness in one of its blood-kin constitutes a "shock". It may resist accepting the notion and keep denying it, by continuing the previously ineffective interventions. Gradually, the family members accept the diagnosis, and sometimes do so with a feeling of relief as they have been suspecting or even dreading the presence of mental illness all along. In any case, the label has a profound effect on the family. Subsequently, the family becomes less tolerant of the individual.

As Sarbaff and Mancuso (1970) put it, deviant behavior is better tolerated by the public as long as it is not labeled as mental illness. Since labeling is usually done to the Chinese by an outsider, it poses an added psychological threat to the family, as it entails public exposure of the family's shame with attendant loss of face. With labeling of the patient as mentally ill, there commences a transition from the stage of intrafamilial coping to the next one, characterized by various extrafamilial interventions. The intrafamilial effort may continue for a while, but with less intensity. Western-trained physicians, psychiatrists or mental health workers of Chinese extraction are often preferred by the family as extrafamilial agents, but in many cases the family may prefer "White physicians" or "White psychiatrists", because they do not want to "wash dirty linen in public" (i.e., bring their plight to the attention of the Chinese community).

The label of mental illness almost instantly and drastically affects the patient and alters his status in the family. He becomes a mental patient ("crazy") with its attendant stigma. The shame and guilt of the family will begin to focus more pointedly on the patient, along with its frustrations, fears and eventual anger. The friendly and warm atmosphere in the family, including tender concern for the sick, is gradually replaced by one of tension, worry and desperation. The attitude to the patient becomes less cordial and more distant. Then finger-pointing or name-calling starts, and the patient will be blamed for some of the things that do not go well for the family. *Feng-tzu* ("lunatic", "madman", "crazy") will be heard with increasing frequency around the house, mixed with sighs, head shaking and even occasional angry stares.

Consulting with outside agencies, physicians or psychiatrists sooner or later leads to the admission of the patient into a mental hospital, often with the help of the police. Despair and exhaustion of the family's tolerance and resources ends the long struggle to contain the patient within the family context. This is replaced by a sense of relief and new hope for "cure" of the patient. The patient's recovery and return from the hospital brings back, at least temporarily, the family's old atmosphere of warmth and mutual concern. Relapse of the psychiatric condition, however, again sets in motion the process of family response and intervention described above. The duration of intrafamilial coping in this second episode is usually shorter and the process of admitting the patient to a mental hospital starts earlier. This cycle of intrafamilial coping — extrafamilial intervention — hospitalization repeats itself, but the phase of intrafamilial coping becomes shorter and shorter and hospitalization becomes longer as the patient's course of illness becomes more chronic. The family's visits to the hospital are in inverse relationship with the number of hospitalizations and also their duration. Rejection is complete when all family contacts cease. Often the hospital finds no one willing to accept the patient for home care even though the patient's condition is sufficiently improved to warrant return home.

It should be noted that the above pattern of help seeking and family intervention primarily applies to psychotic patients with such symptomatology as psychomotor excitement, bizarre behavior, delusions, hallucinations, or negativism, and usually with a protracted course of illness. Other types of mental illness, e.g. depression, neuroses, psychosomatic diseases, seldom come to the attention of psychiatrists or mental health agencies, because either these are not regarded as mental illness, or they are easily treated at home as physical illness by other physicians. Chen's (1977) study of public attitudes toward mental illness revealed that Chinese-Americans are relatively capable of identifying and perceiving mental illness, particularly in the case of violent and acting-out behavior. However, they are less capable of identifying the milder forms of psychosis, neurosis and behavior disorders of children. The notion of low prevalence of depressive illness among Chinese needs re-examination from the point of view of the Chinese concept of mental illness, cultural labeling and somatization. It may be simply due to underreporting by the family or result from a different diagnostic practice through which depressed patients are seen as physically ill as discussed above.

With the advent of modern psychiatry and development of mental health services for Chinese communities, there seems to be growing acceptance of psychiatry especially among Western-educated and second generation Chinese, whose families show willingness to seek psychiatric help at an earlier stage. In the event of treatment failing, the eager and cooperative attitude of the family gradually decreases, leading to frequent no-shows at appointment time. Subsequently, the family is found to be turning to herbalists, other traditional doctors, or religious healers for treatment, with the belief that Western medicine and psychiatry can provide relief, but not cure: "Only our traditional medicine can cure it!" They also see no contradiction in consulting practitioners of Western medicine, while simultaneously seeking help from religious healers. The ensuing course for chronic cases typically follows the sequence described above: intrafamilial coping — extrafamilial intervention — hospitalization. Repeated hospitalizations and exhaustion of family tolerance and resources end in rejection. The fact that access to modern psychiatry does not radically alter the help-seeking behavior of Chinese families in dealing with chronic psychotic patients seems to indicate the pervasiveness as well as the depth of the roots of the cultural forces at work shaping this familial response pattern, in spite of modernization or acceptance of certain Western cultural values. How long this basic pattern of Chinese reaction to mental illness in the family will continue in a changing world, where the younger generation is showing increasing signs of acculturation to Western culture and of gradually parting from their indigenous cultural identity (Sue and Sue 1973; Yee 1973), remains to be seen. We are of the view, however, that it may continue for a long time.

IMPLICATIONS AND QUESTIONS

Understanding the powerful role that Chinese families play in the lives of the mentally ill through the complex psychosocial dynamics that we have discussed has special implications and raises important questions for the practice of psychiatry and mental health for Chinese.

It is obvious that any assistance to Chinese psychiatric patients without involving their families seems futile for diagnostic assessment, the planning of suitable interventions and the execution of treatment and after-care. How to convince resistent families who feel shame and guilt to be involved in this process certainly presents a challenge. A treatise containing process reports of particular cases, successfully treated or otherwise, especially one prepared by workers who understand Chinese language and culture, is a priority task in tackling this difficult problem. With such a document in hand, we would be in a better position to develop culturally appropriate strategies that would yield earlier access to the closely guarded family bastion of the mentally ill. In the writers' experience, trust seems to be the key to unlocking the door to the family that is usually closed to outsiders. Trust can be gained when the family is convinced that the psychiatrist has compassionate understanding of its psychological agony and of the cultural rules governing familial roles and relationships.

Psychotherapy poses a special problem for Chinese patients, as many reports have acknowledged. Not only because Chinese have difficulty in talking about themselves and their families owing to fear of "shaming" the family, but also because they are not at all "psychologically minded" and that makes the work of psychotherapy extremely difficult. For example, the writers saw a patient with the chief complaint of impotence and nocturnal ejaculation, who responded to an enquiry into his marital life with an expression of shock mixed with embarrassment. He normalized everything by saying that there was nothing wrong in his marital relationship. In his view, his marital relationship had nothing to do with his nocturnal ejaculation. According to him, impotence was the result of nocturnal ejaculation, since semen was thought of as the essence of energy and the excretion of it was believed to result in a loss of energy. Obviously the traditional Chinese somatic view of mental illness was guiding his expectation from the therapist. How to develop psychotherapeutic techniques acceptable and effective in working with Chinese who harbor such a hardened, anti-psychotherapeutic cultural orientation is certainly a challenge requiring major concerted effort from clinicians who routinely deliver care to this ethnic group.

The extreme delay of Chinese psychiatric patients in seeking help from psychiatric institutions or mental health agencies is universal (Lin and Lin 1978; Miller and Liu n.d.; Wong 1978) and poses serious problems in many respects. It confines psychiatrists or mental health workers to dealing with only chronic psychotic patients who are on the verge of rejection by the family, if not already rejected (Wong 1978). This not only makes their work difficult, but also extremely unrewarding. The perpetuation of such a situation also maintains the low status of psychiatry and mental health generally in the eyes of Chinese communities. Furthermore, other types of mental disorders, such as depression, neuroses, hysteria, psychosomatic conditions, etc., are being dealt with almost exclusively by non-psychiatric professionals or laymen. How to instill psychiatric knowledge and skills in the training of health professionals like primary care physicians is an immediate and important task. The intensive undergraduate teaching of psychiatry in the medical school curriculum initiated by Lin (1960, 1961) at National Taiwan University marked the first step in this direction. But teaching psychiatry in the context of primary care and general hospital practice requires continuous reinforcement and readjustment to be effective. Conversely, a closer relationship of psychiatry with other medical fields in clinical education and research offers psychiatry a more stable and advantageous base for its development as a clinical discipline. This should not interfere with psychiatry's close interaction with the social sciences, which holds practical significance in improving clinical practice with Chinese and other ethnic groups.

In the search for relevant and effective treatment modalities for Chinese psychiatric patients, one should not overlook the field of psychopharmacology. Since indigenous herbs are the most common and treasured form of treatment, rooted in centuries of tradition, it is puzzling to the writers that psychopharmacological research on traditional herbs has not been more actively pursued. For example, traditional Chinese herbs should be intensively investigated to detect substances that are effective in modern psychiatric use. Careful assessment of differences in effective dose range, side-effects, and mode of action of modern psychotropic drugs in Chinese and Caucasion patients should lead to more discriminating clinical use of these agents in the treatment of psychiatric conditions among Chinese. Takahashi et al. (1975) report, for example, that Japanese patients require lower levels of serum lithium, 0.6–0.7 mEq/liter, for effectively treating manic conditions, when compared to the level of 0.6 to 1.0 mEq/liter or even 1.2 or 1.5 mEq/liter for Western patients. Certain clinical impressions, e.g. that Chinese depressive patients respond to lower doses of Tricyclic antidepressant drugs at the same body weight, deserve careful assessment (Lin and Lin 1978).

Implications for research also deserve special attention. As mentioned in the previous section, the family's perception and interpretation of different types of mental illness, e.g., depression vs. florid psychosis, significantly influences casefinding. It goes without saying that the involvement of family members as informants is essential in comprehensive epidemiological surveys in Chinese society (Lin 1953). Studies of utilization of mental health services for Chinese would have only limited value if the phases of help seeking we have outlined and other sources of delay are not assessed. Studies of attitudes to mental illness and the mentally ill also require careful reference to families that have affected members. For example, it is highly unlikely that simply asking Chinese families their hypothetical attitudes to mental illness, unless they have had to respond to such problems, will provide relevant information; nor will surveys of the attitudes of individuals that do not take into account the family context of beliefs and behavioral norms.

Attention should also be given to how best to train Chinese psychiatrists and mental health professionals. As Wong rightly points out (1978), current training programs in North America are of little practical help to Chinese professionals. Nowhere during the standard psychiatric residency or post-graduate mental health training program is the Chinese trainee exposed to any teaching or supervision specifically focused on treating Chinese patients. Furthermore, many of these trainees are poorly informed and ignorant of their own culture and language, and the press of conforming to universal psychopathological norms means that they then often bend over backwards not to recognize cultural differences. It is of paramount importance to establish at least one center of excellence with qualified teachers for training Chinese mental health professionals to deliver culturally appropriate care while developing a relevant curriculum with data-based cultural teaching material that can be used effectively elsewhere.

CONCLUSION

The reluctance of families to call upon outside help for a troubled person is not unique to Chinese culture, nor are the motivations prompting such reluctance, such as shame, guilt and the understandable desire to protect the individual. However, we feel that the sheer strength of this pattern may be specific to Chinese culture, and therefore, worthy of special note. Practical implications of recognizing this pattern bear on case-finding, modes of intervention and planning of services.

How much and how fast psychiatry and other mental health sciences take up some of the challenges raised above and solve some of these difficult problems might substantially influence their future course of evolution in Chinese communities. It is the writers' view that any applied science performs best in consonance with the psychosocial dynamics of the cultural matrix in which it is destined to grow.

Finally, any study of Chinese family and culture is incomplete without input of relevant data from the People's Republic of China, where one-fourth of the world's population reside. The writers hope that such information will soon become available and that it will further our understanding of mental illness and its treatment in Chinese culture.

REFERENCES

Buck, Pearl S.
    1931 The Good Earth. New York: John Day Co.
Chen, Pei-Ngor
    1970 The Chinese community in Los Angeles. Social Casework 15:591−598.
Chen, Peter W.
    1977 Chinese-Americans View their Mental Health. San Francisco: R. & E. Research
        Associates, Inc.
Ho, D. Y. F.
    1974 Prevention and treatment of mental illness in the People's Republic of China.
        American Journal of Orthopsychiatry 44: 620−623.
Kleinman, A.
    1979 Patients and Healers in the Context of Culture. Berkeley: University of California
        Press; pp. 119−179.

Lee, Ivy
    1973 A Profile of Asians in Sacramento. Mimeographed Report. Washington, D.C.: U.S.
          Department of Health, Education and Welfare. Grant No. IRO/MH 21086–01,
          September 30.
Lin, Tsung-yi
    1953 A study of incidence of mental disorders in Chinese and other cultures. Psychiatry
          15:313–336.
Lin, Tsung-yi
    1960 Undergraduate teaching of psychiatry in the National Taiwan University. British
          Medical Journal ii: 345–
Lin, Tsung-yi
    1961 Evolution of mental health programs in Taiwan. American Journal of Psychiatry
          117:961–   .
Lin, T. Y., Tardiff, K., Donnetz, G., Goresky, W.
    1978 Ethnicity and patterns of help-seeking. Culture, Medicine and Psychiatry 2:3–13.
Lin, T. Y. and Lin, M. C.
    1978 Service delivery issues in Asian-North American communities. American Journal
          of Psychiatry 135:454–456.
Mak, K. Y. and Chen, S. C. L.
    1979 Mental health services and Mainland Chinese in Hong Kong. In Uprooting and
          Mental Health; With particular Reference to East-West Migration. R. Nann, R.
          Seebaran and Mei-chen Lin, eds. Vancouver, Canada: World Federation for Mental
          Health.
Miller, M., Liu, T.
    n.d. Unpublished manuscript.
Needham, J.
    1956 Science and Civilization in China. Cambridge, England: Cambridge University
          Press. Vol. ll:132.
Sarbaff, T. R., Mancuso, J. C.
    1970 Failure of a moral enterprise: Attitudes of the public toward mental illness.
          Journal of Counselling and Clinical Psychology 35:159–173.
Sue, S. and Sue, D. W.
    1973 Chinese personality and mental health. In Asian-Americans: Psychological Per-
          spectives. S. Sue and N. Wagner, eds. Palo Alto, California: Science and Behavior
          Book Inc.
Sue, S. and McKinney, H.
    1975 Asian-Americans in the community mental health care system. American Journal
          of Orthopsychiatry 45: 111–118.
Takahashi, R. et al.
    1975 Comparison of efficiency of lithium carbonate and chlorpromazine in mania.
          Archives of General Psychiatry 32: 1310–1318.
Tseng, W. S.
    1973 The development of psychiatric concepts in traditional Chinese medicine. Archives
          of General Psychiatry 29: 569––575.
Tseng, W. S.
    1972 Psychiatric study of shamanism in Taiwan. Archives of General Psychiatry 26:
          561–565.
Veith, I.
    1966 The Yellow Emperor's Classic of Internal Medicine. Berkeley: University of Cali-
          fornia Press.
Visher, J. S. and Visher, E. B.
    1979 Impressions of psychiatric problems and their management: China, 1977. American
          Journal of Psychiatry 136: 28–32.

Wong, N.
　1978　Psychiatric education and training of Asian and Asian-American psychiatrists. American Journal of Psychiatry 135: 1525–1530.
Yee, A. H.
　1973　Myopic perceptions and textbooks: Chinese-Americans' search for identity. Journal of Social Issues 29: 99–113.

ARTHUR KLEINMAN AND TSUNG-YI LIN

EPILOGUE

In the Introduction to the volume we set out a brief overview of our subject and in our short introductions to each of the sections of the book we summarized each of the chapters and indicated how they contributed to the book's chief themes. Here we wish to list subjects that this volume either has not covered in sufficient depth or discussed at all, but that we believe are important issues for future research on normal and abnormal behavior in Chinese culture. These subjects are meant to complement and extend the specific questions for future research discussed in individual chapters.

Certain psychopathological conditions deserve considerably more descriptive and comparative assessment if we are one day to possess either a Chinese psychiatry adequate for understanding salient mental health problems among Chinese or a truly comparative psychiatry that can relate these problems to similar ones among other populations. The rate of manic-depressive disorder needs to be assessed in different Chinese communities as does its genetic basis. Modern lithium therapy and prophylaxis make this a topic of great practical importance. The prevalence and types of atypical (or reactive) psychoses also need to be much better understood. Is reactive psychosis more common among Chinese than among Western populations? If so, how much more prevalent is it? What are its typical phenomenology, course, and treatment response? Does it differ for rural or urban, educated or illiterate, traditionally-oriented or Western-oriented populations? Are the life event changes and other stresses associated with its onset distinctive for Chinese?

We require prevalence rates for obsessive-compulsive neurosis and other neuroses among Chinese. How do these compare with rates for the same disorders in Western cultures? What do clinical epidemiological assessments tell us about the symptomatology, illness behavior, help seeking, and treatment response of these disorders? Psychiatric problems associated with sexual functioning, aging, rapid social change, migration, acculturation and value alterations, use of leisure time, changing sex roles, and many related stresses of contemporary life require further study. Other relevant research concerns should be drug abuse, crime and juvenile delinquency, maladaptive life styles, and family pathology, including divorce, illegitimacy, child abuse, and related problems. Low risk problems, including alcoholism, homosexuality, anorexia nervosa, and learning disorders in children which are often neglected, deserve to be researched along with high risk problems such as suicide in single, elderly Chinese males in North America. Such research requires careful case finding, clinical description, and cross-cultural comparisons. Epidemiological surveys also should focus on regional variations in rates of mental illness and social deviance across different Chinese communities.

403

A. Kleinman and T.-Y. Lin (eds.), Normal and Abnormal Behavior in Chinese Culture, 403–410.
Copyright © 1980 by D. Reidel Publishing Company.

Effects of migration on mental health and illness are of particular research significance. Studies should focus on migration from the China mainland to well-established Chinese communities in Asia as well as on migration from Hong Kong, Taiwan, and Singapore to overseas Chinese communities in North America. The current massive migration of Vietnamese of Chinese ethnicity raises anew many serious questions about the nature of stresses involved in acculturation, rates of psychopathology of migrants, and how to measure and improve their adaptive response to their new environment. Rural to urban migration, which has been such a common occurrence in contemporary Chinese communities in Asia, requires particular attention as it is an aspect of modernization that virtually all societies undergoing rapid social change have experienced, frequently as severe problems of social dislocation, family breakdown, and personal demoralization. Problems of unemployment and poverty, rapid value change and value conflicts, alterations in family relations and social role that are often associated with rural to urban migration undoubtedly exert important influences on mental health and illness that demand further investigation.

A most important topic not covered in the present volume is treatment of Chinese patients. Can culturally-appropriate therapeutic practices be shown to demonstrate improved outcome? Studies are needed comparing treatment outcome of Chinese patients in traditional psychiatric treatment programs both with matched non-Chinese patients and with matched Chinese patients treated with culturally-appropriate psychotherapy and other therapeutic modalities. For example, does outcome for intercultural psychotherapy differ from outcome when patient and therapist are both Chinese? What are the determinants of such differences? Can these be operationalized into practical psychotherapeutic strategies that can be shown to positively affect care? Are traditional Chinese medicines and folk healing practices effective in the treatment of particular mental illnesses? What toxicities do they possess? Can they be integrated into modern primary health care delivery systems in cost effective ways? As a corollary, can traditional healers be trained in modern psychiatry to provide clinically sophisticated triage and integrated treatment of certain mental disorders? What comparative assessments can be made for the various patterns of traditional and modern treatment provided in different Chinese societies? Physiological research that examines differential pharmacokinetic responses to psychopharmacological agents is also extremely important. As is research on the planning and delivery of community mental health services that takes into account the cultural and familial influences on care reviewed in the preceding chapter.

A particularly important therapeutic and preventive aspect of psychiatry in Chinese settings is the problem of the stigma of mental illness. Research studies should better delineate the nature, extent, and consequences of this stigma. We also are in need of intervention studies that examine different ways of handling the stigma of mental illness among Chinese. For example, can it be shown that preventive mental health programs that better educate patients' families, general practitioners, teachers, community leaders, and the lay public in a modern understanding of psychiatric disorders and treatment have a demonstrable effect on diminishing stigma and its negative consequences? Since psychiatry now possesses effective treatment for many mental illnesses, such educational programs should be evaluated to determine if they improve early case detection, entrance into appropriate care, and compliance with treatment regimens. Community psychiatric research must assess prevention and treatment programs that aim to decrease delays in seeking professional help, rationalize help seeking so that there is more appropriate and cost effective utilization of available treatment resources (modern and traditional), train care-givers to provide culturally sensitive treatment, and break the repeated cycle of intrafamilial care — extrafamilial resort — and eventual rejection of patients by their families described in the preceding chapter. As many of the chapters in this book point out, the strong Chinese cultural tendency for patients to somatize mental illness means that primary care physicians provide most of the professional care for the mentally ill. Hence it is important to assess their skills in recognizing and treating mental illness, and whether these can be improved through suitable training programs.

Since the People's Republic has developed an important health care delivery system that includes services for treating mental illness (see Chapter 17), health services researchers and planners need to determine if any components of this system might be transferable to other Chinese communities to improve psychiatric care. Preventive mental health services, it is generally agreed, should focus on children. A great deal needs to be done in this respect in Chinese societies. Research should determine, for example, the effect of traditional diet and nutrition, birthing practices, pre- and post-natal care on physical and psychological development. Intervention studies can then investigate if providing training in modern mental health principles and skills to midwives, pediatricians, and teachers can improve early detection and treatment of childhood psychiatric disorders. The kinds of school mental health programs advocated by the Soongs in Chapter 9 need to be evaluated in terms of their impact on the traditional milieu of Chinese schools. Do they significantly change the maladaptive effects on personality development that these educational environments often appear to produce? Studies of the aged and aging in different Chinese settings also should be of significance in assessing the need for preventive and treatment programs for this high risk group.

So many other psychiatric issues for future research have been discussed throughout the book that we will not recapitulate these but refer the reader back to the relevant sections of Chapters 8, 13, 15, 17, 18, and 20. An even greater number of researchable issues can be identified for future social science studies of normal behavior and social deviance in Chinese societies. We do not intend to list these in full, but a few examples are worth citing to illustrate the kinds of investigations we regard as crucial.

We are in need of precise and meticulous descriptions of common child rearing practices, such as shaming techniques and the inculcation of core cultural values. Such studies would support more sophisticated cross-cultural comparisons than are presently available in the research literature. Studies of family functioning and relationships in different everyday life settings would provide the needed background to identify characteristic adaptive and maladaptive features of Chinese family life. To the best of our knowledge there is now no such information. But it is essential if we are to determine universal and culture-specific aspects of family pathology and elaborate clinical strategies for dealing with such problems. Basic cognitive, affective, behavioral and interpersonal studies are also important research requirements. For example, a hypothesis has been advanced that Chinese and Caucasian-Americans differ in the coping processes they use to manage dysphoric affects (see the Introduction to this volume and Kleinman 1979). This argument states that the coping processes are universal but that their particular patterns of deployment in typical hierarchies of resort are culture-specific. Such an hypothesis could be fairly easily tested in comparative cross-cultural studies that examine denial, somatization, dissociation, and other relevant coping strategies among key groups of matched subjects — depressed and anxious patients, normal subjects reacting to similar life event changes and other social stressors, etc.

Specific cultural mechanisms that mediate other Chinese psychological processes can be gotten at by experiments that are constructed to measure reactions to common life situations, such as perception of and meanings attributed to pain, ranking of significance of perceived stressors vis-à-vis ranking of similar stressors by subjects from other cultures, coping with particular marital and work problems, and so forth. Perhaps comparative studies of adult development, elicitation of life histories, and analysis of culturally salient methods of managing major life transitions (adolescence, senescense, death) would provide a useful complement to psychocultural experiments. Inasmuch as core psychocultural processes are always embedded in cultural categories, researchers should be aware that only meaning-centered psychological research can offer appropriate methodologies to research these issues (cf. Chapters 8, 13, 17 and 18 above).

We regard the problem of research methods as absolutely central here, because most cross-cultural psychological and sociological studies are organized around research paradigms that prohibit investigation of the semantic and symbolic links between subjective experience and social reality that are the essence of psychocultural phenomena. Hence the kind of behavioral science research we are calling for, like the clinical epidemiological investigation of illness behavior we have already discussed, must be anthropologically informed and meaning centered if we are to understand how Chinese behave and how those patterns of behavior differ from members of other cultures.

One of the great dangers of psychocultural research is the construction of crude behavioral stereotypes that do not adequately reflect either cross-cultural or intracultural differences. Hence any research along the lines suggested above must take into account differences based on social setting, class, value orientation, and individual variation. It is this incredibly complex biopsychosocial web of determinants (see Engel 1977) that makes cross-cultural behavioral science research so difficult. Nonetheless, we believe that important research in this field can and should be conducted, and that a major reason for the lack of parsimony in our current theoretical formulations is that heretofore so little research has been carried out.

The question of appropriate research methodologies for future studies of normal and abnormal behavior among Chinese has several other components. We have tended to emphasize the value of basic descriptions, but at some point, if a field is to mature scientifically, such research must be complemented by hypothesis testing. Several of the chapters in this volume, including this one, have suggested specific hypotheses for future research (see, for example, Chapter 13). Hypotheses to be tested in the field should be derived from descriptive research, refined by relating them to the available research literature, significant in terms of the current state of our empirical knowledge and theoretical constructs, and capable of being tested by available field methods.

Another concern about methodology is that research on Chinese behavioral parameters should not simply represent the importation into Chinese settings of Western psychometric instruments and psychiatric assessment schedules that have been translated into Chinese. It is of course essential to have bilingual assistants do back translations from Chinese to English to test the accuracy of translations. But it is equally important that reliability and validity studies be carried out in Chinese populations, that Chinese response norms be developed as the basis for assessing Chinese individuals' test performances, that culturally irrelevant or biased items be removed, and that where feasible efforts be made to build special measurement instruments appropriate for Chinese culture. Although it is desirable to obtain quantitative data from formal assessment devices that are comparable to findings with the same techniques in other cultures, the first concern of cultural (anthropological) psychiatrists should be that tests are valid for Chinese culture.

The range of different Chinese communities makes comparisons between Chinese in different settings valuable. Such comparisons may reveal differences owing to divergent social structures and experiences of culture change that yield a more precise assessment of universal and culture-specific dimensions of Chinese behavior and psychopathology. Now that it is becoming possible to consider collaborative psychiatric research in the People's Republic, much is to be gained by extending cross-cultural comparisons to Chinese in that setting. Similarly, it is to be hoped that we will quickly move beyond the stage of bicultural comparisons (e.g., Chinese and Caucasian-Americans) to include other relevant cultural groups, such as Japanese and other Asian or non-Western samples, that can provide a more refined range of contrasts of key behavioral patterns than the often crude distinctions generated from two greatly different cultures. For example, the comparison of Chinese and Caucasian-American depressed patients means that somatization among Chinese is often viewed as an aberration, whereas comparisons involving other Asian and non-Western depressives is likely to indicate that it is "psychologization" in the contemporary West that is atypical in cross-cultural perspective. Such comparisons also would enable us to determine differences in styles of somatization of depression among members of different Asian and non-Western groups.

The longitudinal studies carried out by Lin and his colleagues in Taiwan (see Chapter 13) represent a prototype for future longitudinal epidemiological and clinical studies, which are strengthened to the extent they involve the same investigators during the entire course of the research as well as the same stand-ardized instruments and the same conceptual and methodological framework.

One aspect of research on Chinese culture rarely gets discussed: namely, who should do the research. The studies we have outlined obviously require the use of interdisciplinary methods or teams of investigators. But must these investi-gators themselves be ethnic Chinese? Today, there is increasing concern among Chinese, as in other non-Western groups, that anthropologists, psychiatrists, and other behavioral scientists who conduct research among them should attempt to contribute to the solution of culturally salient problems. Sometimes this view overlaps with another that holds that researchers who are themselves Chinese are more likely to be aware of such problems and committed to help solve them. In our view, it is important that all researchers in Chinese settings study problems that are locally salient and work with local communities to make the knowledge gained from such research available for current treatment and preventive pro-grams as well as for future policy planning and implementation. But to our mind it is no guarantee that investigators will act in this way simply because they themselves are Chinese. While Chinese ethnicity certainly provides the investiga-tor with a rich source of intuitive insights about Chinese culture, it may also blind him or her to taken-for-granted aspects of Chinese culture that are more visible to members of other groups. Furthermore, it is well known that Western-ized members of non-Western societies may harbor strong prejudices about the traditional culture that make it difficult for them to objectively assess indigenous beliefs and behaviors. Hence, use of indigenous researchers offers both advantages and disadvantages. We believe the ideal research team of investigators to study behavior in Chinese culture should include both Chinese members (including members of local communities) and members of other cultures, and might in-clude along with professional anthropologists, psychiatrists and psychologists, perhaps lay members as well.

It is quite appropriate for us to end our comments on the question of man-power because this is a very real problem in Chinese societies. As the preceding chapters disclose, the reason why relatively few Chinese have entered the mental health field until very recently is not difficult to discover. There is a substantial cultural barrier. Chinese culture has not only not fostered an interest in psychia-try and behavioral science, but has at times actively discouraged such an interest. Sinologists and China scholars generally have tended, with a few outstanding exceptions, to reflect this bias. Finally, psychiatry itself in Chinese settings has been much more concerned with practical clinical and preventive issues than with research and theory. Indeed for much of this century, psychiatry in Chinese settings has been ethnocentric, medicocentric, and psychocentric and has failed to deal with the clinical scientific consequences of the profound Chinese cultural influences on normal and abnormal behavior that we discussed in the Introduction to the volume.

For these and other reasons a very small number of Chinese have carried out psychiatric or behavioral science research on psychocultural themes and psychopathology. Even research on treatment has been extremely limited. Those few scholars who have been active in this field have often been ground breaking pioneers, self-trained and self-directed, who have opened up different disciplinary approaches to behavior in Chinese culture. They have frequently worked in isolation from other workers attacking the same subject from different disciplinary perspectives. Indeed it is not an exaggeration to refer to these leaders of research as having created distinctive research "schools": some more epidemiological, others more clinical. The contributions of these scholars and their "schools", while not extensive, have been crucial for the elaboration of an indigenized psychiatry appropriate for Chinese settings. The chapters in this book are evidence that such a Chinese psychiatry as well as a Chinese contribution to comparative psychiatry are presently in the making.

In examining past record and present situation as a basis for recommendations about research manpower training, it is our impression that what is needed are greatly expanded resources to support formal research training of psychiatrists and behavioral scientists in research centers where epidemiological, clinical, psychometric, and anthropological conceptual frameworks and research methodologies can be learned as part of ongoing interdisciplinary research projects. Trainees need to be part of comparative cross-culture field studies. But they also need to learn how to handle recent developments in psychiatric and social science theory in as sophisticated ways as are available. We strongly believe the objects of their study must hold real clinical relevance. Rather than set out more specific recommendations, we wish to emphasize that progress in this field is tied to better training and that better training requires identification and support of research centers that specialize in behavioral science and psychiatry studies of Chinese culture, that are either located in Chinese communities or have research field stations there, and that have a multidisciplinary staff of researchers who are working at integrating clinical and social science approaches in the context of specific interdisciplinary field projects.

In closing, we wish again to emphasize to our readers the *exploratory* quality of this volume. We see *Normal and Abnormal Behavior in Chinese Culture* not as a finished product, but an early report of work in progress. We have shared our uncertainties about the present "state of the art" and our goals for the future along with our somewhat limited and provisional knowledge. We have ventured forth on this slippery slope not without some hesitancy and realistic concern for potential dangers. We have dared to do so because we believe that this is a subject of such great significance and so appropriate for the current period that we saw ourselves faced with a charge we could not avoid. It has been our desire both to report on important ground already covered, much of it unfamiliar to our psychiatric and behavioral sciences colleagues, and to open new ground for future work.

REFERENCES

Engel, G. L.
  1977 The need for a new medical model: A challenge for biomedicine. Science 196: 129–136.
Kleinman, A.
  1979 Patients and Healers in the Context of Culture: An Exploration of the Borderland between Anthropology, Medicine, and Psychiatry. Berkeley: University of California Press.

LIST OF CONTRIBUTORS

A. A. Alexander, Department of Psychiatry, University of Wisconsin at Madison.

Martha Li Chiu, Departments of History and East Asian Languages, Harvard University.

Stevan Harrell, Department of Anthropology, University of Washington.

David Y. F. Ho, Department of Psychology, University of Hong Kong.

Andrew C. K. Hsieh, Department of History and Council on East Asian Studies, Yale University.

Marjorie H. Klein, Department of Psychiatry, University of Wisconsin at Madison.

Arthur Kleinman, Division of Cross-Cultural Psychiatry, Department of Psychiatry and Department of Anthropology, University of Washington.

Rance P. L. Lee, Social Research Center, Chinese University of Hong Kong.

Keh-ming Lin, Department of Psychiatry, Harbor General Hospital, University of California at Los Angeles.

Mei-chen Lin, formerly with Strathcona Community Care Team, Vancouver.

Tsung-yi Lin, Department of Psychiatry, University of British Columbia, and Departments of Psychiatry and Mental Health, University of Tokyo (1979–80).

James P. McGough, Department of Sociology and Anthropology, Middlebury College.

David Mechanic, Graduate School of Social Work, Rutgers University.

Thomas A. Metzger, Department of History, University of California at San Diego.

Milton H. Miller, Department of Psychiatry, Harbor General Hospital, University of California at Los Angeles.

William L. Parish, Department of Sociology, University of Chicago.

Hsien Rin, Department of Neurology and Psychiatry, National Taiwan University Hospital.

Gary Seaman, Department of Anthropology, University of Colorado at Boulder.

Ko-ping Soong, formerly with Fu-Jen University, Taiwan.

Wei-tsuen Soong, Children's Mental Health Center, Department of Neurology and Psychiatry, National Taiwan University Hospital, and Department of Psychiatry, University of British Columbia.

Jonathan D. Spence, Department of History and Council on East Asian Studies, Yale University.

Stanley Sue, Department of Psychology, University of Washington.

Eng-Seong Tan, Department of Psychiatry, University of Melbourne.

L. Neal Teng, Department of Psychology, University of Washington.

Mavis Tsai, Department of Psychology, University of Washington.

Ching-lun Wang, Department of Urology, National Taiwan University Hospital.

Jung-kwang Wen, Department of Neurology and Psychiatry, National Taiwan University Hospital.

Richard W. Wilson, International Programs and Department of Political Science, Rutgers University.

CITATION INDEX

Numbers in italics refer to pages on which the complete references are listed.

SUBJECT INDEX

The abbreviation 'PRC' is used for the People's Republic of China

Aborigines, Taiwan, psychopathology, 241–242
Accident-proneness, acculturation and, 297–298
Acculturation, stress and, 296–298
Achievement
  stress and, 279–285
Acupuncture
  for hysteria, 351
  PRC, 336
  in psychiatric treatment, PRC, 337, 342
Administration
  PRC, 62, 207–208
  of religious cults, 67–71
Adoption, 173
  of daughter-in-law, 191–192
  by prostitute, 198
  See Marriage, adopted, daughter-in-law
Age
  advantages, 306
  psychiatric symptoms and, 278–279
Aggression, 19, 297
  expectation of, 151–152
Agriculture, family and, 190
Alcohol, 249
  facial flushing, 49, 304
  use of, 4
  See also ciu-kui (alcohol ghosts); Drinking
Alcoholism, xvii, 49–58, 248–250
  Chinese-Americans and, 304–305
  Hong Kong, 248
  PRC, 349
  prevalence, 333, 360, 361
  research need, 403
  Singapore, 249
  Taipei, 217
  Taiwan, 240–241, 248–249
Alcohol psychosis, 249–250
Amae, xiv
Americans, perceptions of, by Taiwanese, 320–322, 323–324
Amnesties, imperial
  insane murderer and, 85
  for insane prisoners, 88–89
Amok, 380–381, 383
  as schizophrenia, 383
  spread of, 379

transcultural dimension of, 382
Ancestors
  cult of, 65
  filial piety and, 392–393
  mental illness and, 392–393
Ancestral line, 89–90
Anger, righteous, 19
Anthropology, 233
  epidemiological, 254
  ethnocentrism in, 171
  See also Research
Antidepressant drugs, xv, 348, 349, 354, n.4, 398
Antipsychotic medications, PRC, 346
Anxiety, 15
  in culture shock, 326
  in moral development, 123
  patterns, 132
  peer group and, 123
  psychosocial problems and, 334
  somatic distress and, xiii, xiv
  traditional clinics and, 334–335
  values and, 132
  Western and Chinese, xv
Anxiety neurosis, xix
  diagnosis, 333
  in Kuala Lumpur, 245
  in PRC, 349
  Koro as, 383
  prevalence, PRC, 341
Art of the Bed Chamber, The, 358
Aspirations, stress and, 279–285
Assault, sexual, suicide and, 35, 36
Assizes, 92 n.7
Authoritarianism, 7, 8
  behavioral scientists on, 19
  dependency and, 20
  filial piety and, 145
Authority, 7, 8, 11, 63
  opposing, 132
Authority figures, 16, 19
  questioning of, 127
  self-esteem and, 19
Autonomy, 8, 9, 19, 21
  Confucianism and, 8
Ayurvedic medicine, 365
  semen and, 359

420